HEALTH BEHAVIOR AND HEALTH EDUCATION

HEALTH BEHAVIOR AND HEALTH EDUCATION

Theory, Research, and Practice

Second Edition

Karen Glanz

Frances Marcus Lewis

Barbara K. Rimer

Editors

Foreword by J. Michael McGinnis, M.D.

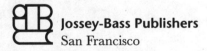

Jossey-Bass Publishers
San Francisco

Substantial discounts on bulk quantities of Jossey-Bass books are available to corporations, professional associations, and other organizations. For details and discount information, contact the special sales department at Jossey-Bass Inc., Publishers (415) 433–1740; Fax (800) 605–2665.

For sales outside the United States, please contact your local Simon & Schuster International Office.

TCF Manufactured in the United States of America on Lyons Falls Pathfinder Tradebook. This paper is acid-free and 100 percent totally chlorine-free.

Library of Congress Cataloging-in-Publication Data

Health behavior and health education / [edited by] Karen Glanz,
  Frances Marcus Lewis, Barbara K. Rimer.—2nd ed.
      p.   cm.—(Jossey-Bass health series)
  Includes bibliographical references and indexes.
  ISBN 0–7879–0310–8 (hardcover : alk. paper)
    1. Health behavior.   2. Health education.   I. Glanz, Karen.
  II. Lewis, Frances Marcus.   III. Rimer, Barbara K.   IV. Series.
  RA776.9.H434   1996
  613—dc20   96–26919

SECOND EDITION
HB Printing   10 9 8 7 6 5 4 3 2 1

CONTENTS

TABLES AND FIGURES

Tables

Figures

FOREWORD

Nothing is more fundamental, or more vexing, to civilization than behaviors that usher in declines in the well-being of individuals, families, or communities that make up a population. Particularly when the adverse consequences of behavioral choices are evident to those making the choices, when fate stares them squarely in the face but has no apparent impact, the problems seem all the less explicable, the solutions all the more evasive.

Behavioral factors have been recognized as prominent contributors to human health prospects throughout recorded history. Today, individual behavioral choices have been documented as the source of perhaps half of all premature deaths that occur in the United States, raising compelling economic and humanitarian challenges to society.

Human motivation is complicated. At the superficial level, the explanation for unwise or destructive behavior seems the result of straightforward choices for short-term pleasure in the trade-offs with long-term consequences. People smoke because of the immediate stimulus to the central nervous system. Alcohol may provide them a sense of easier interaction with their social environment. Overeating is the result of the pleasure from activated taste buds, lethargy the path of least resistance. Imprudent sexual activity is the product of unchecked sensations and instincts conditioned over millennia by the need for species survival. There are few mysteries why people initiate these behaviors. They are actions derivative of immediacy, if not primacy.

Still, over time, knowledge of the longer term or broader social consequences of behavioral choices that yield reflexively to physiological and psychological triggers has prompted most people to alter their choices in ways that are more beneficial to health. Tobacco use has been cut in half in less than a generation in the United States. The shift in consumption of saturated fats to poly- and mono-unsaturated fats has been dramatic. The levels of blood alcohol controlling the steering mechanisms of moving vehicles have dropped considerably, as have the consequences.

Why, in the central nervous system processes that give rise to perceptions and decisions, some people opt in one direction and others take a different tack is the central challenge of the science and art of health promotion. Some of the answers may ultimately come from the neurosciences and molecular biology, as more is learned about the atomic structure of human motivation. Yet just as the nature of behavior is often complicated and sometimes contradictory, so are the factors that give rise to it.

Human behavior is the product of the interaction of multiple factors found in the many facets of our biological, environmental, and cultural exposures. Any one of these factors can be powerful but none acts independently. In the aggregate, the task of those involved in health education research is to tease out the ways in which these factors might interact to yield certain behaviors under different conditions. It is a formidable task, far exceeding the difficulty and complexity of the task of those engaged, for example, in the pursuit of knowledge about the structure of a particular enzyme or the nature of a certain chemical reaction. So thorny is the challenge that in the past, as the authors note, many have based their findings "primarily on precedent, tradition, or intuition."

With the second edition of *Health Behavior and Health Education: Theory, Research, and Practice,* a resource is made available to the community of health education researchers and practitioners that helps bring order to the systematic advance of the discipline. It comes at a timely point, as more is learned about risk factors and their consequences, and as the importance of effective approaches to health-related behavior change assumes new prominence with the growth of managed care delivery systems. In these pages, the editors offer a thorough survey and analysis of the most widely used theories of health behavior, an evaluation of the application of those theories, based on the firsthand experience of the authors involved, and an indication of some of the future directions for both research and practice in health education. In doing so, they lay the groundwork for the sort of progress in understanding and enhancing health behavior that is so vital to improving the human condition throughout the world.

August 1996

J. Michael McGinnis, M.D.
Scholar-in-residence
National Academy of Sciences
Washington, D.C.

PREFACE

A health promotion and education program or intervention is most likely to benefit participants and the community when it is guided by a theory of health behavior. Theories of health behavior identify the targets for change and the methods for accomplishing these changes. Theories also inform the evaluation of change efforts by helping to identify the outcomes to be measured and the timing and methods of study to be used. Such theory-driven health promotion and education efforts stand in contrast to programs based primarily on precedent, tradition, intuition, or principles.

Theory-driven health promotion and education programs and interventions require an understanding of the components of health behavior theory as well as of the operational or practical forms of these theories. The first edition of *Health Behavior and Health Education: Theory, Research, and Practice,* published in 1990, was the first text to provide in-depth analysis of a variety of theories of health behavior relevant to health education in a single volume. It brought together dominant health behavior theories, the research based on those theories, and examples of health education practice derived from the theories tested through evaluation and research processes.

This second edition of *Health Behavior and Health Education* updates and substantially improves upon the earlier volume. Its main purpose is the same: to advance the science and practice of health promotion and education through the informed application of theories of health behavior. Likewise, it serves as the definitive text for students, practitioners, and scientists in health promotion and education in three ways: by analyzing the key components of theories of health behavior relevant to health education, by evaluating current applications of these theories in selected health promotion programs and interventions, and by identifying important future directions for research and practice in health promotion and health education.

This second edition responds to new developments in health behavior theory and in the application of theory in new settings and in new ways. It includes an enhanced focus on the application of theories in diverse settings; a new section on using theory, including the translation of theory into program planning; and new chapters on additional theories of health behavior. One new chapter addresses the challenges of making health behavior theory relevant and useful in populations with varied sociodemographic and cultural backgrounds. Another looks into the future to explore how health promotion theory, research, and practice might advance in the face of increasing globalization, new communication technologies, and health care reform.

Audience

Health Behavior and Health Education speaks to graduate students, practitioners, and scientists who spend part or all of their time in the broad arena of health promotion and health education; this audience will find that this book assists them both to understand relevant theories and to apply them in practical settings. Both practitioners and students will find the text a major reference for the development and evaluation of theory-driven health promotion and education programs and interventions. Researchers should emerge with a recognition of areas where empirical support is deficient and theory testing is required; this book can help them set the research agenda for health promotion and education.

Health Behavior and Health Education is intended to assist all professionals who value the need to influence health behavior positively. Their fields include health promotion and education, medicine, nursing, health psychology, behavioral medicine, nutrition and dietetics, dentistry, pharmacy, social work, exercise science, clinical psychology, and occupational and physical therapy.

Overview of the Book

The chapter authors bring to their contributions to this book an understanding of both theory and its application in a variety of settings that characterize the diverse practice of public health education: for example, worksites, hospitals, ambulatory care settings, schools, and communities. The chapters, written expressly for this book, address theories of behavior at the level of the individual, dyad, group, organization, and community.

This book is organized into six parts. Part One defines key terms and concepts. The next three parts reflect important units in health promotion and education practice: the individual, the interpersonal or group level, and the community or aggregate level. Each of these parts has several chapters. Part Two focuses on theories of individual health behavior, variables *within individuals* that influence their health behavior and response to health promotion and education interventions. Four bodies of theory are reviewed in separate chapters: the Health Belief Model, The Transtheoretical Model, the Theory of Reasoned Action and the Theory of Planned Behavior, and stress and coping. Part Three examines interpersonal theories, which emphasize elements in the *interpersonal* environment that affect individuals' health behavior. Three chapters in this section focus on Social Cognitive Theory, social support and social networks, and patient-provider communication. Part Four covers models for the *community or aggregate level* of change, and the chapters cover community organization, adoption and diffusion of innovations, organizational change, and media communications. Part Five is a new section. It examines using theory, presenting the key components and applications of overarching planning and process models and discussing cultural, gender, and socioeconomic factors moderating the application of theory. The chapters in this section cover the PRECEDE-PROCEED model of health promotion planning; social marketing; ecological models; and cultural, ethnic, and socioeconomic factors. Part Six consists of the final chapter, which presents future directions for theory, research, and practice in health promotion and education.

The major emphasis in *Health Behavior and Health Education* is on the analysis and application of health behavior theories to health promotion and education practice. Each core chapter in Parts Two, Three, and Four begins with a discussion of the background of the relevant theory or model and a presentation of the theory itself, reviews empirical support for the theory, and concludes with a description of two applications. The synthesis chapters provide integrative perspectives on each part of the book. They review related theories and summarize their potential application to the development of health education interventions. Strengths, weaknesses, areas for future development and research, and promising strategies are highlighted.

The chapter authors are established researchers and practitioners who draw on their experience in state-of-the-art research to analyze the theories critically and apply them to health education. This book makes otherwise lofty theories accessible and practical and advances health education in the process.

No single book can be truly comprehensive and still be concise and readable. Our decisions about which theories to include were made with both an appreciation of the evolution of health promotion and education and a vision of its future (see Chapter Two). We purposely chose to emphasize theories and conceptual frameworks that encompass a range from the individual to the societal level. Of necessity, some promising evolving theories were not included.

The first edition of *Health Behavior and Health Education* grew out of our own experiences, frustrations, and needs as well as our desire to synthesize the diverse literatures and to draw clearly the linkages between theory, research, and the practice of health promotion and education. We have sought to show how theory, research, and practice interrelate and to make each element accessible and practical. In this second edition, we have attempted to respond to changes in the science and practice of health promotion and to update the coverage of rapidly evolving areas.

Acknowledgments

We owe deep gratitude to all the authors whose work is represented here. They worked diligently with us to produce an integrated volume, and we greatly appreciate their willingness to tailor their contributions to realize the vision of the book. Their collective depth of knowledge and experience across the broad range of theories and topics far exceeds the expertise that we can claim among ourselves. We also wish to acknowledge authors who contributed to the first edition of this text; although some of them did not write chapters for this edition, their intellectual contributions formed an important foundation for it. In addition, the readers of the first edition confirmed for us that there is a need for a book of this type and offered constructive suggestions for improving this edition, for which we are most grateful.

Susan Curry, Brian Flynn, and Celette Skinner provided timely and insightful reviews of the chapters at a crucial stage in the book's development. The staff at Jossey-Bass provided valuable support to us in development, production, and marketing from the time the first edition was released through completion of this edition. Our editors at Jossey-Bass, Becky McGovern and Barbara Hill, provided encouragement, assistance, and exceptional guidance throughout.

We are also indebted to our colleagues and students who, over the years, have taught us the importance of both health behavior theories and their cogent and precise representation. These people have challenged us to stretch, adapt, and continue to learn throughout our years of work at Stanford University, the University of Michigan, Johns Hopkins University, Temple University, the University of Washington, Fox Chase Cancer Center, Duke University, and the University of Hawai'i.

We particularly want to acknowledge the following individuals: Noel Chrisman, Elizabeth Cohen, Lee Cronbach, Sanford Dornbush, Anna Farmer, Jorge Fernandes, Larry Green, Jennifer Heisler, Beverly Horn, Ruby Isom, Mae Isonaga, Rebecca Kang, Marshall Kreuter, Brick Lancaster, Bob Marshall, Bill Rakowski, Rommel Silverio, and Morris Zelditch.

Technology, although perhaps not warranting or appreciating acknowledgment, played a central role in the development of this text. We learned to value the Internet, portable computers, and well-functioning fax machines—tools that enabled us to cross boundaries of time, distance, and large bodies of water and that were unavailable when we worked on the first edition of *Health Behavior and Health Education*.

Completion of this manuscript would not have been possible without the continual and dedicated assistance of Gwen Ramelb.

We also wish to express our thanks to our colleagues, friends, staffs, and families, whose patience, good humor, and encouragement sustained us through our work on this book.

August 1996

Karen Glanz
Honolulu, Hawai'i

Frances Marcus Lewis
Seattle, Washington

Barbara K. Rimer
Durham, North Carolina

Me ka pumehana for the akamai ones—whose kōkua and
pōmaika'i have inspired me to try to live with pono—
and in honor of the memory of my mother, Jean.

K.G.

To the living angels in my life: Laurel Mae, Millie,
Stormy, Deloris Jane, John Gregg, Steven, and David.

F.M.L.

Thanks to my husband, Bernard Glassman,
my parents, Joan and Irving Rimer, and my earliest and
longest mentor, Ruby Isom, for the support that
makes this kind of undertaking possible.

B.K.R.

THE EDITORS

Karen Glanz is professor (researcher) at the Cancer Research Center of Hawai'i at the University of Hawai'i in Honolulu and adjunct professor at the University of Hawai'i School of Public Health. From 1979 to 1993, she was professor in the Department of Health Education at Temple University in Philadelphia. She received her B.A. degree (1974) in Spanish and her M.P.H. (1977) and Ph.D. (1979) degrees in health behavior and health education, all from the University of Michigan.

Glanz's research and academic interests have been in the areas of health promotion program development and evaluation, cancer prevention and control, ethnic differences in health behavior, nutrition behavior and education, medical education, and employee health promotion. In 1984, she received the Early Career Award of the Public Health Education Section of the American Public Health Association (APHA), and in 1992, she was a co-recipient (with Frances Lewis and Barbara Rimer) of the Mayhew Derryberry Award for outstanding contributions to theory and research in health education, also from the Public Health Education and Health Promotion Section of APHA. Glanz's scholarly contributions consist of more than 130 journal articles and book chapters. With colleagues, she has published most recently in the *Journal of the American Medical Association, American Journal of Public Health, Health Education Quarterly, American Journal of Health Promotion, Academic Medicine, Public Health Reports,* and *Annals of Behavioral Medicine.*

Glanz was visiting professor at Teachers College, Columbia University, in 1982 and spent 1987 to 1988 as a visiting scholar in the division of epidemiology at the University of Minnesota School of Public Health. She was visiting professor at the School of Public Health at Queensland University of Technology in Brisbane, Australia, in 1994 and 1995.

Frances Marcus Lewis is professor in the School of Nursing at the University of Washington. She received her B.S.N. degree, graduating summa cum laude (1967), from Loretto Heights College in Denver and her M.N. degree (1968) from the University of Washington. She received her Ph.D. (1977) in sociology of education from Stanford University and completed her postdoctoral training (1978) in health education at the Johns Hopkins University School of Hygiene and Public Health.

Lewis's research interests are primarily in the areas of theory-based health education intervention and program evaluation, psychosocial adjustment of the family to chronic illness, community-based health promotion, and women's health. Currently, Lewis is principal investigator for two large-scale intervention studies that aim to enhance health outcomes in women and families affected by breast cancer. Her scholarly contributions include more than fifty professional papers and numerous book chapters. Her recent publications, with colleagues, include articles in the *Journal of Behavioral Medicine, Social Science and Medicine, Journal of the Medical Women's Association, Patient Education and Counseling, Cancer Practice, Health Care International for Women, Oncology Nursing Forum,* and *Cancer.*

In 1992, Lewis was a co-recipient (with Karen Glanz and Barbara Rimer) of the Mayhew Derryberry Award for outstanding contributions to theory and research in health education, from the Public Health Education and Health Promotion Section of APHA. Lewis is a member of the American Academy of Nursing, has served as a member of several peer review committees for the National Institutes of Health, and was recently named a fellow of the Japanese Society for the Promotion of Science.

Barbara K. Rimer is director of cancer prevention, detection, and control research at the Duke Comprehensive Cancer Center at Duke University in Durham, North Carolina, a position she has held for the past five years. She is also professor of community and family medicine at the Duke University School of Medicine. Rimer is the chair of the National Cancer Advisory Board, the first woman and the first behavioral scientist in that position. Prior to assuming her present position at Duke University, she was a scientist and director of behavioral research at Fox Chase Cancer Center in Philadelphia for ten years. She received her B.A. degree (1970) in English, her M.P.H. degree (1973) in health education and health administration from the University of Michigan, and her Ph.D. degree (1982) in health education from the Johns Hopkins University School of Hygiene and Public Health.

Rimer's research has focused on identifying and overcoming, through cost-effective, acceptable interventions, people's barriers to cancer prevention and early detection. Much of her research has been directed at minorities.

In 1992, Rimer was a co-recipient (with Karen Glanz and Frances Lewis) of the Mayhew Derryberry Award for outstanding contributions to theory and research in health education, from the Public Health Education and Health Promotion Section of APHA. She presently serves or has recently served on the editorial boards of several journals, including *Health Education Quarterly, Preventive Medicine,* and *Health Education Research.* She recently served as guest editor of a special issue of the *Annals of Behavioral Medicine* on breast cancer control. Rimer is the author or coauthor of more than 140 scientific articles. With colleagues, she has published most recently in *Journal of the National Cancer Institute, American Journal of Public Health, Health Psychology,* and *Annals of Behavioral Medicine.*

THE CONTRIBUTORS

David B. Abrams is professor of psychiatry and human behavior and director of the Center for Behavioral and Preventive Medicine at the Brown University School of Medicine and the Miriam Hospital in Providence, Rhode Island.

Tom Baranowski is professor in the Department of Behavioral Science at the University of Texas M.D. Anderson Cancer Center.

Karen M. Emmons is assistant professor at the Dana-Farber Cancer Institute in Boston and in the Department of Health and Social Behavior at the Harvard University School of Public Health.

Kerry E. Evers is research assistant at the Cancer Prevention Research Center at the University of Rhode Island.

John R. Finnegan, Jr., is associate professor in the Division of Epidemiology at the University of Minnesota School of Public Health.

Andrea Carlson Gielen is associate professor of social and behavioral sciences in the Department of Health Policy and Management at the Johns Hopkins University School of Hygiene and Public Health in Baltimore.

Robert M. Goodman is associate professor of public health and director of the Center for Community Research at the Bowman Gray School of Medicine at Wake Forest University in North Carolina.

Judith A. Hall is professor in the Department of Psychology at Northeastern University in Boston.

Deborah M. Hardcastle is research psychologist in the Department of Psychological Medicine at the University of Sydney, Australia.

Catherine A. Heaney is assistant professor in the Division of Health Behavior and Health Promotion at the School of Public Health at Ohio State University.

Barbara A. Israel is professor and chair of the Department of Health Behavior and Health Education at the School of Public Health, University of Michigan.

Danuta Kasprzyk is senior research scientist at the Centers for Public Health Research and Evaluation, Battelle Memorial Institute in Seattle and affiliate assistant professor in the Department of Psychosocial and Community Health at the University of Washington School of Nursing.

Michelle C. Kegler is assistant professor of health promotion sciences at the College of Public Health at the University of Oklahoma.

Gerjo Kok is professor in health education and scientific director of the research institute HEALTH at the University of Maastricht, the Netherlands, and holds an endowed chair for AIDS prevention and health education from the Dutch AIDS Foundation.

R. Craig Lefebvre is chief technical officer and vice president for health communications at Prospect Associates in Rockville, Maryland.

Caryn Lerman is associate professor of medicine and psychiatry and director of bio-behavioral research in the Lombardi Cancer Center at the Georgetown University Medical Center in Washington, D.C.

Laura A. Linnan is project director at the Center for Behavioral and Preventive Medicine at the Miriam Hospital and the Brown University School of Medicine in Providence, Rhode Island.

Eileen M. McDonald is instructor in the Department of Health Policy and Management at the Johns Hopkins University School of Hygiene and Public Health in Baltimore, and codirector of the master's degree program in health education.

Meredith Minkler is professor and chair of community health education in the School of Public Health at the University of California, Berkeley.

Daniel E. Montaño is senior research scientist at the Centers for Public Health Research and Evaluation, Battelle Memorial Institute in Seattle and affiliate assistant professor in the Department of Psychosocial and Community Health at the University of Washington School of Nursing and the Department of Health Services at the University of Washington School of Public Health.

Brian Oldenburg is professor and head of the School of Public Health and director of the Center for Public Health Research at the Queensland University of Technology, in Brisbane, Australia.

Neville Owen is professor of human movement science at Deakin University in Burwood, Australia.

Guy S. Parcel is professor of behavioral sciences and pediatrics at the Houston Health Sciences Center at the University of Texas and director of the Center for Health Promotion Research and Development at the University of Texas School of Public Health.

Rena J. Pasick is associate director for prevention sciences at the Northern California Cancer Center.

Cheryl L. Perry is professor in the Division of Epidemiology of the University of Minnesota School of Public Health.

James O. Prochaska is professor of clinical and health psychology and director of the Cancer Prevention Research Center at the University of Rhode Island.

Colleen A. Redding is assistant research professor at the Cancer Prevention Research Center and adjunct professor of psychology at the University of Rhode Island.

Lisa Rochlin is a senior adviser with Promoting Public Causes, a Washington, D.C.–based organization dedicated to providing communications expertise to non-profit organizations.

Irwin M. Rosenstock is emeritus professor of health behavior at the University of Michigan and at California State University, Long Beach.

Debra L. Roter is professor of health policy and management and associate chair of the faculty of social and behavioral sciences at the Johns Hopkins University School of Hygiene and Public Health in Baltimore.

James F. Sallis is professor in the Department of Psychology at San Diego State University and faculty member in the Department of Pediatrics, University of California, San Diego, School of Medicine.

Allan Steckler is professor of health behavior and health education and associate dean at the School of Public Health, University of North Carolina at Chapel Hill.

Victor J. Strecher is director of cancer prevention and control at the University of Michigan Comprehensive Cancer Center and professor in the Department of Health Behavior and Health Education at the University of Michigan School of Public Health.

Stephen H. Taplin is associate professor of family medicine at the University of Washington School of Medicine and associate investigator in the Center for Health Studies, Group Health Cooperative of Puget Sound.

K. Viswanath is assistant professor in the School of Journalism at Ohio State University.

Nina Wallerstein is associate professor in the Department of Family and Community Medicine at the University of New Mexico School of Medicine.

HEALTH BEHAVIOR AND
HEALTH EDUCATION

PART ONE

HEALTH BEHAVIOR
AND HEALTH EDUCATION:
THE FOUNDATIONS

CHAPTER ONE

THE SCOPE OF HEALTH PROMOTION AND HEALTH EDUCATION

The Editors

The range of health promotion and education activities today is nearly limitless. Health promotion specialists and health professionals may counsel people at risk for AIDS about safe sex; help children avoid tobacco, alcohol, and drugs; assist adults to stop smoking; help patients manage and cope with their illnesses; and organize communities or advocate policy changes aimed at fostering health improvement. Health education and health promotion professionals work all over the world in a variety of settings including schools, worksites, medical sites, and communities. They may also forge and test the fundamental theories that drive research and practice in health promotion and education. A premise of *Health Behavior and Health Education* is that a dynamic exchange between theory, research, and practice produces effective health education.

Perhaps never before have those concerned with health behavior and health education been faced with more challenges and opportunities than they are today. Kanfer and Schefft (1988) observed that "as science and technology advance, the greatest mystery of the universe and the least conquered force of nature remains the human being and his actions and human experiences." The body of research in health behavior and health education has grown rapidly over the past two decades, and health education is recognized increasingly as a way to meet public health objectives and improve the success of public health and medical interventions. Although this increasing literature improves the scientific base of health education, it also challenges those in the field to master and be facile with an almost overwhelming body of knowledge.

Health education and health promotion are eclectic, rapidly evolving, and reflective of an amalgamation of approaches, methods, and strategies drawn from social and health sciences. They employ the theoretical perspectives, research findings, and practice tools of such diverse disciplines as psychology, sociology, anthropology, communications, nursing, and marketing. Health education also requires knowledge produced by the fields of epidemiology, statistics, and medicine. This reliance on other disciplines requires the individual health education professional to synthesize large and diverse literatures.

Many types of professionals contribute to and conduct health promotion and education programs and research. Health education practice is strengthened by the close collaboration among professionals of different disciplines, each concerned with the behavioral and social intervention process and each contributing a unique perspective. Psychology brings to health education a rich legacy of over one hundred years of research and practice on the differences between individuals and on human motivation, learning, persuasion, and attitude and behavioral change (Matarazzo and others, 1984). Physicians are important collaborators and are in key roles to effect change in individuals' health behavior. Likewise, nurses and social workers bring to health education their particular expertise in working with individual patients and patients' families to facilitate learning, adjustment, and behavioral change. Other health, education, and human service professionals contribute their special expertise as well. Increasingly, there will be partnerships with genetic counselors and other specialists in this rapidly developing field.

Health, Disease, and Health Behavior: The Changing Context

The major causes of death in the United States and other developed countries today are chronic diseases such as heart disease, cancer, and stroke (U.S. Department of Health, Education and Welfare, 1979). Behavioral factors, particularly tobacco use, diet and activity patterns, alcohol consumption, sexual behavior, and avoidable injuries are among the most prominent contributors to mortality (McGinnis and Foege, 1993). The resurgence of infectious diseases including foodborne illnesses and tuberculosis and the emergence of new infectious diseases such as antibiotic-resistant infections and HIV and AIDS (human acquired immunodeficiency syndrome) are also largely affected by human behaviors (Lederberg, Shope, and Oakes, 1992; Glanz and Yang, 1996). Substantial suffering, premature mortality, and medical costs can be avoided by positive changes in individuals' behavior.

During the past twenty years, there has been a dramatic increase in public, private, and professional interest in preventing disability and death through lifestyle changes and participation in screening programs. Much of this interest in health promotion and disease prevention has been stimulated by the epidemiological transition from infectious to chronic diseases as leading causes of death, the aging of the population, rapidly escalating health care costs, and data linking individual behaviors to increased risk of morbidity and mortality. More recent developments, such as the AIDS epidemic, have also contributed. Even as epidemiologists' efforts to better specify the links between diet, lifestyle, and environmental factors and disease approach the limits of science, they continue to generate headlines, draw public attention (Taubes, 1995), and influence public policy (Marshall, 1995).

Landmark reports in Canada and the United States during the 1970s and 1980s heralded the commitment of governments to health promotion (Lalonde, 1974; U.S. Department of Health, Education, and Welfare, 1979; Epp, 1986). In the United States, federal initiatives for public health education and monitoring populationwide behavioral patterns were spurred by the development of the health objectives published in *Promoting Health and Preventing Disease: Health Objectives for the Nation* (U.S. Department of Health and Human Services, 1980) and the succeeding health objectives identified in *Healthy People 2000: National Health Promotion and Disease Prevention Objectives* (U.S. Department of Health and Human Services, 1991). Increased interest in behavioral determinants of health and disease has drawn attention to the importance of health behavior change and spawned numerous training programs and public and commercial service programs.

Data systems now make it possible to track trends in risk factors, health behaviors, and health-promoting policies in the United States. The data show that indeed, there have been positive changes in several areas of concern (U.S. Department of Health and Human Services, 1995). Blood pressure control has improved and mean population blood cholesterol levels have declined. Alcohol-related motor vehicle deaths have decreased, and deaths due to automobile crashes and to falls and drowning are down. Fewer adults are using tobacco products and living sedentary lifestyles. Average daily intake of dietary fat has dropped from 36 percent to 34 percent of total energy, and the use of seat belts is up from 42 percent in 1988 to 67 percent in 1994. The proportion of women aged forty and older who have had breast examinations and mammograms more than doubled between 1988 and 1994. Restrictive smoking policies and laws have become widespread, as have worksite health promotion programs. The collective efforts of those in health promotion and education have indeed made a difference. Although this progress is encouraging, much work remains to be done in these areas.

Not all the news is favorable, either. More adults than before are overweight. More adolescents are sexually active. Teenaged girls have been remarkably resistant to messages about smoking prevention. The incidence of tuberculosis, a disease thought to have been eradicated, has risen. Drug abuse–related emergency room visits are more common, and the incidence of diagnosed cases of AIDS has increased dramatically (U.S. Department of Health and Human Services, 1995). Further, ethnic minorities and those in poverty experience a disproportionate burden of preventable disease and disability (Adler and others, 1994), and for many conditions, the gap between disadvantaged and affluent groups is widening (U.S. Department of Health and Human Services, 1991).

Changes in the health care system provide new supports and opportunities for health promotion and education. Respect for patients' rights is now recognized as fundamental to the practice of medicine (National Health Council, 1995; Levinsky, 1996). At the same time, patients' access to information about their health care institutions and providers remains limited. Insurance carriers and managed care systems can impose barriers that impede patients' exercise of their right to make treatment decisions (Weston and Lauria, 1996; Levinsky, 1996). The advent of managed health care and health care financing reform poses new challenges as the drive for cost containment affects the entire health care system (Shore and Beigel, 1996). Although increased accountability often results in cost savings and fewer unnecessary services, little is known about its effects on the health of patients and the overall quality of care (Iglehart, 1996). Clinical prevention and behavioral interventions may grow in importance under managed care when their cost effectiveness is demonstrated and recognized (Sobel, 1994), but the impact of fiscal constraint is sure to be negative, at least in the short run.

Health Promotion, Health Education, and Health Behavior

Scope and Evolution of Health Promotion and Education

In the field of health education during the 1970s and 1980s, the emphasis on individuals' behaviors as determinants of their health status eclipsed attention to the broader social determinants of health. Advocates of system-level changes to improve health then called for renewal of a broad vision of health promotion (Minkler, 1989; Terris, 1992). These calls for moving health education toward social action are well within the tradition of health education and are consistent with its increased concern with social, economic, and political forces.

Over the past thirty years, outstanding leaders in health education have repeatedly stressed the importance of political, economic, and social factors as determinants of health. Mayhew Derryberry (1960) noted that "health education . . . requires careful and thorough consideration of the present knowledge, attitudes, goals, perceptions, social status, power structure, cultural traditions, and other aspects of whatever public is to be addressed." In 1966, Dorothy Nyswander wrote of the importance of attending to social justice and individuals' sense of control and self-determination. These ideas were reiterated later when William Griffiths (1972) stressed that "health education is concerned not only with individuals and their families, but *also with the institutions and social conditions* that impede or facilitate individuals toward achieving optimum health" (emphasis added).

The view that health education is an instrument of social change has been renewed and invigorated during the past decade. Advocacy, policy change, and organizational change have been adopted as central activities of public health education and health promotion. This volume purposefully includes chapters on community and societal influences on health behavior, and strategies to effect community and social policy changes. In this context, definitions of health education and health promotion can be recognized and discussed as overlapping and intertwined.

Definitions

Health education and health promotion have been defined in many ways. According to Griffiths (1972), *health education* "attempts to close the gap between what is known about optimum health practice and that which is actually practiced." Simonds (1976) defined health education as aimed at "bringing about behavioral changes in individuals, groups, and larger populations from behaviors that are presumed to be detrimental to health, to behaviors that are conducive to present and future health."

Subsequent definitions of health education have emphasized voluntary, informed behavioral changes. In 1980, Green defined health education as "any combination of learning experiences designed to facilitate voluntary adaptations of behavior conducive to health" (Green, Kreuter, Deeds, and Partridge, 1980). The Role Delineation Project defined health education as "the process of assisting individuals, acting separately or collectively, to make informed decisions about matters affecting their personal health and that of others" (National Task Force on the Preparation and Practice of Health Educators, 1985).

Health education evolved from three settings: communities, schools, and patient care sites. Kurt Lewin's pioneering work in group process and his developmental field theory during the 1930s and 1940s form the intellectual roots of much of today's health education practice. One of the earliest models developed to explain health behavior, the Health Belief Model, was developed during the 1950s to explain behavior related to tuberculosis screening (Hochbaum, 1958).

Health education includes not only instructional activities and other strategies to change individual health behavior but also organizational efforts, policy directives, economic supports, environmental activities, and community-level programs. Two key ideas from an ecological perspective help direct the identification of personal and environmental leverage points for health promotion and education interventions (Glanz and Rimer, 1995). First, behavior is viewed as being affected by, and affecting, *multiple levels of influence.* Five levels of influence for health-related behaviors and conditions have been identified: (1) intrapersonal, or individual factors; (2) interpersonal factors; (3) institutional, or organizational, factors; (4) community factors; and (5) public policy factors (McLeroy, Bibeau, Steckler, and Glanz, 1988). The second key idea is that there is *reciprocal causation* between individuals and their environments: that is, behavior both influences *and* is influenced by the social environment (Stokols, 1992; Glanz and Rimer, 1995).

Health education covers the continuum from disease prevention and promotion of optimal health to the detection of illness to treatment, rehabilitation, and long-term care. Health education is delivered in almost every conceivable setting—universities, schools, hospitals, pharmacies, grocery stores and shopping centers, community organizations, voluntary health agencies, worksites, churches, prisons, health maintenance organizations, migrant labor camps, advertising agencies, and health departments at all levels of government. These diverse settings are discussed later in this chapter.

Health promotion is a term of more recent origin than health education. As defined by Green, it is "any combination of health education and related organizational, economic, and environmental supports for behavior of individuals, groups, or communities conducive to health" (Green and Kreuter, 1991).

Another, slightly different definition is suggested by O'Donnell (1989): "Health promotion is the science and art of helping people change their lifestyle to move toward a state of optimal health. . . . Lifestyle change can be facilitated by a combination of efforts to enhance awareness, change behavior, and create environments that support good health practices." Definitions arising in Europe and Canada have another emphasis again (Kolbe, 1988; Hawe, Degeling, and Hall, 1990). For example, the *Ottawa Charter for Health Promotion* defines health promotion as "the process of enabling people to increase control over, and to improve, their health . . . a commitment to dealing with the challenges of reducing inequities, extending the scope of prevention, and helping people to cope with their circumstances . . . creating environments conducive to health, in which people are better able to take care of themselves" (Epp, 1986).

Although some may argue that greater precision of terminology can be achieved by drawing a clear distinction between health education and health promotion, to do so is to ignore long-standing tenets of health education and its broad social mission. Clearly, health educators have long used more than "educational" strategies. In fact, the terms health promotion and health education are often used interchangeably in the United States (Breckon, Harvey, and Lancaster, 1994). In some countries, such as Australia, health education is considered a much narrower endeavor than health promotion. Nevertheless, although the term health promotion emphasizes efforts to influence the broader social context of health behavior, the two terms remain closely linked and overlapping and share a common historical and philosophical foundation. They are often used in combination, as in the title of this chapter. In most cases, we consider the two terms too closely related to distinguish between them.

Health Behavior

The central concern of health promotion and health education is health behavior. It is included or suggested in every definition of health promotion and education and is the crucial dependent variable in most research on the impact of health education intervention strategies. Positive informed changes in health behavior are typically the ultimate aims of health promotion and education programs; if behaviors change but health is not subsequently improved, the result is a paradox that must be resolved by examining other issues, such as the link between behavior and health status.

In the broadest sense, *health behavior* refers to the actions of individuals, groups, and organizations and to those actions' determinants, correlates, and consequences, including social change, policy development and implementation, improved coping skills (see Chapter Six), and enhanced quality of life (Parkerson and others, 1993). This is similar to the working definition of health behavior that Gochman proposed (although his definition emphasized individuals): it includes not only observable, overt actions but also the mental events and feeling states that can be reported and measured. Gochman (1982) defined health behavior as "those personal attributes such as beliefs, expectations, motives, values, perceptions, and other cognitive elements; personality characteristics, including affective and emotional states and traits; and overt behavioral patterns, actions, and habits that relate to health maintenance, to health restoration, and to health improvement."

Gochman's definition is consistent with and embraces the definitions of specific categories of overt health behavior proposed by Kasl and Cobb in their seminal articles (1966a, 1966b). Kasl and Cobb define three categories of health behavior:

1. *Preventive health behavior.* Any activity undertaken by an individual who believes himself to be healthy, for the purpose of preventing or detecting illness in an asymptomatic state.

2. *Illness behavior.* Any activity undertaken by an individual who perceives himself to be ill, to define the state of his health, and to discover a suitable remedy (Kasl and Cobb, 1966a).

③ *Sick-role behavior.* Any activity undertaken by an individual who considers himself to be ill, for the purpose of getting well. It includes receiving treatment from medical providers, generally involves a whole range of dependent behaviors, and leads to some degree of exemption from one's usual responsibilities (Kasl and Cobb, 1966b).

Settings and Audiences for Health Promotion and Education

During the past century and more specifically during the past few decades, the scope and methods of health promotion and education have broadened and diversified dramatically. This section briefly reviews the range of settings and audiences for health promotion and education today.

Settings: Where Are Health Promotion and Education Provided?

Today, health promotion and education can be found nearly everywhere. The settings for health promotion are important because they represent channels for delivering programs and access to specific populations and gatekeepers, they usually have existing communication systems for diffusion of programs, and they facilitate development of policies and organizational change to support positive health practices (Mullen and others, 1995). Five major settings are particularly relevant to health promotion and education: schools, communities, worksites, health care sites, and the consumer marketplace.

Schools. Health education in the schools includes classroom teaching, teacher training, and changes in the school environment that support healthy behaviors (Parcel, Simons-Morton, and Kolbe, 1988). To support long-term health enhancement initiatives, theories of organizational change are applied to encourage adoption of comprehensive smoking control programs in schools (see Chapter Fourteen). Diffusion theory and the Theory of Reasoned Action have been used to analyze factors associated with adoption of AIDS prevention curricula in Dutch schools (see Chapter Thirteen).

Communities. Community-based health education draws on social relationships and organizations to reach large populations through media and interpersonal strategies. Models of community organization enable program planners both to gain support for and to design suitable health messages and delivery mechanisms (see Chapter Twelve). Community interventions in churches, clubs, and neighborhoods have been used to encourage healthful nutrition, reduce risk of cardiovascular disease, and use peer influence to promote breast cancer detection among minority women (see Chapters Eight and Nine).

Worksites. Since its emergence in the mid-1970s, worksite health promotion has grown and spawned new tools for health educators. Because people spend so much time at work, the workplace is both a source of stress and a source of social support (Israel and Schurman, 1990). Effective worksite programs can harness social support as a buffer to stress, with the goal of improving worker health and health practices. Today, many businesses, particularly large corporations, provide health promotion programs for their employees (Office of Disease Prevention and Health Promotion, 1992). Strategies aimed at both high-risk individuals and entire populations have been used in programs to reduce individuals' risk of cancer (Tilley and others, 1995; Sorensen and others, 1996) and cardiovascular disease (Glasgow and others, 1995).

Health Care Sites. Health education for high-risk persons, patients, their families, and the surrounding community and in-service training for health care providers are all part of health care today. The changing nature of health service delivery has stimulated greater emphasis on health education in physicians' offices, health maintenance organizations, public health clinics, and hospitals (Strecher and others, 1994; Walsh and McPhee, 1992; King and others, 1993). Primary care settings, in particular, provide an opportunity to reach a substantial number of people (Campbell and others, 1993; Glanz and others, 1990). Health education in these settings focuses on preventing and detecting disease, helping people make decisions about genetic testing, and managing acute and chronic illnesses.

Consumer Marketplace. The advent of home health and self-care products and the use of "health" appeals to sell consumer goods have created new opportunities for health education *and* for misleading consumers about the potential health effects of items they can purchase (Glanz and others, 1995). Social marketing, with its roots in consumer behavior theory, is used increasingly by health educators to enhance the salience of health messages and to improve their persuasive impact (see Chapter Eighteen). Theories of Consumer Information Processing provide a framework for understanding why people do or do not pay attention to, understand, and make use of nutrient labels on packaged food products (Rudd and Glanz, 1990).

Audiences: Who Are the Recipients of Health Promotion and Education?

For health promotion and education to be effective, they should be designed with an understanding of the recipients, or target audiences: their health and social characteristics and their beliefs, attitudes, values, skills, and past behaviors. These audiences consist of people who may be reached as individuals, in groups, through organizations, or in communities or sociopolitical entities. They may be health professionals, clients, people at risk for disease, or patients. This section discusses two dimensions along which the potential audiences can be characterized: sociodemographic characteristics and life cycle stages.

Sociodemographic Characteristics. Socioeconomic status has been linked with both health status and health behavior, with less affluent persons consistently experiencing higher morbidity and mortality (Adler and others, 1994). Various sociodemographic characteristics such as gender, age, race, marital status, place of residence, employment, and educational level characterize health education audiences. These factors, although generally not *modifiable* within the bounds of health education programs, are useful in guiding the tailoring of strategies and educational material and in identifying channels through which to reach consumers. Printed educational materials should be appropriate to and, ideally, tailored to the educational and reading levels of particular target audiences and be consistent with their ethnic and cultural backgrounds. Chapter Twenty examines the role of cultural and sociodemographic factors in health behavior theory, research, and practice.

Life Cycle Stage. Health promotion and health education are provided for people at every stage of the life cycle, from childbirth education, whose beneficiaries are not yet born, to self-care education and rehabilitation for the very old. Developmental perspectives help guide the choice of intervention and research methods. Children may have misperceptions about health and illness, such as that illnesses are a punishment for bad behavior (Armsden and Lewis, 1993). Knowledge of children's cognitive development provides a framework for adults to understand these beliefs and ways to respond to them. Adolescents may feel invulnerable to accidents and chronic diseases. The Health Belief Model (see Chapter Three) is a useful framework for understanding the factors that may predispose youth to engage in unsafe sexual practices. Older adults may attribute symptoms of cancer to the inexorable process of aging. Beliefs such as this must be considered in designing, implementing, and evaluating programs (Rimer and others, 1983; Keintz, Rimer, Fleisher, and Engstrom, 1988).

Progress in Health Promotion and Health Behavior Research

Over the past two decades, research programs have been established to identify and test the most effective methods for achieving individual behavioral change. More precise quantification of personal health behaviors and improved health outcomes have grown out of the partnerships between behavioral health scientists and biomedical health experts (Green and Lewis, 1986; Epstein, 1992). In the past few years, the findings of several large health behavior intervention studies have been published. Some major trials have yielded disappointing results, thereby increasing the dilemmas involved in applying theory, research, and theory-testing research in health promotion and education practice.

In the late 1970s and early 1980s, three large community cardiovascular disease intervention studies were begun in California, Minnesota, and Rhode Island (Matarazzo and others, 1984; Winkleby, 1994). Each study addressed smoking, hypertension, high-fat diets, obesity, and physical inactivity—all widespread risk factors that many practitioners were tackling. The multicomponent risk reduction programs in these trials used mass media and interpersonal education programs for the public, professionals, and those at high risk. Community organization strategies were used to create institutional and environmental support for the programs, and theoretically derived program-planning strategies emphasized community participation (Winkleby, 1994).

All three studies have now reported their findings for risk factor changes. The Stanford Five-City Project in California found strong positive secular trends—that is, changes in control communities that could not be attributed to intervention—and significant improvements in blood pressure and smoking favoring the treatment communities (Farquhar and others, 1990). Findings from the Minnesota Heart Health Program recently were released, and they also documented strong secular trends in risk factors in all communities, but only modest, short-lived, and nonsignificant positive changes in risk factors in the intervention communities (Luepker and others, 1994). Results of the Pawtucket Heart Health Program included a greater downward trend in smoking in the control city, and small insignificant differences favoring the intervention community in blood cholesterol and blood pressure (Carleton and others, 1995). Two large worksite trials of multicomponent nutrition and smoking interventions yielded similar findings—modest or nonsignificant intervention effects and apparent favorable secular trends in control sites (Glasgow and others, 1995; Sorensen and others, 1996).

These studies produced a wealth of knowledge about health behavior, and many of the short-term targeted interventions within the larger studies were found to be effective (Winkleby, 1994). Nonetheless, the results cast doubt on the presumed effectiveness of population-based intervention strategies over the long term, especially against the backdrop of a dynamic, changing environment. Still, the lack of significant communitywide impacts in these studies should not be assumed to disprove the conceptual foundations of the intervention methods. An alternative view, for example, is to regard the interventions used in these studies as contributors to the substantial secular trend in chronic disease prevention (Winkleby,

1994). Also, more attention must be paid to finding ways to reach the people who have resisted previous messages and programs.

An important lesson from both the community and worksite studies relates to the methodological limitations of large, complex multicomponent trials (Koepsell, Diehr, Cheadle, and Kristal, 1995). Randomized designs can mask subgroup effects, and the main findings do not tell the whole story. Treatment effects may diminish or appear quite limited when analyzed using conservative methods that consider large units of randomization and analysis, such as schools, worksites, and communities (Rooney and Murray, 1996).

Although randomized controlled trials are the most rigorous test of health behavior interventions, the past decade has been marked by an increase in carefully designed evaluation research in health promotion that combines quantitative and qualitative methods. Recently published evaluations of community-based AIDS prevention projects (Janz and others, 1996) and coalitions for prevention of alcohol, tobacco and other drug abuse (Butterfoss, Goodman, and Wandersman, 1996) exemplify new applications of community research methodologies that offer in-depth process information across multiple programs in diverse settings.

The challenge of understanding and improving health behavior is a central challenge for health policy today and is "one of the most complex tasks yet confronted by science. To competently address that challenge, the . . . research community must simply do more and do it better" in certain key areas of behavioral research (McGinnis, 1994). A coordinated and focused effort will be essential to resolving many of the most vexing health issues facing this society (Regier, 1994). The integration of the best available knowledge from theory, research, and health promotion and education practice can help advance that agenda in the next decade.

Health Behavior and Education Foundations and the Importance of Theory, Research, and Practice

This chapter has discussed the dynamic nature of health promotion and education today in the context of changing patterns of disease and trends in health care, health promotion, and disease prevention. It has provided definitions of health education, health promotion, and health behavior and described the broad and diverse parameters of this maturing field. Health behavior research has experienced great progress, but disappointing findings raise new questions and pose methodological, theoretical, and substantive challenges. The interrelationships and importance of theory, research, and practice are set against a backdrop of the growing and complex challenges in health promotion, health education, and health behavior.

References

Adler, N. E., and others. "Socioeconomic Status and Health: The Challenge of the Gradient." *American Psychologist*, 1994, *49*(1), 15–24.

Armsden, G., and Lewis, F. M. "The Child's Adaptation to Parental Medical Illness: Theory and Clinical Implications." *Patient Education and Counseling*, 1993, *22*, 153–165.

Breckon, D. J., Harvey, J. R., and Lancaster, R. B. *Community Health Education: Settings, Roles and Skills for the 21st Century.* Gaithersburg, Md.: Aspen, 1994.

Butterfoss, F. D., Goodman, R. M., and Wandersman, A. "Community Coalitions for Prevention and Health Promotion: Factors Predicting Satisfaction, Participation, and Planning." *Health Education Quarterly*, 1996, *23*(1), 65–79.

Campbell, M., and others. "Improving Dietary Behavior: The Effectiveness of Tailored Messages in Primary Care Settings." *American Journal of Public Health*, 1993, *84*(5), 783–787.

Carleton, R. A., and others. "The Pawtucket Heart Health Program: Community Changes in Cardiovascular Risk Factors and Projected Disease Risk." *American Journal of Public Health*, 1995, *85*(6), 777–785.

Derryberry, M. "Health Education: Its Objectives and Methods." *Health Education Monographs*, 1960, *8*, 5–11.

Epp, L. *Achieving Health for All: A Framework for Health Promotion in Canada.* Toronto: Health and Welfare Canada, 1986.

Epstein, L. H. "Role of Behavior Theory in Behavioral Medicine." *Journal of Consulting and Clinical Psychology*, 1992, *60*(4), 493–498.

Farquhar, J. W., and others. "Effect of Community-Wide Education on Cardiovascular Disease Risk Factors: The Stanford Five-City Project." *Journal of the American Medical Association*, 1990, *264*, 359–365.

Glanz, K., and Rimer, B. K. *Theory at a Glance: A Guide for Health Promotion Practice.* NIH publication no. 95–3896. Bethesda, Md.: National Institutes of Health, National Cancer Institute, 1995.

Glanz, K., and Yang, H. "Communicating About Risk of Infectious Diseases." *Journal of the American Medical Association*, 1996, *275*(3), 253–256.

Glanz, K., and others. "Patient Reactions to Nutrition Education for Cholesterol Reduction." *American Journal of Preventive Medicine*, 1990, *60*(6), 311–317.

Glanz, K., and others. "Environmental and Policy Approaches to Cardiovascular Disease Prevention Through Nutrition: Opportunities for State and Local Action." *Health Education Quarterly*, 1995, *22*(4), 512–527.

Glasgow, R. E., and others. "Take Heart: Results from the Initial Phase of a Work-Site Wellness Program." *American Journal of Public Health*, 1995, *85*(2), 209–216.

Gochman, D. S. "Labels, Systems, and Motives: Some Perspectives on Future Research." *Health Education Quarterly*, 1982, *9*, 167–174.

Green, L. W., and Kreuter, M. W. *Health Promotion Planning: An Educational and Environmental Approach.* (2nd ed.) Mountain View, Calif.: Mayfield, 1991.

Green, L. W., Kreuter, M. W., Deeds, S. G., and Partridge, K. B. *Health Education Planning: A Diagnostic Approach.* Mountain View, Calif.: Mayfield, 1980.

Green, L. W., and Lewis, F. M. *Measurement and Evaluation in Health Education and Health Promotion.* Mountain View, Calif.: Mayfield, 1986.

Griffiths, W. "Health Education Definitions, Problems, and Philosophies." *Health Education Monographs*, 1972, *31*, 12–14.

Hawe, P., Degeling, D., and Hall, J. *Evaluating Health Promotion: A Health Worker's Guide.* Sydney: MacLennan and Petty, 1990.

Hochbaum, G. M. *Public Participation in Medical Screening Programs: A Sociopsychological Study.* PHS publication no. 572. Bethesda, Md.: U.S. Department of Health and Human Services, Public Health Service, 1958.

Iglehart, J. "Managed Care and Mental Health." *New England Journal of Medicine,* 1996, *334*(2), 131–135.

Israel, B. A., and Schurman, S. J. "Social Support, Control, and the Stress Process." In K. Glanz, F. M. Lewis, and B. K. Rimer (eds.), *Health Behavior and Health Education: Theory, Research, and Practice.* San Francisco: Jossey-Bass, 1990.

Janz, N. K., and others. "Evaluation of 37 AIDS Prevention Projects: Successful Approaches and Barriers to Program Effectiveness." *Health Education Quarterly,* 1996, *23*(1), 80–97.

Kanfer, F. H., and Schefft, B. *Guiding the Process of Therapeutic Change.* Champaign, Ill.: Research Press, 1988.

Kasl, S. V., and Cobb, S. "Health Behavior, Illness Behavior, and Sick-Role Behavior: I. Health and Illness Behavior." *Archives of Environmental Health,* 1966a, *12,* 246–266.

Kasl, S. V., and Cobb, S. "Health Behavior, Illness Behavior, and Sick-Role Behavior: II. Sick-Role Behavior." *Archives of Environmental Health,* 1966b, *12,* 531–541.

Keintz, M., Rimer, B., Fleisher, L., and Engstrom, P. F. "Educating Older Adults About Their Increased Cancer Risk." *Gerontologist,* 1988, *28,* 487–490.

King, E., and others. "Promoting Mammography Through Progressive Interventions." *American Journal of Public Health,* 1993, *84*(1), 1644–1656.

Koepsell, T., Diehr, P., Cheadle, A., and Kristal, A. "Invited Commentary: Symposium on Community Intervention Trials." *American Journal of Epidemiology,* 1995, *142,* 1–6.

Kolbe, L. J. "The Application of Health Behavior Research: Health Education and Health Promotion." In D. S. Gochman (ed.), *Health Behavior: Emerging Research Perspectives.* New York: Plenum, 1988.

Lalonde, M. *A New Perspective on the Health of Canadians: A Working Document.* Toronto: Health and Welfare Canada, 1974.

Lederberg, J., Shope, R., and Oakes, S. (eds.). *Emerging Infections: Microbial Threats to Health in the United States.* Washington, D.C.: National Academy Press, 1992.

Levinsky, N. "Social, Institutional, and Economic Barriers to the Exercise of Patients' Rights." *New England Journal of Medicine,* 1996, *334*(8), 532–534.

Luepker, R. V., and others. "Community Education for Cardiovascular Disease Prevention: Risk Factor Changes in the Minnesota Heart Health Program." *American Journal of Public Health,* 1994, *84,* 1383–1393.

Marshall, J. R. "Editorial: Improving Americans' Diet—Setting Public Policy with Limited Knowledge." *American Journal of Public Health,* 1995, *85*(12), 1609–1611.

Matarazzo, J. D., and others (eds.). *Behavioral Health: A Handbook of Health Enhancement and Disease Prevention.* New York: Wiley, 1984.

McGinnis, J. M. "The Role of Behavioral Research in National Health Policy." In S. Blumenthal, K. Matthews, and S. Weiss (eds.), *New Research Frontiers in Behavioral Medicine: Proceedings of the National Conference.* Bethesda, Md.: National Institutes of Health, Health and Behavior Coordinating Committee, 1994.

McGinnis, J. M., and Foege, W. H. "Actual Causes of Death in the United States." *Journal of the American Medical Association,* 1993, *270*(18), 2207–2212.

McLeroy, K. R., Bibeau, D., Steckler, A., and Glanz, K. "An Ecological Perspective on Health Promotion Programs." *Health Education Quarterly,* 1988, *15,* 351–377.

Minkler, M. "Health Education, Health Promotion, and the Open Society: A Historical Perspective." *Health Education Quarterly*, 1989, *16*, 17–30.

Mullen, P. D., and others. "Settings as an Important Dimension in Health Education/Promotion Policy, Programs, and Research." *Health Education Quarterly*, 1995, *22*, 329–345.

National Health Council. *Putting Patients First: Patients' Rights and Responsibilities.* Washington, D.C.: National Health Council, 1995.

National Task Force on the Preparation and Practice of Health Educators. *A Framework for the Development of Competency-Based Curricula.* New York: National Task Force on the Preparation and Practice of Health Educators, 1985.

Nyswander, D. "The Open Society: Its Implications for Health Educators." *Health Education Monographs*, 1966, *1*, 3–13.

O'Donnell, M. P. "Definition of Health Promotion. Part III: Expanding the Definition." *American Journal of Health Promotion*, 1989, *3*, 5.

Office of Disease Prevention and Health Promotion, Public Health Service. *National Survey of Worksite Health Promotion Programs.* Washington, D.C.: Office of Disease Prevention and Health Promotion, Public Health Service, 1992.

Parcel, G. S., Simons-Morton, B., and Kolbe, L. J. "Health Promotion: Integrating Organizational Change and Student Learning Strategies." *Health Education Quarterly*, 1988, *15*, 435–450.

Parkerson, G., and others. "Disease-Specific Versus Generic Measurement of Health-Related Quality of Life in Insulin Dependent Diabetic Patients." *Medical Care*, 1993, *31*, 629–637.

Regier, D. "Health Care Reform: Opportunities and Challenge." In S. Blumenthal, K. Matthews, and S. Weiss (eds.), *New Research Frontiers in Behavioral Medicine: Proceedings of the National Conference.* Bethesda, Md.: National Institutes of Health, Health and Behavior Coordinating Committee, 1994.

Rimer, B. K., and others. "Planning a Cancer Control Program for Older Citizens." *Gerontologist*, 1983, *23*, 384–389.

Rooney, B., and Murray, D. M. "A Meta-Analysis of Smoking Prevention Programs After Adjustment for Errors in the Unit of Analysis." *Health Education Quarterly*, 1996, *23*(1), 48–64.

Rudd, J., and Glanz, K. "How Individuals Use Information for Health Action: Consumer Information Processing." In K. Glanz, F. M. Lewis, and B. K. Rimer (eds.), *Health Behavior and Health Education: Theory, Research, and Practice.* San Francisco: Jossey-Bass, 1990.

Shore, M., and Beigel, A. "The Challenges Posed by Managed Behavioral Health Care." *New England Journal of Medicine*, 1996, *334*(2), 116–118.

Simonds, S. "Health Education in the Mid-1970s: State of the Art." In *Preventive Medicine USA.* New York: Prodist, 1976.

Sobel, D. "Mind Matters, Money Matters: The Cost-Effectiveness of Clinical Behavioral Medicine." In S. Blumenthal, K. Matthews, and S. Weiss (eds.), *New Research Frontiers in Behavioral Medicine: Proceedings of the National Conference.* Bethesda, Md.: National Institutes of Health, Health and Behavior Coordinating Committee, 1994.

Sorensen, G., and others. "Working Well: Results from a Worksite-Based Cancer Prevention Trial." *American Journal of Public Health*, 1996, *86*, 939–947.

Stokols, D. "Establishing and Maintaining Healthy Environments: Toward a Social Ecology of Health Promotion." *American Psychologist*, 1992, *47*(1), 6–22.

Strecher, V. J., and others. "The Effects of Computer-Tailored Smoking Cessation Messages in Family Practice Settings." *Journal of Family Practice*, 1994, *39*(3), 262–270.

Taubes, G. "Epidemiology Faces Its Limits." *Science*, July 14, 1995, *269*, 164–169.

Terris, M. "Concepts of Health Promotion: Dualities in Public Health Theory." *Journal of Public Health Policy*, Autumn 1992, pp. 267–276.

Tilley, B., and others. "Planning the Next Step: A Screening Promotion and Nutrition Intervention Trial in the Work Site." *Annals of the New York Academy of Sciences*, 1995, *768*, 292–295.

U.S. Department of Health, Education, and Welfare. *Healthy People: The Surgeon General's Report on Health Promotion and Disease Prevention.* PHS publication no. 79–55071. Bethesda, Md.: U.S. Department of Health, Education, and Welfare, Public Health Service, 1979.

U.S. Department of Health and Human Services. *Promoting Health and Preventing Disease: Health Objectives for the Nation.* Washington, D.C.: U.S. Government Printing Office, 1980.

U.S. Department of Health and Human Services. *Healthy People 2000: National Health Promotion and Disease Prevention Objectives.* DHHS publication no. PHS 91–50213. Washington, D.C.: U.S. Government Printing Office, 1991.

U.S. Department of Health and Human Services. *Healthy People 2000 Review: 1994.* DHHS publication no. PHS 95–12561. Washington, D.C.: U.S. Government Printing Office, 1995.

Walsh, J., and McPhee, S. "A Systems Model of Clinical Preventive Care: An Analysis of Factors Influencing Patient and Physician." *Health Education Quarterly*, 1992, *19*, 157–176.

Weston, B., and Lauria, M. "Patient Advocacy in the 1990s." *New England Journal of Medicine*, 1996, *334*(8), 543–544.

Winkleby, M. A. "The Future of Community-Based Cardiovascular Disease Intervention Studies." *American Journal of Public Health*, 1994, *84*, 1369–1372.

CHAPTER TWO

LINKING THEORY, RESEARCH, AND PRACTICE

The Editors

Theory, Research, and Practice: Interrelationships

Aristotle distinguished between *theoria* and *praxis*. *Theoria* signifies those sciences and activities that are concerned with knowing for its own sake, whereas *praxis* corresponds to the ways in which people now commonly speak of action or doing. This contrast between theory and practice (Bernstein, 1971) permeates Western philosophical and scientific thought from Aristotle to Marx and on to Dewey and other contemporary twentieth-century philosophers. Dewey attempted to resolve the dichotomy by focusing on the similarities and continuities between theoretical and practical judgments and inquiries. He described "experimental knowing" essentially as an art that involves a conscious, directed manipulation of objects and situations. "The craftsman perfects his art, not by comparing his product to some 'ideal' model, but by the cumulative results of experience—experience which benefits from tried and tested procedures but always involves risk and novelty" (Bernstein, 1971). Dewey thus described empirical investigation, that is, research, as the ground between theory and practice and the testing of theory in action.

Although the perception of theory and practice as a dichotomy has a long tradition in intellectual thought, we follow in Dewey's tradition and focus on the similarities and continuities rather than on the differences. Theory, research, and practice are a continuum along which the skilled professional can move with ease.

Theory and research are not solely the province of the academic, just as practice is not solely the field of the practitioner. Researchers and practitioners may differ in their priorities, but the relationship between research and its application can and should move in both directions (D'Onofrio, 1992; Freudenberg and others, 1995). "The search for truth and for an ultimate understanding of the forces that make humans think, feel, and act as they do is the long-term goal" (Kanfer and Schefft, 1988).

The task of health promotion and education is both to understand health behavior and to transform knowledge about behavior into useful strategies for health enhancement. Research in health promotion and education has an inherently applied cast; it is motivated and driven by service to existing or anticipated health concerns of individuals, groups, communities, and societies (Green and others, 1994; Kok and others, 1996). Researchers need to test their theories iteratively in the real world (Rosenstock, 1990). When they do so, theory, research, and practice begin to converge. The theories in this book are examined in light of their applicability and not as *basic* health behavior research.

Health Behavior and Health Education aims to help educators, whatever their background, understand some of the most important theoretical underpinnings of health promotion and education and use theory to inform research and practice. To function effectively in the increasingly complex world of health education, individuals need a broad-based understanding of theory, research, and practice. "Clearly, application of well-defined and carefully tested theories to the program development process holds tremendous advantages for health educators in terms of coherence, effectiveness, and evaluation of interventions" (van Ryn and Heaney, 1992).

We believe that "there is nothing so useful as a good theory" (Lewin, 1935). Each chapter in *Health Behavior and Health Education* demonstrates the practical value of theory; each synthesizes what was learned through conceptually sound research and practice; and each draws the linkages between theory, research, and practice.

Professionals charged with responsibility for health education are, by and large, interventionists. They are action oriented. They use their knowledge to design and to implement programs to improve health. This is true whether they are working to encourage positive changes in individual or community behavior. It is equally true of most health education research. Such research is conducted primarily in the real world, not in isolated laboratories. Usually, in the process of attempting to change behavior or policies, researchers must do precisely what practitioners do—develop and deliver interventions. At some level, both practitioners and researchers are accountable for results, whether these are measured in terms of participants' satisfaction with programs or changes in awareness, knowledge, attitudes, beliefs, and health behaviors; institutional norms; community integration; or more distal results including morbidity, mortality, and quality of life. Health educators may assess these results anecdotally (Burdine and McLeroy, 1992), or they may conduct more rigorous evaluations.

The design of interventions that yield desirable changes can best be done with an understanding of theories of behavioral change and an ability to use them skillfully in practice. Most health educators work in situations in which resources are limited, a circumstance that makes judgments about the choice of intervention very important. There may be no second chance to reach a critical target audience.

A synthesis of theory, research, and practice will advance what is known about health behavior. A health educator without a theory is like a mechanic or a mere technician, whereas the professional who understands theory and research comprehends the *why?* and can design and craft well-tailored interventions. He or she does not blindly follow a cookbook recipe but constantly creates the recipe anew, depending on the circumstances (Kreuter, 1988). In health promotion and education, the circumstances include the nature of the target audience, setting, resources, goals, and constraints (Fishbein and others, 1991; Prochaska, DiClemente, and Norcross, 1992; Green and others, 1994).

An understanding of theory also guides the health promoter to measure more carefully and astutely in order to assess the impact of interventions. Learning from successive interventions strengthens not only the knowledge base of the individual health professional but also, over time, such cumulative learning contributes to the knowledge base of all. Along their continuum, theory, research, and practice nurture and are nurtured by each other.

The health educator in a health maintenance organization who understands the relevance of The Transtheoretical Model or Social Cognitive Theory may be able to design better interventions to help patients lose weight or stop smoking. The community health educator who understands principles of social marketing and media communication can make far better use of the mass media than one who does not. A working knowledge of community organization can help the educator identify and mobilize key individuals and groups to develop or maintain a health promotion program. The physician who understands interpersonal influence can communicate more effectively with patients. The health psychologist who understands The Transtheoretical Model of Stages of Change will know how to design better smoking cessation and exercise interventions and how to tailor them to the needs of his or her patients.

What Is Theory?

A *theory* is a set of interrelated concepts, definitions, and propositions that presents a *systematic* view of events or situations by specifying relations among variables in order to *explain* and *predict* the events or situations. The notion of *generality*, or broad application, is important, as is *testability* (Green, 1991; van Ryn and Heaney, 1992). Theories are by their nature *abstract:* that is, they do not have a specified content or topic area (Glanz and Rimer, 1995). Like an empty coffee cup, they have a shape and boundaries but nothing concrete inside. They come alive only when they are filled with practical topics, goals, and problems.

A fully developed formal theory—more an ideal than a reality—is a completely closed deductive system of propositions that identifies interrelationships among concepts and is a systematic view of the phenomena at issue (Kerlinger, 1986; Blalock, 1969). In reality, there is no such system in the social sciences or in health promotion and education; it can only be approximated (Blalock, 1969). Theory has been defined in a variety of ways, each consistent with Kerlinger's definition. Table 2.1 summarizes several definitions of theory.

Theories can help investigators during the various stages of planning, implementing, and evaluating an intervention. Program planners can use theories to shape the pursuit of answers to why, what, and how. That is, theories can guide the search for *why* people are not following public health and medical advice or not caring for themselves in healthy ways. They can pinpoint *what* one needs to know before developing and organizing an intervention program. They can provide insight into *how* to shape program strategies to reach people and organizations and

TABLE 2.1. DEFINITIONS OF THEORY.

Definition	Source
A set of interrelated constructs (concepts), definitions, and propositions that presents a systematic view of phenomena by specifying relations among variables, with the purpose of explaining and predicting phenomena	Kerlinger, 1986, p. 9
A systematic explanation for the observed facts and laws that relate to a particular aspect of life	Babbie, 1989, p. 46
A formal and abstract statement about a selected aspect of reality	Kar, 1986, pp. 157–158
Knowledge writ large in the form of generalized abstractions applicable to a wide range of experiences	McGuire, 1983, p. 2
A set of relatively abstract and general statements that collectively purport to explain some aspect of the empirical world	Chafetz, 1978, p. 2
An abstract, symbolic representation of what is conceived to be reality—a set of abstract statements designed to "fit" some portion of the real world	Zimbardo, Ebbesen, and Maslach, 1977, p. 53

make an impact on them. They can also identify *what* should be monitored, measured, or compared in a program evaluation (Glanz, Lewis, and Rimer, 1990; Glanz and Rimer, 1995).

Thus, theories and models *explain* behavior and suggest ways to achieve behavioral *change*. Explanatory theories, often called *theories of the problem*, help describe and identify why a problem exists. They guide the search for such modifiable factors as knowledge, attitudes, self-efficacy, social support, and lack of resources. Change theories, or *theories of action*, guide the development of interventions. They also form the basis for evaluation, pushing the evaluator to make explicit her or his assumptions about how a program should work (Green and Lewis, 1986; Glanz and Rimer, 1995). These two types of theory often have different foci but are quite complementary (Fishbein and others, 1991).

Even though various theoretical models of health behavior may reflect the same general ideas (Cummings, Becker, and Maile, 1980; Fishbein and others, 1991; Weinstein, 1993), each theory employs a unique vocabulary to articulate the specific factors considered to be important. The *why* tells investigators about the processes through which changes occur in the target variables. Theories also vary in the extent to which they have been conceptually developed and empirically tested. Bandura (1986) points out that "theories are interpreted in different ways depending on the stage of development of the field of study. In advanced disciplines, theories integrate laws; in less advanced fields, theories specify the determinants governing the phenomena of interest." The term theory must be used in the latter sense in *Health Behavior and Health Education* because the field this book addresses is still relatively young.

Concepts, Constructs, and Variables

Concepts are the major components of a theory; they are its building blocks or primary elements. Concepts can vary in the extent to which they have meaning or can be understood outside the context of a specific theory. When concepts have been developed or adopted for use in a particular theory, they are called *constructs* (Kerlinger, 1986). The term *subjective normative belief*, for example, is a construct within Ajzen and Fishbein's Theory of Reasoned Action (1980); the specific construct can be understood only within the context of that theory. Another example of a construct is the term *perceived susceptibility* in the Health Belief Model (see Chapter Three).

Variables are the empirical counterparts or operational forms of constructs (Green and Lewis, 1986). They specify how a construct is to be measured in a specific situation. It is important to keep in mind that *variables* should be matched to *constructs* when identifying what should be assessed in the evaluation of a theory-driven program.

Principles

Theories go beyond principles. Principles are general guidelines for action (Green and Lewis, 1986). They are broad and nonspecific and may actually distort realities or results based on research. Principles may be based on precedent or history, *or* they may be based on research. At their worst, principles are so broad that they invite multiple interpretations and are therefore unreliable. At their weakest, principles are like horoscopes: anyone can derive whatever meaning he or she wants from them. At their best, principles are based on accumulated research. They provide hypotheses and serve as practitioners' most informed hunches about how or what they should do to obtain a desired outcome in a target population.

Models

Health behavior and the guiding concepts for influencing it are far too complex to be explained by a single unified theory. *Models* draw on a number of theories to help people understand a specific problem in a particular setting or context. Models are often informed by more than one theory as well as by empirical findings (Earp and Ennett, 1991). Several models that support program-planning processes are widely used in health promotion and education: Green and Kreuter's PRECEDE-PROCEED model (1991; see Chapter Seventeen), social marketing (see Chapter Eighteen), and ecological planning approaches (Green and others, 1994; McLeroy, Bibeau, Steckler, and Glanz, 1988; see Chapter Nineteen). New frameworks to integrate various theories and incorporate multilevel influences have also been proposed by Stokols (1992), Winett (1995), and Flay and Petraitis (1994; Petraitis, Flay, and Miller, 1995).

Paradigms for Theory and Research in Health Promotion and Education

A paradigm is a basic schema that organizes people's broadly based view of something (Babbie, 1989). Paradigms are widely recognized scientific achievements that, for a time, provide model problem-solving approaches to a community of practitioners and scientists. Paradigms include theory, application, and instrumentation and comprise models that represent coherent traditions of scientific research (Kuhn, 1962). Paradigms gain status when they are more successful at solving pressing problems than are their competitors (Kuhn, 1962).

Paradigms create boundaries within which the search for answers occurs; they do not answer particular questions, but they do direct the search for answers to questions (Babbie, 1989). Paradigms circumscribe or delimit what is important to examine in a given field of inquiry. The collective judgments of scientists define the dominant paradigm that constitutes the body of science (Wilson, 1952).

In the fields of health promotion and education and health behavior (and in this text), the dominant paradigm that supports the largest body of theory and research is that of *logical positivism*, or *logical empiricism*. This basic view, developed in the Vienna Circle from 1924 to 1936, has two central features: (1) an emphasis on the use of induction, or sensory experience, feelings, and personal judgments, as the source of knowledge; and (2) the view that deduction is the standard for verification or confirmation of theory, so that theory must be tested through empirical methods and systematic observation of phenomena (Runes, 1984). Logical empiricism reconciles the deductive and inductive extremes; it prescribes that the researcher begin with a hypothesis deduced from a theory and then test it, subjecting it to the jeopardy of disconfirmation through empirical test (McGuire, 1983; Thompson, 1985).

An alternative worldview in health promotion and education relies more heavily on induction and is often identified as a predominantly *constructivist* paradigm. This perspective argues that the organization and explanation of events must be revealed through a process of discovery rather than organized into prescribed conceptual categories before a study begins (Lewis, forthcoming). Therefore, data collection methods such as standardized questionnaires and predetermined response categories have a limited place. Ethnography, phenomenology, and grounded theory are examples of approaches using a constructivist paradigm (Strauss, 1987; Mullen and Iverson, 1986). It has become increasingly common in the field for work to originate within a constructivist paradigm and then shift toward a focus on answering specific research questions using methodologies from the logical positivist paradigm.

Lewin's metatheory stipulates the rules to be followed for building good theory; this metatheory is consistent with logical positivism but focuses on Lewin's view that the function of social psychology is to further understanding of the interrelationships between the individual and the social environment (Gold, 1992). Lewin's metatheory is an orientation distinct from his specific Field Theory (Gold, 1992), and it has been influential in health behavior theory since the earliest attempts to use social science to solve public health problems (Rosenstock, 1990). Key rules of Lewin's metatheory require analysis that starts with the situation as a whole, contemporaneity, a dynamic approach, a constructive method, the mathematical representation of constructs and variables, and a psychological approach that explains both inner experiences and overt actions from the actor's perspective (Lewin, [1942] 1951). The latter rule implies a single level of analysis requiring *closed theory* and poses a serious limitation to solving the problems of contemporary health promotion. It raises the issue—one that individuals concerned with health behavior often grapple with—that they must often trade off theoretical elegance in favor of relevance (Gold, 1992).

While the paradigms described here focus on basic schemata for development and application of knowledge, health promotion and education are also concerned with approaches to solving social problems, in other words, how to bring about change. Considerable scholarly and practitioner effort has been devoted to developing techniques that change behavior. While this effort grew out of a desire to produce a better world, techniques that "push" people to change have been experienced by many as manipulative, reducing freedom of choice, and sustaining a balance of power in favor of the "change agent" (Kipnis, 1994). A paradigm shift has occurred whereby most behavioral techniques today (for example, social support, empowerment, and personal growth) are based on *reducing restraints against change* and promoting informed decision making, rather than on pushing people to change. Nevertheless, as Kipnis (1994) notes, even when health promotion (or social psychology) uses these techniques for the elimination of injustice, the inherent exercise of power remains a problem.

New paradigms for understanding, studying, and applying knowledge about human behavior continue to arise and may be influential in the future of applied social sciences in health promotion and education. Sperry (1993) suggests that a "cognitive revolution" that explains conscious behavior as based on subjective mental states is increasingly blending free will and determinism and regarding subjective human values as the underlying key to world change. Barton (1994) notes that models based on concepts of chaos, nonlinear dynamics, and self-organization provide a new paradigm for understanding systems and system change. He advocates their use and predicts that these models will increase in stature as professionals and scientists find that linear equations cannot adequately describe or explain what occurs in natural systems.

Trends in the Use of Health Behavior Theories and Models

Theories that gain recognition in a discipline shape the field, help define the scope of practice, and influence the training and socialization of its professionals. No single theory or conceptual framework dominates research or practice in health promotion and education today. Instead, a multitude of theories exist from which to choose. In a review of 116 theory-based articles published between 1986 and 1988 in two major health education journals, which we conducted during planning for the first edition of this book, we found fifty-one distinct theoretical formulations. At that time, the three most frequently mentioned theories were Social

Learning Theory, the Theory of Reasoned Action, and the Health Belief Model (Glanz, Lewis, and Rimer, 1990). In all likelihood, all the theories included in the first edition of this book gained greater visibility.

Since 1990, several publications have described experts' views of the dominant theoretical models used in health promotion and education today. There appears to be consensus that the Health Belief Model, Social Cognitive Theory, and the Theory of Reasoned Action are widely used (Freudenberg and others, 1995; Fishbein and others, 1991; van Ryn and Heaney, 1992; Earp and Ennett, 1991; Glanz and Rimer, 1995; Weinstein, 1993). Other frequently noted theories and models include The Transtheoretical Model, diffusion of innovations, the empowerment model, and ecological models (Freudenberg and others, 1995; van Ryn and Heaney, 1992; Glanz and Rimer, 1995). In one effort to identify a small set of variables "believed to account for most of the variance in any given behavior" and cutting across specific theories, Fishbein and others (1991) proposed eight key variables: intention, ability/skill, norms, environmental constraints, anticipated outcomes, self-standards, emotion, and self-efficacy.

Along with the published observations about *which* theories are being used, concerns have been raised about *how* these theories are used (or not used) in research and practice. A common refrain is that researchers may not understand how to measure and analyze constructs of health behavior theories (Fishbein and others, 1991; Wallston, 1991; Green, 1991). Considerable conceptual confusion—among both researchers and practitioners—about interrelationships between related theories and variables has also been observed (Rosenstock, Strecher, and Becker, 1988; Weinstein, 1988; Wallston, 1991). Clearly, the need for clarification and illustration of applied theory continues to be a priority.

Selection of Theories for This Book

Our selection of theories and models to be included in the second edition of *Health Behavior and Health Education* has been based on the published information summarized in the previous section, supplemented by an extensive analysis of the health behavior literature. We reviewed all issues of twenty-four journals in health education, medicine, and behavioral sciences published from mid-1992 to mid-1994. In the first stage of the review, we counted the total number of articles and identified those articles relevant to health behavior and health promotion and education. The second stage of review included only the thirteen journals in which at least 20 percent of all articles were relevant to health behavior and health promotion and education. Out of the 1,174 relevant articles, 526, or 44.8 percent, used one or more theories or models (based on a liberal definition of theory use).

Sixty-six different theories and models were identified, and twenty-one of these were mentioned eight times or more. As Table 2.2 shows, 67 percent of the total instances of theory use in the 497 articles that used one or more of the twenty-one most common theories or models were accounted for by the first eight theories or models: the Health Belief Model, Social Cognitive Theory, self-efficacy, the Theory of Reasoned Action and the Theory of Planned Behavior, community organization, The Transtheoretical Model/Stages of Change, social marketing, and social support and social networks. The results of this analysis probably represent recent research and publication prepared over the past seven or eight years, given the time lag between completing program planning and research and publication in peer-reviewed journals. Nevertheless, the most often cited theories and models emerged with great clarity in this review. For example, the marked increase in publications using The Transtheoretical Model and its central construct of the Stages of Change illustrates the rapid emergence of that model, with its emphasis on readiness to change and its postulate that behavioral change is a process rather than an event (Prochaska, DiClemente, and Norcross, 1992).

Thirteen of the most often cited theories and models are the focus of chapters in this second edition of *Health Behavior and Health Education*. These theories have been selected to provide readers with a range of theories representing different units of intervention, for example, the individual, the group, and the community. Some have also been chosen because, like the Health Belief Model, Social Cognitive Theory, and the Theory of Reasoned Action, they represent dominant theories of health behavior and health promotion and education. Others, like social marketing and community organization, were chosen for their practical value in applying theoretical formulations in a way that has demonstrated usefulness to professionals concerned with health behavior change.

Our selection of theories resulted from our review and also reflects some difficult editorial decisions. Three criteria that are consistent with and confirmatory of our review also helped us to define the content of this book. First, we determined that the theory must meet basic standards of adequacy for research and practice, thus having the potential for effective use by health education practitioners. Second, *current* health behavior and health promotion and education research must use the theory. (That is why, for example, we include the Health Belief Model rather than Lewin's Field Theory.) The third criterion is that there must be at least promising, if not substantial, empirical evidence supporting the theory's validity in predicting or changing health behavior.

In some cases, a purpose rather than a theory is the identifying title for a chapter—as in the case of Chapter Ten ("Patient-Provider Communication"), which describes theories of interpersonal communication and influence and illustrates their utility for health education. Chapter Twelve ("Improving Health

TABLE 2.2. MOST COMMONLY USED THEORIES AND MODELS IN 497 ARTICLES: 1992 TO 1994.

Theory or Model	Number of Articles Using the Theory or Model[a]
Health Belief Model	100
Social Cognitive Theory/Social Learning Theory	74
Self-efficacy	74
Theory of Reasoned Action/Theory of Planned Behavior	66
Community organization	50
Stages of Change/The Transtheoretical Model	50
Social marketing	44
Social support, social networks	37
PRECEDE-PROCEED model	28
Diffusion of innovations	27
Stress and coping	24
Relapse prevention	23
Economic models	21
Information processing	21
Health Locus of Control	21
Patient-provider interaction	18
Empowerment	17
Protection Motivation Theory	10
Behavioral theory	10
Communication theory, persuasive communication	9
Decision making	8

[a]Total article count is greater than the number of articles because some articles use more than one theory.

Through Community Organization and Community Building") is named for the resultant intervention strategies rather than for the convergent theoretical bases that form the foundation for community organization work. The chapters in Part Five present the PRECEDE-PROCEED model for program planning, social marketing, and ecological models, and each chapter draws on multiple theories to understand health behavior and assist in development of effective intervention programs and strategies.

We recognize the lack of consensus regarding the definition and classification of theories. We have taken a liberal, ecumenical stance toward theory. And we concede that the lowest common denominator of the theoretical models herein might be that they are all *conceptual or theoretical frameworks,* or broadly conceived perspectives used to organize ideas. Nevertheless, the term theory accurately signals the spirit of this book and describes the goal to be attained in developing frameworks and one set of tools for refining health education research and practice.

Fitting Theory to Research and Practice: Building Bridges and Forging Links

Effective health promotion and education depends on practitioners' marshaling the most appropriate theory and practice strategies for a given situation. Different theories are best suited to different units of practice, such as individuals, groups, and organizations. For example, when one is attempting to overcome women's personal barriers to obtaining mammograms, the Health Belief Model may be useful. The Transtheoretical Model may be especially useful when one is developing smoking cessation interventions. When one is trying to change physicians' mammography practices by instituting reminder systems, organizational change theories are more suitable. The choice of a suitable theory or theories should begin with identifying the problem, goal, and units of practice (van Ryn and Heaney, 1992; Hochbaum, Sorenson, and Lorig, 1992; Prochaska, DiClemente, and Norcross, 1992), *not* with selecting a theoretical framework because it is intriguing, familiar, or in vogue.

The adequacy of a theory most often is assessed in terms of three criteria: (1) its *logic*, that is, its *internal consistency* in not yielding mutually contradictory derivations, (2) the extent to which it is *parsimonious*, that is, broadly relevant while using a manageable number of concepts, and (3) its *plausibility* in fitting with prevailing theories in the field (McGuire, 1983).

Theories are further judged in the context of practitioners' and researchers' activities. Practitioners apply the pragmatic criterion of *usefulness* to a theory. They ask whether it is consistent with everyday observations (Burdine and McLeroy, 1992; Glanz and Rimer, 1995). Researchers make scientific judgments of a theory's *ecological validity*, the extent to which it conforms to observable reality when empirically tested (McGuire, 1983). All of us need to test our theories iteratively in the real world (Rosenstock, 1990). When we do so, theory, research, and practice begin to converge.

Health education theory is eclectic and derivative. Adaptations and refinements of theories of health behavior and health education occur in response to both scientists' and practitioners' concerns. A circularity links theory and practice. As Roberts (1959) astutely noted three decades ago, "the theoretical base of our profession must be augmented and modified by continuing, careful analysis of documented practice and from collaborative action research."

Practitioners of health promotion and education at once benefit from and are challenged by the eclectic and derivative nature of their endeavor: a multitude of theoretical frameworks and models from the social sciences are available for their use, but the best choices and direct translations may not be immediately evident. There is an inherent danger in a book like this: one can begin to think that the links between theory, research, and health promotion practice are easily forged. They are not. For the unprepared, the choices can be overwhelming, but for those who understand the commonalities and differences among theories of health behavior and health education, a growing knowledge base can provide a firm foundation upon which to build. We hope that *Health Behavior and Health Education* will provide and strengthen that foundation for readers.

Science is by definition cumulative, and the same applies to the scientific base that supports long-standing as well as innovative health promotion interventions. The gift of theory is that it provides conceptual underpinnings for well-crafted research and informed practice. "The scientist values research by the size of its contribution to that huge, logically articulated structure of ideas which is already, though not half built, the most glorious accomplishment of mankind" (Medawar, 1967).

In this book, we aim to demystify theory and to communicate theory and theoretically inspired research alongside their implications for practice. We encourage informed criticism of theories—only through rigorous scrutiny will theories improve. The ultimate test of the ideas and the information presented here rests on their use over time. Like any long-term behavior, this testing will require social support, supportive environments, and periodic reinforcement. The benefits will be mutually for practitioners, researchers, and the participants in health promotion programs.

As this chapter and the preceding one demonstrate, health promotion and health behavior are concerns of ever increasing importance to the well-being of humankind worldwide. As scholars, researchers, and practitioners, all of us grapple with the complexities of human beings and society. We press forward within the limits of current methodologies while striving to build a cumulative body of knowledge in a fast-changing world. The results of some efforts are disappointing, but this should motivate, not deter, us in pursuing high-quality work. Continual dialogue between theory, research, and practice involves compromise, creativity, healthy criticism, appreciation of others' skills, and a willingness to cooperate to learn and to set high standards. "We must learn to honor excellence in every socially accepted human activity, however humble the activity, and to scorn shoddiness, however exalted the activity. An excellent plumber is infinitely more admirable than an incompetent philosopher. The society that scorns excellence in plumbing because plumbing is a humble activity and tolerates shoddiness in philosophy because it is an exalted activity will have neither good plumbing nor good philosophy. Neither its pipes nor its theories will hold water" (Gardner, 1984).

Limitations of This Book

No text can be all-inclusive. This is certainly true of *Health Behavior and Health Education*. Some theories and frameworks presented in the first edition of this book do not appear in this edition: Consumer Information Processing (Rudd and Glanz, 1990), Multiattribute Utility Theory (Carter, 1990), Attribution Theory (Lewis and Daltroy, 1990), and media advocacy (Wallack, 1990). These theories and frameworks remain important, but we found them to be less widely used than those included in the present edition. Interested readers should refer to the first edition of this book (Glanz, Lewis, and Rimer, 1990) and to other sources (Glanz and Rimer, 1995) to read about these frameworks.

There are other important theories and conceptual frameworks that could not be included because of space limitations. These include Self-Regulation Theory (Leventhal, Zimmerman, and Gutmann, 1984), Protection Motivation Theory (Rogers, 1975), and more familiar classical theories such as Field Theory (Lewin, 1935) and cognitive consistency (Festinger, 1957). Some of these, however, are described in discussions of the historical origins of the various theories in this book. Others, such as the Precaution Adoption Model (Weinstein, 1993) are discussed in the synthesis and perspectives chapters (Chapters Seven, Eleven, Sixteen, and Twenty-One).

This book is not intended to be a how-to guide or manual for program planning and development in health promotion and education. Other books in health promotion and education, nursing, medicine, psychology, and nutrition serve that purpose, and readers should seek out key sources in each discipline for more on the nuts and bolts of practice. In addition, this volume will be most useful when it is part of a problem-oriented learning program (Hochbaum, Sorenson, and Lorig, 1992; van Ryn and Heaney, 1992), whether in formal professional education settings or in continuing education venues (Glanz and Rimer, 1995).

Neither is this volume intended to serve as an in-depth treatise on research methods in health behavior and health education. Instead, it demonstrates through a modest number of examples how theories are put into operation. The reader who wishes more guidance regarding applied research for studies of health promotion and education will find ample resources in books on social science research methodology and measurement.

We the editors hope that readers will emerge with a critical appreciation of theory and with the curiosity to pursue not only the theories presented in *Health Behavior and Health Education* but other promising theories as well. This book should be regarded as a starting point, not the end.

Theories—or conceptual frameworks—can be, and *are,* useful because they enrich, inform, and complement the practical technologies of health promotion and education. Thus, the readers of this book should "pass with relief from the tossing sea of Cause and Theory to the firm ground of Result and Fact" (Churchill, 1898). As the ocean meets the shore, so we hope you will find that theory, research, and practice in health promotion and education stretch out to converge in a single landscape.

References

Ajzen, I., and Fishbein, M. *Understanding Attitudes and Predicting Social Behavior.* Englewood Cliffs, N.J.: Prentice Hall, 1980.

Babbie, E. *The Practice of Social Research.* (5th ed.) Belmont, Calif.: Wadsworth, 1989.

Bandura, A. *Social Foundations of Thought and Action: A Social Cognitive Theory.* Englewood Cliffs, N.J.: Prentice Hall, 1986.

Barton, S. "Chaos, Self-Organization, and Psychology." *American Psychologist,* 1994, *49*(1), 5–14.

Bernstein, R. *Praxis and Action.* Philadelphia: University of Pennsylvania Press, 1971.

Blalock, H. M., Jr. *Theory Construction: From Verbal to Mathematical Constructions.* Englewood Cliffs, N.J.: Prentice Hall, 1969.

Burdine, J. N., and McLeroy, K. R. "Practitioners' Use of Theory: Examples from a Workgroup." *Health Education Quarterly,* 1992, *19*(3), 315–330.

Carter, W. "Health Behavior as a Rational Process: Theory of Reasoned Action and Multiattribute Utility Theory." In Glanz, K., Lewis, F. M., and Rimer, B. K. (eds.), *Health Behavior and Health Education: Theory, Research, and Practice.* San Francisco: Jossey-Bass, 1990.

Chafetz, J. *A Primer on the Construction of Theories in Sociology.* Itasca, Ill.: Peacock, 1978.

Churchill, W. *The Malakand Field Force.* 1898.

Cummings, K. M., Becker, M. H., and Maile, M. C. "Bringing the Models Together: An Empirical Approach to Combining Variables Used to Explain Health Actions." *Journal of Behavioral Medicine,* 1980, *3*(2), 123–145.

D'Onofrio, C. N. "Theory and the Empowerment of Health Education Practitioners." *Health Education Quarterly,* 1992, *19*(3), 385–403.

Earp, J. A., and Ennett, S. T. "Conceptual Models for Health Education Research and Practice." *Health Education Research,* 1991, *6*(2), 163–171.

Festinger, L. *A Theory of Cognitive Dissonance.* Stanford, Calif.: Stanford University Press, 1957.

Fishbein, M., and others. *Factors Influencing Behavior and Behavior Change; Final Report—Theorist's Workshop.* Washington, D.C.: American Cancer Society, 1991.

Flay, B., and Petraitis, J. "The Theory of Triadic Influence: A New Theory of Health Behavior with Implications for Preventive Interventions." *Advances in Medical Sociology,* 1994, *4,* 19–44.

Freudenberg, N., and others. "Strengthening Individual and Community Capacity to Prevent Disease and Promote Health: In Search of Relevant Theories and Principles." *Health Education Quarterly,* 1995, *22*(3), 290–306.

Gardner, J. *Excellence.* (Rev. ed.) New York: Norton, 1984.

Glanz, K., Lewis, F. M., and Rimer, B. K. (eds.). *Health Behavior and Health Education: Theory, Research, and Practice.* San Francisco: Jossey-Bass, 1990.

Glanz, K., and Rimer, B. K. *Theory at a Glance: A Guide for Health Promotion Practice.* NIH publication no. 95–3896. Bethesda, Md.: National Institutes of Health, National Cancer Institute, 1995.

Gold, M. "Metatheory and Field Theory in Social Psychology: Relevance or Elegance?" *Journal of Social Issues,* 1992, *48*(2), 67–78.

Green, L. W. "Everyone Has a Theory, Few Have Measurement." *Health Education Research,* 1991, *6*(2), 249–250.

Green, L. W., and Kreuter, M. W. *Health Promotion Planning: An Educational and Environmental Approach.* (2nd ed.) Mountain View, Calif.: Mayfield, 1991.

Green, L. W., and Lewis, F. M. *Evaluation and Measurement in Health Education and Health Promotion.* Mountain View, Calif.: Mayfield, 1986.

Green, L. W., and others. "Can We Build On, or Must We Replace, the Theories and Models in Health Education?" *Health Education Research,* 1994, *9*(3), 397–404.

Hochbaum, G. M., Sorenson, J. R., and Lorig, K. "Theory in Health Education Practice." *Health Education Quarterly,* 1992, *19*(3), 295–313.

Kanfer, F. H., and Schefft, B. *Guiding the Process of Therapeutic Change.* Champaign, Ill.: Research Press, 1988.

Kar, S. B. "Introduction: Theoretical Foundations of Health Education and Promotion." *Advances in Health Education and Promotion,* 1986, *1*, 157–163.

Kerlinger, F. N. *Foundations of Behavioral Research.* (3rd ed.) Austin, Tex.: Holt, Rinehart and Winston, 1986.

Kipnis, D. "Accounting for the Use of Behavior Technologies in Social Psychology." *American Psychologist,* 1994, *49*(3), 165–172.

Kok, G., and others. "Social Psychology and Health Education." In W. Stroebe and M. Hewstone (eds.), *European Review of Social Psychology.* Vol. 7. New York: Wiley, 1996.

Kreuter, M. "The Practical Outcomes of Theory-Based Health Education Practice." Paper presented at the American Public Health Association annual meeting, Boston, Nov. 14, 1988.

Kuhn, T. S. *The Structure of Scientific Revolution.* Chicago: University of Chicago Press, 1962.

Leventhal, H., Zimmerman, R., and Gutmann, M. "Compliance: A Self-Regulation Perspective." In D. Gentry (ed.), *Handbook of Behavioral Medicine.* New York: Guilford Press, 1984.

Lewin, K. *A Dynamic Theory of Personality.* New York: McGraw-Hill, 1935.

Lewin, K. "Field Theory and Learning." In K. Lewin, *Field Theory in Social Science: Select Theoretical Papers* (D. Cartwright, ed.). New York: HarperCollins, 1951. (Originally published 1942.)

Lewis, F. "Whom and from What Paradigm Should Health Promotion Serve?" *Health Education Quarterly,* forthcoming.

Lewis, F. M., and Daltroy, L. "How Causal Explanations Influence Health Behavior: Attribution Theory." In K. Glanz, F. M. Lewis, and B. K. Rimer (eds.), *Health Behavior and Health Education: Theory, Research, and Practice.* San Francisco: Jossey-Bass, 1990.

McGuire, W. J. "A Contextualist Theory of Knowledge: Its Implications for Innovation and Reform in Psychological Research." *Advances in Experimental Social Psychology,* 1983, *16*, 1–47.

McLeroy, K. R., Bibeau, D., Steckler, A., and Glanz, K. "An Ecological Perspective on Health Promotion Programs." *Health Education Quarterly,* 1988, *15*, 351–377.

Medawar, P. B. *The Art of the Soluble.* New York: Methuen, 1967.

Mullen, P. D, and Iverson, D. "Qualitative Methods." In L. W. Green and F. M. Lewis, *Measurement and Evaluation in Health Education and Health Promotion*. Mountain View, Calif.: Mayfield, 1986.

Petraitis, J., Flay, B., and Miller, T. "Reviewing Theories of Adolescent Substance Use: Organizing Pieces in the Puzzle." *Psychological Bulletin*, 1995, *117*(1), 67–86.

Prochaska, J. O., DiClemente, C. C., and Norcross, J. C. "In Search of How People Change: Applications to Addictive Behaviors." *American Psychologist*, 1992, *47*(9), 1102–1114.

Roberts, B. J. "Decision Making: An Illustration of Theory Building." Presidential address, 10th annual meeting of the Society of Public Health Educators, Atlantic City, N.J., Oct. 18, 1959.

Rogers, R. W. "A Protection Motivation Theory of Fear Appeals and Attitude Change." *Journal of Psychology*, 1975, *91*, 93–114.

Rosenstock, I. M. "The Past, Present, and Future of Health Education." In Glanz, K., Lewis, F. M., and Rimer, B. K. (eds.), *Health Behavior and Health Education: Theory, Research, and Practice*. San Francisco: Jossey-Bass, 1990.

Rosenstock, I. M., Strecher, V. J., and Becker, M. H. "Social Learning Theory and the Health Belief Model." *Health Education Quarterly*, 1988, *15*(2), 175–183.

Rudd, J., and Glanz, K. "How Individuals Use Information for Health Action: Consumer Information Processing." In K. Glanz, F. M. Lewis, and B. K. Rimer (eds.), *Health Behavior and Health Education: Theory, Research, and Practice*. San Francisco: Jossey-Bass, 1990.

Runes, D. *Dictionary of Philosophy*. Lanham, Md.: Rowman & Littlefield, 1984.

Sperry, R. W. "The Impact and Promise of the Cognitive Revolution." *American Psychologist*, 1993, *48*(8), 878–885.

Stokols, D. "Establishing and Maintaining Healthy Environments: Toward a Social Ecology of Health Promotion." *American Psychologist*, 1992, *47*(1), 6–22.

Strauss, A. L. *Qualitative Analysis for Social Scientists*. Cambridge, England: Cambridge University Press, 1987.

Thompson, J. L. "Practical Discourse in Nursing: Going Beyond Empiricism and Historicism." *Advances in Nursing Sciences*, 1985, *7*, 59–71.

van Ryn, M., and Heaney, C. A. "What's the Use of Theory?" *Health Education Quarterly*, 1992, *19*(3), 315–330.

Wallack, L. "Media Advocacy: Promoting Health Through Mass Communication." In K. Glanz, F. M. Lewis, and B. K. Rimer (eds.), *Health Behavior and Health Education: Theory, Research, and Practice*. San Francisco: Jossey-Bass, 1990.

Wallston, K. A. "The Importance of Placing Measures of Health Locus of Control Beliefs in a Theoretical Context." *Health Education Research*, 1991, *6*(2), 251–252.

Weinstein, N. D. "The Precaution Adoption Process." *Health Psychology*, 1988, *7*(4), 355–386.

Weinstein, N. D. "Testing Four Competing Theories of Health-Protective Behavior." *Health Psychology*, 1993, *12*(4), 324–333.

Wilson, E. B. *An Introduction to Scientific Research*. New York: McGraw-Hill, 1952.

Winett, R. A. "A Framework for Health Promotion and Disease Prevention Programs." *American Psychologist*, 1995, *50*(5), 341–350.

Zimbardo, P. G., Ebbesen, E. B., and Maslach, C. *Influencing Attitudes and Changing Behavior*. (2nd ed.) Reading, Mass.: Addison-Wesley, 1977.

PART TWO

MODELS OF INDIVIDUAL HEALTH BEHAVIOR

Barbara K. Rimer

Individuals are one of the essential units of health education and health behavior theory, research, and practice. This does not mean that the individual is the only or necessarily the most important unit of intervention. But all other units, whether they are groups, organizations, worksites, communities, or larger units, are composed of individuals. To explain human behavior and to influence it, those concerned with health behavior and health education must understand the individual.

A wide range of health professionals, including health educators, physicians, psychologists, and nurses, focus all or most of their efforts on changing the health behavior of individuals. To intervene effectively and to make informed judgments about how to measure the success of such interventions, health professionals must have an understanding of the role of the individual in health behavior. This section of *Health Behavior and Health Education* helps the reader achieve a greater understanding of theories that focus primarily on individual health behavior.

Lewin's seminal Field Theory (1935) was one of the early and most far-reaching theories of behavior, and most contemporary theories of health behavior owe a major intellectual debt to Lewin. During the 1940s and 1950s, researchers began to learn more about how individuals make decisions concerning health and what determines health behavior. Rosenstock and Hochbaum, from their vantage point at the U.S. Public Health Service, began their pioneering work to understand why individuals participated in screening programs for tuberculosis. In Chapter Three,

Strecher and Rosenstock review the evolution of the Health Belief Model that resulted from that work. In the last twenty years, considerable progress has been made in understanding the determinants of individuals' health-related behaviors and ways to stimulate positive behavior changes. Value expectancy theories, which include both the Health Belief Model and the Theory of Reasoned Action (Chapter Five), matured during this time. Together with theories of stress, coping, and health behavior and The Transtheoretical Model, they form the basis for Part Two of this book.

Strecher and Rosenstock explain in Chapter Three that the Health Belief Model is used to understand why people accept preventive health services and why they do or do not adhere to other kinds of health care regimens. The Health Belief Model has spawned literally hundreds of health education research studies and provided the conceptual basis for many interventions and research studies in the years since it was formulated. It has been used across the health continuum, from prevention to detection to illness and sick-role behavior (Becker and Maiman, 1975; Janz and Becker, 1984). It is among the most widely applied theoretical foundations for the study of health behavior change. The Health Belief Model is appealing and useful to a wide range of professionals concerned with behavioral change. Physicians, dentists, nurses, psychologists, and health educators have all used the Health Belief Model in designing and evaluating interventions to alter health behavior.

In Chapter Five, Montaño, Kasprzyk, and Taplin discuss two value expectancy theories, the Theory of Reasoned Action (TRA) and the Theory of Planned Behavior (TPB). This family of theories has had a major influence on both research and practice in health behavior and health education. The Theory of Reasoned Action and the Theory of Planned Behavior, as developed by Fishbein and Ajzen (1975), propose that behavioral intentions and behaviors result from a rational process of decision making. These theories have been used to intervene in many health behaviors, including having mammograms, smoking, controlling weight, family planning, and selecting commercial products in response to the marketing of those products (Jaccard and Davidson, 1972; Ajzen and Fishbein, 1980; McCarty, 1981; Lowe and Frey, 1983). Recently, these theories have been used by AIDS researchers in developing interventions to help people at high risk to lower their risk of infection.

Montaño, Kasprzyk, and Taplin show how the TRA was used to guide the development of a mammography program, identifying the factors that influence women's decisions about receiving mammograms. A second example focuses on prediction of condom use. Overall, the authors conclude that TRA and TPB serve as excellent frameworks for identifying the determinants of behavior.

Two new chapters have been added to this section to reflect trends in the use of health behavior theory. The first of these trends is the use of The Transtheoretical Model (TTM), developed by Prochaska and DiClemente (Prochaska, DiClemente, Velicer, and Rossi, 1993). Over a relatively short time, this theory has achieved widespread use and acceptance by researchers and practitioners in health education and health behavior. In the previous edition of this book, TTM was included as a developing theory, but it has developed to the point that it now serves as one of the behavioral foundations of health education and health behavior theory, research, and practice. In Chapter Four, Prochaska, Redding, and Evers present the key components of the theory: the concepts of stage, decisional balance, and pros and cons. They discuss the fact that to have a public health impact, increasingly it will be necessary for practitioners to use proactive strategies that reach out to people, rather than relying on reactive strategies that ultimately reach few individuals. The TTM is particularly useful for guiding the development of proactive interventions.

In their examples, Prochaska, Redding, and Evers show how the TTM has been used in the development of both smoking cessation interventions and multiple risk factor interventions for minority adolescents. This chapter should be of value to both researchers and practitioners and, we hope, will encourage additional testing of this interesting theory.

In Chapter Six, Lerman and Glanz cover theories of stress and coping and health behavior. While those in health education may be less familiar with these theories than with the other theories discussed in this book, these theories are extremely important. Stress, as most readers will know through personal experience, can contribute to illness both directly and indirectly. Lerman and Glanz review the major theories in this area and make them accessible to practitioners and researchers. They focus especially on one of these theories, the Transactional Model of Stress and Coping. This theory is useful not only in understanding how people respond to stressors but also in developing interventions to improve coping. In their examples, Lerman and Glanz show how the Transactional Model has been used in developing interventions for first-degree relatives of breast cancer patients as well as for people coping with HIV/AIDS.

Taken together, these four chapters provide researchers and practitioners alike with an introduction to widely used theories of health education and health behavior. The different theories are suitable to different problems and populations, and some are easier to use and apply than others. But each has made an important contribution to our understanding of health behavior. Each deserves to be read, studied, and considered. The distinguished authors have provided chapters that should be accessible to a wide range of health professionals.

References

Ajzen, I., and Fishbein, M. *Understanding Attitudes and Predicting Social Behavior.* Englewood Cliffs, N.J.: Prentice Hall, 1980.

Becker, M. H., and Maiman, L. A. "Sociobehavioral Determinants of Compliance with Health and Medical Care Recommendations." *Medical Care,* 1975, *13,* 10–24.

Fishbein, M., and Ajzen, I. *Belief, Attitude, Intention and Behavior: An Introduction to Theory and Research.* Reading, Mass.: Addison-Wesley, 1975.

Jaccard, J. J., and Davidson, A. R. "Toward an Understanding of Family Planning Behaviors: An Initial Investigation." *Journal of Applied Social Psychology,* 1972, *2,* 228–235.

Janz, N. K., and Becker, M. H. "The Health Belief Model: A Decade Later." *Health Education Quarterly,* 1984, *11,* 1–47.

Lewin, K. *A Dynamic Theory of Personality.* New York: McGraw-Hill, 1935.

Lowe, R. H., and Frey, J. D. "Predicting Lamaze Childbirth Intentions and Outcomes: An Extension of the Theory of Reasoned Action to a Joint Outcome." *Basic and Applied Social Psychology,* 1983, *4,* 353–372.

McCarty, D. "Changing Contraceptive Usage Intention: A Test of the Fishbein Model of Intention." *Journal of Applied Social Psychology,* 1981, *11,* 192–211.

Prochaska, J. O., DiClemente, C. C., Velicer, W. F., and Rossi, J. S. "Standardized, Individualized, Interactive, and Personalized Self-Help Programs for Smoking Cessation." *Health Psychology,* 1993, *12*(5), 399–405.

CHAPTER THREE

THE HEALTH BELIEF MODEL

Victor J. Strecher
Irwin M. Rosenstock

For over four decades, the Health Belief Model (HBM) has been one of the most widely used conceptual frameworks in health behavior. The HBM has been used both to explain change and maintenance of health behavior and as a guiding framework for health behavior interventions. The HBM has been expanded, broken down into components, compared to other frameworks, and analyzed using a wide array of multivariate analytical techniques. Over the most recent two decades, further research has been conducted to specify measures of health beliefs and relationships between these beliefs.

This chapter reviews the ideas within the HBM that remain vital. We also examine other psychosocial constructs that further explain relationships within the HBM. However, we decided not to supply a review of recent HBM research findings, as has been done for the two previous decades (Becker, 1974; Janz and Becker, 1984). Even recent research concerning the HBM continues to emphasize individual health beliefs, placing them in multivariate analyses, and looking at their predictive qualities. This type of analysis does little to further specify measurement of or relationships between health beliefs. Although there are certainly new, interesting results to review, what is most needed is a consideration of three aspects of the HBM: its components, the relationships between those components, and how to use the HBM to examine issues of public health concern.

We begin by describing the origins of the HBM and its place in psychosocial theory. Issues related to the measurement of and relationships between HBM constructs, areas that we believe have received only minimal attention, are then discussed in some detail. Finally, we discuss how the HBM may be used to explain and intervene in cigarette smoking behavior and in AIDS-related behavior. These examples were selected because they represent two very different behaviorally based public health problems in today's society.

Origins of the Health Belief Model

The Health Belief Model was developed initially in the 1950s by a group of social psychologists in the U.S. Public Health Service in an effort to explain the widespread failure of people to participate in programs to prevent or to detect disease (Hochbaum, 1958; Rosenstock, 1960, 1966, 1974). Later, the model was extended to apply to people's responses to symptoms (Kirscht, 1974) and to their behavior in response to diagnosed illness, particularly their compliance with medical regimens (Becker, 1974). Although the model evolved gradually in response to very practical programmatic concerns that will be described presently, its basis in psychological theory is provided here as an aid to understanding its rationale and its strengths and weaknesses.

During the early 1950s, academic social psychology was engaged in developing an approach to understanding behavior that grew out of a confluence of learning theories derived from two major sources: Stimulus Response (S-R) Theory (Thorndike, 1898; Watson, 1925; Hull, 1943) and Cognitive Theory (Tolman, 1932; Lewin, 1935, 1936, 1951; Lewin, Dembo, Festinger, and Sears, 1944).

In simple terms, S-R theorists believe that learning results from events (termed *reinforcements*) that reduce physiological drives that activate behavior. Skinner (1938) formulated the widely accepted hypothesis that the frequency of a behavior is determined by its consequences (or reinforcements). For Skinner, the mere temporal association between a behavior and an immediately following reward is sufficient to increase the probability that the behavior will be repeated. Such behaviors are termed *operants;* they operate on the environment to bring about changes resulting in reward or reinforcement. In this view, no mentalistic concepts such as reasoning or thinking are required to explain behavior.

Cognitive theorists, in contrast, emphasize the role of subjective hypotheses or expectations held by the subject (see, Lewin, Dembo, Festinger, and Sears, 1944). In this perspective, behavior is a function of the subjective value of an outcome and of the subjective probability, or expectation, that a particular action will achieve that outcome. Such formulations are generally termed *value expectancy* theories. Mental processes such as thinking, reasoning, hypothesizing, or expecting are critical components of all cognitive theories. Cognitive theorists, along with behaviorists, believe that reinforcements, or consequences of behavior, are important, but for cognitive theorists, reinforcements operate by influencing expectations, or hypotheses, regarding the situation rather than by influencing behavior directly (Bandura, 1977b).

The HBM is a value expectancy theory. When value expectancy concepts were gradually reformulated in the context of health-related behavior, the translations were (1) the desire to avoid illness or to get well (value) and (2) the belief that a specific health action available to a person would prevent (or ameliorate) illness (expectancy). The expectancy was further delineated in terms of the individual's estimate of personal susceptibility to and severity of an illness and of the likelihood of being able to reduce that threat through personal action.

The development of the HBM grew out of real concerns with the limited success of various programs of the Public Health Service in the 1950s. One such early example was the failure of large numbers of eligible adults to participate in tuberculosis (TB) screening programs provided at no charge in mobile X-ray units conveniently located in various neighborhoods. Program operators were concerned to explain people's behavior by illuminating those factors that were facilitating or inhibiting positive responses.

Beginning in 1952, Hochbaum (1958) studied probability samples of more than 1,200 adults in three cities that had conducted recent TB screening programs in mobile X-ray units. He assessed these individuals' "readiness" to obtain X-rays, which included assessing their beliefs that they were susceptible to tuberculosis and their beliefs in the personal benefits of early detection. Perceived susceptibility to tuberculosis itself comprised two elements: first, the respondents' beliefs about whether contracting tuberculosis was a realistic (not merely a mathematical) possibility for them personally and, second, the extent to which they accepted the fact that a person may have tuberculosis in the absence of all symptoms.

The measure of perceived personal benefits of early detection also included two elements: whether respondents believed that X-rays could detect tuberculosis prior to the appearance of symptoms and whether they believed that early detection and treatment would improve the prognosis. Among the group of people who exhibited both beliefs, that is, belief in their own susceptibility to tuberculosis and the belief that overall benefits would accrue from early detection, 82 percent had had at least one voluntary chest X-ray during a specified period preceding the interview. Of the group exhibiting neither of these beliefs, only 21 percent had obtained a voluntary X-ray during the criterion period. In short, four out of five people who exhibited both beliefs (susceptibility and benefits) took the predicted action while four of five people who accepted neither of the beliefs had not taken the action. Hochbaum thus demonstrated with considerable precision that a particular action to screen for a disease was associated strongly with the two interacting variables of perceived susceptibility and perceived benefits.

Components of the HBM

Over the years since Hochbaum's survey, many investigations have expanded and clarified the model and have extended its application beyond screening behaviors to include preventive actions, illness behaviors, and sick-role behaviors (see summaries in Rosenstock, 1974; Kirscht, 1974; Becker, 1974; Becker and Maiman, 1980; Janz and Becker, 1984). In general, it now is believed that individuals will take action to ward off, to screen for, or to control an ill-health condition if they regard themselves as susceptible to the condition, if they believe it to have potentially serious consequences, if they believe that a course of action available to them would be beneficial in reducing either their susceptibility to or the severity of the condition, and if they believe that the anticipated barriers to (or costs of) taking the action are outweighed by its benefits. The definitions in Table 3.1 and the following commentary specify the key variables in greater detail.

Perceived Susceptibility

The dimension of perceived susceptibility measures an individual's subjective perception of his or her risk of contracting a health condition. For cases of medically established illness, the dimension has been reformulated to include the individual's acceptance of the diagnosis, personal estimates of resusceptibility, and susceptibility to illness in general.

Perceived Severity

Perceived severity addresses feelings concerning the seriousness of contracting an illness or of leaving it untreated. Perceived severity includes evaluation of both medical and clinical consequences (such as death, disability, and pain) and possible social consequences (such as effects of the condition on work, family life, and social relations). The combination of susceptibility and severity has been labeled the *perceived threat*.

Perceived Benefits

Although acceptance of personal susceptibility to a condition also believed to be serious (that is, susceptibility to a perceived threat) produces a force leading to behavior, the particular course of action taken will depend upon beliefs regarding the effectiveness of the various available actions in reducing the disease threat, termed the perceived benefits of taking health action. Other factors include non-heath-related benefits (for example, quitting smoking to save money or getting a

TABLE 3.1. KEY CONCEPTS AND DEFINITIONS OF THE HEALTH BELIEF MODEL.

Concept	Definition	Application
Perceived susceptibility	One's opinion of chances of getting a condition.	Define population(s) at risk, risk levels.
		Personalize risk based on a person's characteristics or behavior.
		Make perceived susceptibility more consistent with individual's actual risk.
Perceived severity	One's opinion of how serious a condition and its sequelae are.	Specify consequences of the risk and the condition.
Perceived benefits	One's opinion of the efficacy of the advised action to reduce risk or seriousness of impact.	Define action to take: how, where, when; clarify the positive effects to be expected.
Perceived barriers	One's opinion of the tangible and psychological costs of the advised action.	Identify and reduce perceived barriers through reassurance, correction of misinformation, incentives, assistance.
Cues to action	Strategies to activate one's "readiness."	Provide how-to information, promote awareness, employ reminder systems.
Self-efficacy	One's confidence in one's ability to take action.	Provide training, guidance in performing action.
		Use progressive goal setting.
		Give verbal reinforcement.
		Demonstrate desired behaviors.
		Reduce anxiety.

mammogram to please a family member). Thus, an individual exhibiting an optimal level of beliefs in both susceptibility and severity would not be expected to accept any recommended health action unless that action were perceived as potentially efficacious.

Perceived Barriers

The potentially negative aspects of a particular health action, the perceived barriers, may act as impediments to undertaking the recommended behavior. A kind of nonconscious cost-benefit analysis occurs, wherein the individual weighs the action's expected effectiveness against perceptions that it may be expensive, dangerous (having negative side effects or iatrogenic outcomes), unpleasant (painful, difficult, or upsetting), inconvenient, time consuming, and so forth. Thus, "the combined levels of susceptibility and severity [provide] the energy or force to act and the perception of benefits (less barriers) [provide] a preferred path of action" (Rosenstock, 1974).

Cues to Action

Various early formulations of the HBM discussed the concept of *cues* that trigger action. Hochbaum (1958), for example, thought that the readiness to take action (perceived susceptibility and perceived benefits) could be potentiated only by other factors and particularly by cues such as bodily events and environmental events, for example, media publicity, that instigate action. He did not, however, study the role of cues empirically. Cues to action may ultimately prove to be important, but they have not been systematically studied. Indeed, even though the concept of cues as trigger mechanisms is appealing, it has been difficult to study in explanatory surveys; a cue might be as fleeting as a sneeze or the barely conscious perception of a poster.

Other Variables

Diverse demographic, sociopsychological, and structural variables may affect an individual's perceptions and thus indirectly influence health-related behavior. Specifically, sociodemographic factors, particularly educational attainment, are believed to have an indirect effect on behavior by influencing the perception of susceptibility, severity, benefits, and barriers.

Self-Efficacy

In 1977, Bandura introduced the concept of self-efficacy, or efficacy expectation, as distinct from outcome expectation (Bandura, 1977a, 1977b, 1986), which we believe must be added to the HBM in order to increase its explanatory power (Rosenstock, Strecher, and Becker, 1988). Outcome expectation, defined as a person's estimate that a given behavior will lead to certain outcomes, is quite similar to the HBM concept of perceived benefits. Self-efficacy is defined as "the conviction that one can successfully execute the behavior required to produce the outcomes" (Bandura, 1977a). We view lack of efficacy as a perceived barrier to taking a recommended health action.

It is not difficult to see why self-efficacy was never explicitly incorporated into early formulations of the HBM. The original focus of the early model was on circumscribed, usually one-shot, preventive actions, such as accepting a screening test or an immunization, actions that generally were simple behaviors for most people to perform. It is likely that most prospective members of target groups for the programs examined had adequate self-efficacy for performing the simple behaviors the programs required; therefore, that dimension was not even recognized.

The situation is vastly different, however, when practitioners work with lifestyle behaviors requiring long-term changes. The problems involved in modifying lifelong habits of eating, drinking, exercising, smoking, and sexual practices are obviously far more difficult to surmount than those involved in accepting a one-time immunization or a screening test. It requires a good deal of confidence that one can, in fact, alter such lifestyles before successful change is possible. Thus, for behavioral change to succeed, people must (as the original HBM theorizes) feel threatened by their current behavioral patterns (perceived susceptibility and severity) and believe that change of a specific kind will be beneficial by resulting in a valued outcome at an acceptable cost, but they must also feel themselves competent (self-efficacious) to overcome perceived barriers to taking action. A growing body of literature supports the importance of self-efficacy in accounting for initiation and maintenance of behavioral change (Bandura, 1977a; Bandura, 1986; Marlatt and Gordon, 1985; Strecher, DeVellis, Becker, and Rosenstock, 1986).

The Health Belief Model, originally developed to explain health-related behavior, focused on cognitive variables. Efforts to change cognitions about health matters, however, have often involved attempts to arouse individuals' fear through threatening messages (Leventhal, 1970). According to Protection Motivation Theory (Rogers, 1975), the most persuasive communications are those that arouse fear while enhancing perceptions central to the HBM of the severity of an event, the likelihood of exposure to that event, and the efficacy of responses to that threat. Rogers (1983) also has incorporated self-efficacy into his theory. This view of the joint role of fear and reassurance in persuasive communications is generally accepted.

The Health Belief Model components and their linkages are summarized in Figure 3.1.

**FIGURE 3.1. HEALTH BELIEF MODEL
COMPONENTS AND LINKAGES.**

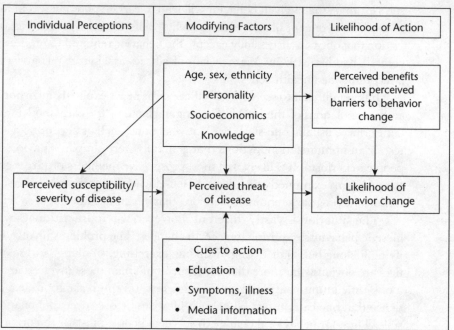

Evidence for and Against the Model

In 1974, *Health Education Monographs* devoted an entire issue to the Health Belief Model and personal health behavior (Becker, 1974). That issue summarized findings from research on the HBM to understand why individuals did or did not engage in a wide variety of health-related actions, and it provided considerable support for the model in explaining behavior pertinent to prevention and behavior in response to symptoms or to diagnosed disease.

During the decade following publication of that monograph, the HBM continued to be a major organizing framework for explaining and predicting acceptance of health and medical care recommendations. Accordingly, an updated critical review was made of HBM studies conducted between 1974 and 1984. This review also combined the new results with earlier findings to permit an overall assessment of the model's performance (Janz and Becker, 1984). Space limitations permit only a brief summary of the findings of the detailed reviews of 1974 and 1984; the interested reader should consult the original sources for details.

Included in the 1984 review were such preventive health and screening behaviors as receiving influenza inoculations, practicing breast self-examination, attending screening programs for Tay-Sachs disease carrier status and high blood pressure, using a seat belt, exercising, paying attention to nutrition, stopping smoking, visiting physicians for checkups, and fearing apprehension while driving under the influence of alcohol. Sick-role behaviors included compliance with antihypertensive regimens, diabetic regimens, end-stage renal disease regimens, medication regimens for parents caring for children with otitis media or with asthma, and weight loss regimens.

Summary results provide substantial empirical support for the HBM, with findings from prospective studies at least as favorable as those obtained from retrospective research. The component of perceived barriers was the most powerful single predictor among the HBM dimensions across all studies and behaviors. Although both perceived susceptibility and perceived benefits were important overall, perceived susceptibility was a stronger predictor of preventive health behavior than sick-role behavior, but the reverse was true for perceived benefits. Overall, perceived severity was the least powerful predictor; however, this dimension was strongly related to sick-role behavior.

One of the most important deficits in the research on the HBM has been inconsistent measurement of HBM concepts. The vast majority of studies using the HBM reported in the literature have failed to establish validity or reliability prior to model testing (Rosenstock, Strecher, and Becker, 1994). Another prevalent problem in HBM research is the confusion about the relationships among HBM components. Some researchers have attempted to establish each of the four major concepts—susceptibility, seriousness, benefits, and barriers—as independent, and others have tried multiplicative approaches. Investigators have been most successful when looking at models that measure direct as well as conditional effects of variables on behavior (Rosenstock, Strecher, and Becker, 1994).

Measuring HBM Constructs

The relationship between theory and measurement cannot be underestimated. Measuring abstract concepts presents a clear challenge to social researchers. Application of constructs requires researchers to be familiar with the theory as well as the processes needed for operationalizing concepts relevant to measurement issues. One mistake often made in using theory to guide instrument development is failure to recognize that the construct measuring the theory may be inconsistent with the theory. Flaws in measurement procedures result in flaws in the conclusions about the theory. Thus, it is imperative that researchers using the HBM be mindful of procedures related to developing valid and reliable health belief measures.

Scale development takes a great deal of knowledge, planning, and work and is an ongoing, iterative process. Even when valid and reliable measures are used, they must be revalidated with each data collection. Validity and reliability are sample specific and may change depending on sample characteristics.

Another issue related to measurement of the HBM constructs is temporality. Most studies have used cross-sectional data with no attempt to determine whether attitudes did in fact precede behavior. If health beliefs and behavior were measured concurrently, belief-behavior relationships might well turn out to be spurious. Janz and Becker (1984) have addressed this issue, recommending that cross-sectional studies be eschewed in favor of predictive studies.

Using the HBM to Address Public Health Concerns

As stated earlier, the Health Belief Model was developed in an effort to address public health concerns. Initially, the HBM was focused on issues related to screening and compliance. Since those initial uses, however, the HBM has been used as both an explanatory and an intervention tool with a broad spectrum of health-related behaviors. In this section, we discuss use of the HBM in two important areas: cigarette smoking behavior and AIDS-related behaviors, addressing how key HBM components are associated with these behaviors.

The HBM and Cigarette Smoking Behavior. The Health Belief Model is not widely used in cigarette smoking research. This may be a result of consistent findings that the majority of cigarette smokers already perceive a general health threat from smoking. In a survey of over 2,000 adult current smokers, ex-smokers, and people who had never smoked (Brownson and others, 1992), 83 percent of current smokers believed that smoking was harmful to health. This percentage was lower, but not much lower, than the 91 percent of people who had never smoked and the 92 percent of ex-smokers in the survey who believed that smoking was harmful. Findings such as these support the common thinking that smokers already perceive a health threat, making a central construct of the Health Belief Model not relevant. Moreover, it is possible that increasing the perceived threat through fear arousal may increase frequency of cigarette smoking and decrease likelihood of cessation, because smoking is often linked with stress and emotional arousal.

Although smokers and nonsmokers may have similar beliefs regarding the harmful nature of smoking in general, personal susceptibility may differ. In a survey of 120 ex-smokers and current smokers, Weinberger, Greene, Mamlin, and Jerin (1981) found that ex-smokers viewed smoking as a serious health problem and felt personally susceptible to adverse consequences due to smoking. Moderate smokers in this survey regarded smoking as a serious health problem but were less likely to feel personally susceptible.

Recent research conducted among 2,785 patients of community-based family practitioners (Strecher, Kreuter, and Kobrin, 1995) found that smokers were more likely to perceive a heightened personal risk of heart attack, cancer, and stroke than nonsmokers. However, a much larger proportion of smokers compared to nonsmokers tended to *underestimate* their actual risk of heart attack, cancer, and stroke. In other words, smokers tend to perceive a health risk, but they underestimate the *magnitude* of that health risk.

Perceived benefits and barriers have received far less examination in their relation to cigarette smoking. In Brownson and others' study (1992), smokers and nonsmokers did not differ in their belief that quitting smoking would result in health benefits. Strecher and colleagues (1985) combined susceptibility to smoking-related illness from continued smoking with susceptibility to illness from quitting smoking (a susceptibility/benefit measure similar to the outcome expectations concept developed by Bandura, 1977a) in a study of Veterans Administration Medical Center patients who smoked. This measure was strongly associated with a desire to quit smoking, and interacted with a measure of self-efficacy in predicting subsequent smoking cessation.

In a study of 308 patients with newly diagnosed pulmonary disease, Peterson, Wanklin, and Baskerville (1984) combined four health beliefs largely focusing on perceived threat and benefits concepts. This combined measure was strongly related to subsequent smoking cessation among smokers who considered their habit related to tension reduction. However, health beliefs were not associated with cessation among smokers who considered their habit related to addiction. This finding suggests that health beliefs may be one component of the smoking habit but by no means the only factor on which to intervene (Henningfield and others, 1994).

It is important that perceived benefits not be viewed strictly in the context of health. Perceived benefits of quitting smoking can include positive reinforcement from family and friends, cost savings from not buying cigarettes, and greater control of one's life. Immediate functional benefits of quitting (for example, greater energy and vitality) should also be considered. As Dubos (1965) stated, "the words health and disease are meaningful only when defined in terms of a given person functioning in a given physical and social environment." Research by Curry, Wagner, and Grothaus (1991) suggests the importance of determining whether the subject perceives the motive for changing to be intrinsic (that is, from an internal reason) or extrinsic (that is, from an external reason). This distinction should receive further research attention.

Barriers to quitting smoking can include fear of stress or anxiety when refraining from cigarettes, fear of significant weight gain (often what is "significant" to a patient is only a few pounds), pressure from other smokers to relapse, and a general fear of relapse (Strecher and others, 1994). Forming a single construct from these barriers is challenging. Velicer and colleagues (1993) have made significant advances in making use of the *pros* and *cons* of smoking by first determining whether the pro or con exists, then determining a valence, or degree, to which it is a pro or a con. Pros and cons are similar to benefits and barriers and have been found to be predictive of movement through stages of behavioral change readiness.

Lack of self-efficacy is strongly related to the barriers component of the HBM (Rosenstock, Strecher, and Becker, 1988). We hypothesize that self-efficacy will be a stronger predictor of behavioral change among those with a strong perception of threat and of the benefits of taking recommended health action. This suggestion is consistent with the work of Witte (1991, 1992, 1994). As Witte (1992) states, "regardless of whether the efficacy construct is explicitly addressed in a fear appeal study, every fear appeal message has an inherent level of efficacy that may inadvertently influence study outcomes. . . . [P]ositive linear findings should be found in studies with strong efficacy depictions, and boomerang findings should be found in studies with weak or missing efficacy depictions."

We did not find cigarette smoking studies that examined the HBM as an entire model: that is, examined behavioral outcomes based on prespecified combinations of HBM components. However, we would predict a number of contingent outcomes and hope to see more research examining such relationships in the future.

The HBM and AIDS-Protective Behaviors.

Catania, Kegeles, and Coates (1990) have suggested that, for individuals who exhibit high-risk behaviors, perceived susceptibility is required before commitment to changing these risky behaviors can occur. Is perceived susceptibility associated with AIDS-protective behaviors? In a longitudinal study of gay men's AIDS-protective behavior, Aspinwall and colleagues (1991) found decreases in numbers of sexual partners (anonymous and known) chiefly among seronegative men who had earlier perceived themselves to be at increased risk of contracting HIV. Cross-sectional studies (for example, Hays, Kegeles, and Coates, 1990; Hingson, Strunin, Berlin, and Heeren, 1990; Allard, 1989; Basen-Engquist, 1992) also have found significant susceptibility-behavior associations. Countering these findings, however are a number of longitudinal studies (for example, McKusick and others, 1990; Montgomery and others, 1989) and cross-sectional studies (for example, Catania and others, 1992; Walter and others, 1992).

Variations in results are related to the measures used to assess susceptibility. A number of articles we reviewed used a behavioral anchor in their susceptibility measures: for example, they asked the question: "*If you do not practice safer sex,* how likely are you to become infected with the AIDS virus?" as opposed to asking simply: "How likely are you to become infected with the AIDS virus?" Recent research by Ronis (1992) suggests that susceptibility questions should be clearly conditional on action or inaction. Unconditional susceptibility measures can lead to a pattern of personalized interpretation: for example, respondents may indicate that their risk of infection is great largely *because* they are not practicing safer sex.

Perceptions of AIDS severity must address the perceived costs of being HIV-positive and of having AIDS. Perceived seriousness, in this case, refers to personal evaluations of the probable biomedical, financial, and social consequences of contracting HIV and having AIDS. Some might argue that asking about AIDS severity would be a waste of respondent time—everyone would report that AIDS is an extremely severe disease. Unfortunately, most measures in the research literature do not focus directly on the importance of AIDS severity (Rosenstock, Strecher, and Becker, 1994). When perception of threat from AIDS is high, the HBM would hypothesize that AIDS-protective behavior decisions become largely a function of perceptions of benefits minus perceived barriers to behavioral change. If the perception of AIDS threat is not high, strong perceived benefits of AIDS-protective behavior may still influence behavioral change. For example, a person who uses condoms because his partner prefers them may adopt and maintain condom-use behavior regardless of his perception of AIDS threat. Although there are perceived benefits in this example, they are not directly related to AIDS-protective behavior but rather to the benefits of pleasing one's partner. If the perceptions of AIDS threat and benefits are not high, it is not likely that low perceived barriers would necessarily influence AIDS-preventive behavior.

Of the possible perceived benefits, *response efficacy,* or the perception that adopting and maintaining AIDS-preventive behaviors will reduce AIDS risk, is one of the most commonly researched. Measures of response efficacy have been associated with AIDS-preventive behaviors in cross-sectional and longitudinal studies (for example, Hingson, Strunin, Berlin, and Heeren, 1990; Allard, 1989; Aspinwall and others, 1991—the latter study finding a relationship only among HIV-positive men without a primary sexual partner). Other benefits of AIDS-preventive behaviors have been examined by Catania and others (1992). Enjoyment of condom use distinguished gay and bisexual men who always used condoms from those who did not.

Relationships between perceived barriers and AIDS-preventive behaviors have been mixed across both longitudinal and cross-sectional studies. Unfortunately, a number of the studies we reviewed included questionable measures of barriers. Montgomery and others (1989), for example, used barriers measures that included knowledge of the virus and modes of transmission, ever being paid for sex, and belief in a vaccine or a potential cure; the study did not include lack of sexual enjoyment as a barrier. These measures were unrelated to subsequent AIDS-protective behavior changes. Another negative study (Allard, 1989) used only two "barriers to [AIDS] treatment"—items not at all relevant to preventive practices.

Studies using more relevant barriers measures tended to find results in the expected direction. Basen-Engquist (1992) found strong associations in the expected direction between perceived barriers and both intention to use condoms and actual condom use. Seven barriers were aggregated to form a single scale; among these barriers were "embarrassment caused by practicing safer sex, moral implications of condom use, and satisfaction involved in practicing safer sex." Aspinwall and colleagues (1991) used barrier measures that included importance, temptation, and difficulty of refraining from sex with numerous partners. This study found that gay men without primary partners who reported strong barriers reported higher numbers of anonymous sexual partners at follow-up. Baseline reports of strong barriers to changing unprotected anal receptive intercourse also predicted subsequent unprotected anal receptive intercourse with partners whose HIV status was unknown.

As these studies suggest, the concepts of benefits and barriers are rather open ended and can include wide domains of factors—emotional, physical, and social. Researchers must continue determining just which benefits and barriers exist and which benefits and barriers have the greatest influence on AIDS-preventive behaviors.

The cue-to-action construct is, both in general and in the area of AIDS prevention, the least-studied construct in the Health Belief Model. This is unfortunate because a good deal of anecdotal evidence supports the importance of brief though salient cues that stimulate a decision to act. Cues to action were examined in the studies of Hingson, Strunin, Berlin, and Heeren (1990) and Aspinwall and others (1991). Hingson, Strunin, Berlin, and Heeren asked respondents among a general population of adolescents whether they had read or heard about AIDS from media sources; whether they had ever discussed AIDS with a family member, teacher, or physician; and whether they knew someone with AIDS. Having discussed AIDS with friends or with a physician was positively associated with condom use. However, knowledge of someone with AIDS was *negatively* associated with condom use. Aspinwall and colleagues (1991) asked survey participants how many close friends had AIDS-related complex (ARC), how many had AIDS, and how many had died from AIDS or ARC in the past year. A summed index of these potential cues to action did not predict AIDS-protective behavior changes.

Recommendations for Further Research

The following recommendations detail goals and principles for studies using the Health Belief Model.

1. Test the Health Belief Model as a model, or at minimum, as a combination of constructs, not as a collection of equally weighted variables operating simultaneously. Good examples of careful examinations of Health Belief Model constructs include the work of Ronis (1992) and of Witte (1994). It makes little sense to put health belief variables into a multivariate analysis, select the "strongest swimmers," and claim that these are the factors on which to intervene. The following hypotheses serve as a starting point for testing the Health Belief Model as a model:

> Perceived threat is a sequential function of perceived severity and perceived susceptibility. A heightened state of severity is required before perceived susceptibility becomes a powerful predictor. Perceived susceptibility, under the state of high perceived severity, will be a stronger predictor of intention to engage in health-related behaviors than it will be a predictor of actual engagement in health-related behaviors.

> Perceived benefits and barriers will be stronger predictors of behavioral change when perceived threat is high than when it is low. Under conditions of low perceived threat, benefits of and barriers to engaging in health-related behaviors will not be salient. The only exception to this may be that when certain benefits of the recommended behavior are perceived to be high (for example, a partner's encouragement for safe sex), perceived threat may not need to be high.

> Self-efficacy, a factor now included in the Health Belief Model, will be a strong predictor of many health-related behaviors. It will be a particularly strong predictor of behaviors that require significant skills to perform.

> Cues to action will have a greater influence on behavior in situations where perceived threat is great. The cue to action construct is a little-studied phenomenon, so little is known about what cues to action exist or their relative impact.

2. Specify the measures used to study belief constructs in publications. An important reason for variance in results between studies probably is large variation among the specific measures used. When the actual questions were included in the articles we examined, or could be uncovered in some manner, a disconcertingly large proportion did not appear to be good indicators of HBM constructs.

3. Delay aggregating items measuring benefits, barriers, and cues to action into general constructs; such items are often unrelated to one another and have low inter-item correlations. To the practitioner charged with creating programs that will contain health messages, analysis of single items can often offer more relevant information than a general grouped construct.

4. Include a behavioral anchor when measuring perceived susceptibility. For example, a behaviorally anchored question for AIDS-preventive behavior would ask, "*If you do not practice safer sex,* how likely are you to become infected with the AIDS virus?" as opposed to, "How likely are you to become infected with the AIDS virus?" (See recent research by Ronis, 1992, cited earlier in this chapter, which finds strong evidence for the importance of asking susceptibility questions that are conditional on action or inaction.)

Conclusion and Recommendations for Practice

This chapter has described both strengths and limitations in the Health Belief Model as formulated to date. It is hoped that future theory-building or theory-testing research will direct efforts more toward strengthening the HBM where it is weak than toward repeating what has already been established. More work is needed on experimental interventions to modify health beliefs and health behaviors than on surveys to reconfirm already established correlations. More work is also needed to specify and measure factors that need to be added to the HBM to increase its predictive power. The addition of self-efficacy to the traditional HBM should improve explanation and prediction, particularly in the area of lifestyle practices.

It is timely for professionals who are attempting to influence health behavior to make use of the health belief variables, including self-efficacy, in their program planning, both in needs assessment and in program strategies. Programs to deal with a health problem should be based, in part, on knowledge of how many and which members of a target population feel susceptible to a particular health outcome, believe the health outcome to constitute a serious health problem, and believe the threat of having the health outcome could be reduced by changing their behavior at an acceptable psychological cost. Moreover, health professionals should also assess the extent to which clients possess adequate self-efficacy to carry out the prescribed action(s), sometimes over long periods of time.

The collection of data on health beliefs, along with other data pertinent to the group or community setting, permits the planning of more effective programs than would otherwise be possible. Interventions can then be targeted to the specific needs identified. This is true whether one is dealing with the problems of individual patients, of groups of clients, or of entire communities. In planning programs to influence the behavior of large groups of people for long periods of time, the role of the HBM (including self-efficacy) must be considered in context. Permanent changes in behavior can rarely be wrought solely by direct attacks on belief systems. Moreover, where the behavior of large groups is the target, interventions at societal levels (for example, through social networks, work organizations, physical environments, and legislatures) along with interventions at the individual level will likely prove more effective than single-level interventions alone. Yet all of us should never lose sight of the fact that a crucial way station on the road to improved health directs our attention toward the beliefs and behavior of each of a series of individuals.

References

Allard, R. "Beliefs About AIDS as Determinants of Preventive Practices and of Support for Coercive Measures." *American Journal of Public Health,* 1989, *79,* 448–452.

Aspinwall, L., and others. "Psychosocial Predictors of Gay Men's AIDS Risk-Reduction Behavior." *Health Psychology,* 1991, *10*(6) 432–444.

Bandura, A. "Self-Efficacy: Toward a Unifying Theory of Behavior Change." *Psychological Review,* 1977a, *84,* 191–215.

Bandura, A. *Social Learning Theory.* Englewood Cliffs, N.J.: Prentice Hall, 1977b.

Bandura, A. *Social Foundations of Thought and Action: A Social Cognitive Theory.* Englewood Cliffs, N.J.: Prentice Hall, 1986.

Basen-Engquist, K. "Psychosocial Predictors of 'Safer Sex' Behaviors in Young Adults." *AIDS Education & Prevention,* 1992, *4,* 120–134.

Becker, M. H. (ed.). "The Health Belief Model and Personal Health Behavior." *Health Education Monographs,* 1974, *2* (entire issue).

Becker, M. H., and Maiman, L. A. "Strategies for Enhancing Patient Compliance." *Journal of Community Health,* 1980, *6,* 113–135.

Brownson, R. C., and others. "Demographic and Socioeconomic Differences in Beliefs About the Health Effects of Smoking." *American Journal of Public Health,* 1992, *82*(1), 99–103.

Catania, J., and others. "Condom Use in Multi-Ethnic Neighborhoods of San Francisco: The Population-Based AMEN (AIDS in Multi-Ethnic Neighborhoods) Study." *American Journal of Public Health,* 1992, *82*(2), 284–287.

Catania, T., Kegeles, J, and Coates, T. "Psychosocial Predictors of People Who Fail to Return for Their HIV Test Results." *AIDS,* 1990, *4*(3), 261–262.

Curry, S. J., Wagner, E. G., and Grothaus, L. C. "Evaluation of Intrinsic and Extrinsic Motivation Interventions with a Self-Help Smoking Cessation Program." *Journal of Consulting and Clinical Psychology,* 1991, *59,* 318–324.

Dubos, R. *Man Adapting.* New Haven, Conn.: Yale University Press, 1965.

Hays, R., Kegeles, S., and Coates, T. "High HIV Risk-Taking Among Young Gay Men." *AIDS,* 1990, *4*(9), 901–907.

Henningfield, J. E., and others. "Smoking and the Workplace: Realities and Solutions." *Journal of Smoking-Related Disease,* 1994, *5* (supp. 1), 261–270.

Hingson, R. H., Strunin, L., Berlin, B., and Heeren, T. "Beliefs About AIDS, Use of Alcohol and Drugs, and Unprotected Sex Among Massachusetts Adolescents." *American Journal of Public Health,* 1990, *80*(3), 295–299.

Hochbaum, G. M. *Public Participation in Medical Screening Programs: A Sociopsychological Study.* PHS publication no. 572. Washington, D.C.: U.S. Government Printing Office, 1958.

Hull, C. L. *Principles of Behavior.* Englewood Cliffs, N.J.: Appleton-Century-Crofts, 1943.

Janz, N. K., and Becker, M. H. "The Health Belief Model: A Decade Later." *Health Education Quarterly,* 1984, *11,* 1–47.

Kirscht, J. P. "The Health Belief Model and Illness Behavior." *Health Education Monographs,* 1974, *2,* 387–408.

Leventhal, H. "Findings and Theory in the Study of Fear Communications." In L. Berkowitz (ed.), *Advances in Experimental Social Psychology,* Vol. 5. Orlando, Fla.: Academic Press, 1970.

Lewin, K. *A Dynamic Theory of Personality.* New York: McGraw-Hill, 1935.

Lewin, K. *Principles of Topological Psychology.* New York: McGraw-Hill, 1936.

Lewin, K. "The Nature of Field Theory." In M. H. Marx (ed.), *Psychological Theory.* New York: Macmillan, 1951.

Lewin, K., Dembo, T., Festinger, L., and Sears, P. S. "Level of Aspiration." In J. Hunt (ed.), *Personality and the Behavior Disorders.* Somerset, N.J.: Ronald Press, 1944.

Marlatt, G. A., and Gordon, J. R. (eds.). *Relapse Prevention.* New York: Guilford Press, 1985.

McKusick, L., and others. "Longitudinal Predictors of Reductions in Unprotected Anal Intercourse Among Gay Men in San Francisco: The AIDS Behavioral Research Project." *American Journal of Public Health,* 1990, *80*(8), 978–983.

Montgomery, S., and others. "The Health Belief Model in Understanding Compliance with Preventive Recommendations for AIDS: How Useful?" *AIDS Education and Prevention,* 1989, *1*(4), 303–323.

Peterson, L. L., Wanklin, J. M., and Baskerville, J. C. "The Role of Health Beliefs in Compliance with Physician Advice to Quit Smoking." *Social Science and Medicine,* 1984, *19*(5), 573–580.

Rogers, R. W. "A Protection Motivation Theory of Fear Appeals and Attitude Change." *Journal of Psychology,* 1975, *91,* 93–114.

Rogers, R. W. "Cognitive and Psychological Factors in Fear Appeals and Attitude Change: A Revised Theory of Protection Motivation." In J. Cacioppo and R. Petty (eds.), *Social Psychophysiology.* New York: Guilford Press, 1983.

Ronis, D. "Conditional Health Threats: Health Beliefs, Decisions, and Behaviors Among Adults." *Health Psychology,* 1992, *11*(2) 127–134.

Rosenstock, I. M. "What Research in Motivation Suggests for Public Health." *American Journal of Public Health,* 1960, *50,* 295–301.

Rosenstock, I. M. "Why People Use Health Services." *Milbank Memorial Fund Quarterly,* 1966, *44,* 94–124.

Rosenstock, I. M. "Historical Origins of the Health Belief Model." *Health Education Monographs,* 1974, *2,* 328–335.

Rosenstock, I. M., Strecher, V. J., and Becker, M. H. "Social Learning Theory and the Health Belief Model." *Health Education Quarterly,* 1988, *15*(2), 175–183.

Rosenstock, I. M., Strecher, V. J., and Becker, M. H. "The Health Belief Model and HIV Risk Behavior Change." In J. Peterson and R. DiClemente (eds.), *Preventing AIDS: Theory and Practice of Behavioral Interventions.* New York: Plenum, 1994.

Skinner, B. F. *The Behavior of Organisms.* Englewood Cliffs, N.J.: Appleton-Century-Crofts, 1938.

Strecher, V. J., DeVellis, B. M., Becker, M. H., and Rosenstock, I. M. "The Role of Self-Efficacy in Achieving Health Behavior Change." *Health Education Quarterly,* 1986, *13,* 73–91.

Strecher, V. J., Kreuter, M. W., and Kobrin, S. C. "Do Cigarette Smokers Have Unrealistic Perceptions of Their Heart Attack, Cancer and Stroke Risks?" *Journal of Behavioral Medicine,* 1995, *18*(1), 45–54.

Strecher, V. J., and others. "Psychosocial Aspects of Changes in Smoking Cessation Behavior." *Patient Education and Counseling,* 1985, *7*(3), 249–262.

Strecher, V. J., and others. "The Effects of Computer-Tailored Smoking Cessation Messages in Family Practice Settings." *Journal of Family Practice,* 1994, *39*(3), 262–270.

Thorndike, E. L. "Animal Intelligence: An Experimental Study of the Associative Processes in Animals." *Psychological Monographs,* 1898, *2* (entire issue 8).

Tolman, E. C. *Purposive Behavior in Animals and Men.* Englewood Cliffs, N.J.: Appleton-Century-Crofts, 1932.

Velicer, W. F., and others. "An Expert System Intervention for Smoking Cessation." *Addictive Behaviors,* 1993, *18,* 269–290.

Walter, H., and others. "Factors Associated with AIDS Risk Behaviors Among High School Students in an AIDS Epicenter." *American Journal of Public Health,* 1992, *82*(4) 528–532.

Watson, J. B. *Behaviorism.* New York: Norton, 1925.

Weinberger, M., Greene, J. Y., Mamlin, J. J., and Jerin, M. J. "Health Beliefs and Smoking Behavior." *American Journal of Public Health,* 1981, *71*(11), 1253–1255.

Witte, K. "Preventing AIDS Through Persuasive Communications: Fear Appeals and Preventive Action Efficacy." Unpublished doctoral dissertation, University of California, Irvine, 1991.

Witte, K. "Putting the Fear Back into Fear Appeals: The Extended Parallel Process Model." *Speech Communication Association,* 1992, *59,* 328–349.

Witte, K. "Fear Control and Danger Control: A Test of the Extended Parallel Process Model (EPPM)." *Communication Monographs,* 1994, *61,* 113–134.

CHAPTER FOUR

THE TRANSTHEORETICAL MODEL
AND STAGES OF CHANGE

James O. Prochaska
Colleen A. Redding
Kerry E. Evers

The Transtheoretical Model uses stages of change to integrate processes and principles of change from across major theories of intervention, hence the name *trans*theoretical. This model emerged from a comparative analysis of leading theories of psychotherapy and behavioral change. The search was for a systematic integration in a field that had fragmented into more than three hundred theories of psychotherapy (Prochaska, [1979] 1984). The comparative analysis identified only ten processes of change among these theories, such as consciousness raising from the Freudian tradition, contingency management from the Skinnerian tradition, and helping relationships from the Rogerian tradition.

In an empirical analysis of self-changers compared to smokers taking professional treatments, we assessed how frequently each group used each of the ten processes (DiClemente and Prochaska, 1982). Research participants said that they used different processes at different times in their struggles with smoking. These naïve subjects were describing a phenomenon that was not included in current therapy theories. They were revealing that behavioral change unfolds through a series of stages (Prochaska and DiClemente, 1983).

From the initial studies of smoking, the stage model rapidly expanded in scope to include investigations and applications of a broad range of health and mental health behaviors. These behaviors focus on alcohol and substance abuse, anxiety and panic disorders, delinquency, eating disorders and obesity, high-fat diets (Glanz and others, 1994), HIV/AIDS prevention, mammograms, cervical cancer screening, compliance with medication regimes, unplanned pregnancy prevention, pregnancy and smoking, radon testing, sedentary lifestyles, sun exposure (Rossi, Blais, Redding, and Weinstock, 1995), and physicians who practice preventive medicine. Over time, these studies have expanded, validated, applied, and challenged the core constructs of The Transtheoretical Model.

Core Constructs

This section defines core constructs including the stages of change, the processes of change, and some critical assumptions underlying the model.

Stages of Change

The *stage construct* is important, in part, because it represents a temporal dimension. The Transtheoretical Model conceives behavioral change as a process involving progress through a series of five stages (see Table 4.1).

Precontemplation is the stage in which people have no intention to take action in the foreseeable future, usually measured as the next six months. People may be in this stage because they are uninformed or underinformed about the consequences of their behavior, or they may have tried to change a number of times and have become demoralized about their abilities to change. Both uninformed and underinformed groups tend to avoid reading, talking, or thinking about their high-risk behaviors. They are often characterized in other theories as resistant or unmotivated clients or as not ready for therapy or health promotion programs. The fact is traditional health promotion programs were not ready for such individuals and were not motivated to match their needs.

Contemplation is the stage in which people intend to change within the next six months. They are now aware of the pros of changing but are also acutely aware of the cons. This balance between the costs and benefits of changing can produce profound ambivalence that can keep people stuck in this stage for long periods of time. We often characterize this phenomenon as chronic contemplation or behavioral procrastination. These people are also not ready for traditional action-oriented programs.

Preparation is the stage in which people intend to take action in the immediate future, usually measured as the next month. They typically have already taken some significant action in the past year. These individuals have a plan of action such as joining a health education class, consulting a counselor, talking to their physician, buying a self-help book, or relying on a self-change approach. These

TABLE 4.1. TRANSTHEORETICAL MODEL CONSTRUCTS.

Constructs	Description
Stages of change	
Precontemplation	Has no intention to take action within the next 6 months
Contemplation	Intends to take action within the next 6 months
Preparation	Intends to take action within the next 30 days and has taken some behavioral steps in this direction
Action	Has changed overt behavior for less than 6 months
Maintenance	Has changed overt behavior for more than 6 months
Decisional balance	
Pros	The benefits of changing
Cons	The costs of changing
Self-efficacy	
Confidence	Confidence that one can engage in the healthy behavior across different challenging situations
Temptation	Temptation to engage in the unhealthy behavior across different challenging situations
Processes of change	
Consciousness raising	Finding and learning new facts, ideas, and tips that support the healthy behavioral change
Dramatic relief	Experiencing the negative emotions (fear, anxiety, worry) that go along with unhealthy behavioral risks
Self-reevaluation	Realizing that the behavioral change is an important part of one's identity as a person
Environmental reevaluation	Realizing the negative impact of the unhealthy behavior or the positive impact of the healthy behavior on one's proximal social and physical environment
Self-liberation	Making a firm commitment to change
Helping relationships	Seeking and using social support for the healthy behavioral change
Counterconditioning	Substituting healthier alternative behaviors and cognitions for the unhealthy behaviors
Contingency management	Increasing the rewards for the positive behavioral change and decreasing the rewards of the unhealthy behavior
Stimulus control	Removing reminders or cues to engage in the unhealthy behavior and adding cues or reminders to engage in the healthy behavior
Social liberation	Realizing that the social norms are changing in the direction of supporting the healthy behavioral change

are the people who should be recruited for such action-oriented programs as smoking cessation, weight loss, or exercise.

Action is the stage in which people have made specific overt modifications in their lifestyles within the past six months. Because action is observable, behavioral change often has been equated with action. But in The Transtheoretical Model, action is only one of six stages. Not all modifications of behavior count as action in this model. People must attain the criterion that scientists and professionals agree is sufficient to reduce risk of disease. In smoking, for example, only total abstinence counts. In watching one's diet, there is a consensus that no more than 30 percent, and preferably close to 20 percent, of calories should be consumed from fat.

Maintenance is the stage in which people work to prevent relapse, but they do not apply change processes as frequently as do people in action. They are less tempted to relapse and increasingly more confident that they can continue their changes. Based on temptation and self-efficacy data from a variety of sources (for example, U.S. Department of Health and Human Services, 1990), we estimate that maintenance lasts from six months to about five years.

Termination is a sixth stage that applies to some behaviors, especially the addictions. This is a stage in which individuals have no temptation and 100 percent self-efficacy. No matter whether they are depressed, anxious, bored, lonely, angry, or stressed, they are sure they will not return to their old unhealthy habit as a way of coping. It is as if they never acquired the habit in the first place. In a study of former smokers and alcoholics, we found that less than 20 percent of each group had reached the criteria of no temptation and total self-efficacy (Snow, Prochaska, and Rossi, 1992). Termination may not be appropriate for some behaviors, such as cancer screening or dietary fat reduction.

Processes of Change

Processes of change are the covert and overt activities that people use to progress through the six stages. Processes of change provide important guides for intervention programs, because the processes are like independent variables that people need to apply to move from stage to stage. Ten processes have received the most empirical support in our research to date.

Consciousness raising involves increased awareness about the cases that relate to a particular problem behavior and about its consequences and cures. Interventions that can increase awareness include feedback, confrontations, interpretations, bibliotherapy, and media campaigns.

Dramatic relief initially produces increased emotional experiences followed by reduced affect if appropriate action is taken. Psychodrama, role-playing, grieving, personal testimonies, and media campaigns are examples of techniques that can move people emotionally.

Self-reevaluation combines both cognitive and affective assessments of one's self-image with and without a particular unhealthy habit, such as one's image as a couch potato and one's different image as an active person. Clarifying values, having healthy role models, and using mental imagery are techniques that can move people evaluatively.

Environmental reevaluation combines both affective and cognitive assessments of how the presence or absence of a personal habit effects one's social environment, such as assessment of the effect of smoking on others. It can also include the awareness that one can serve as a positive or negative role model for others. Empathy training, documentaries, and family interventions can lead to such assessments.

Self-liberation is both the belief that one can change and the commitment and recommitment to act on that belief. New Year's resolutions, public testimonies, and multiple rather than single choices can enhance what the public calls willpower.

Helping relationships combine caring, trust, openness, and acceptance as well as support for the healthy behavior change. Rapport building, therapeutic alliances, counselor calls, and buddy systems can be sources of social support.

Counterconditioning requires the learning of healthy behaviors that can substitute for problem behaviors. Relaxation, assertion, desensitization, nicotine replacement, and positive self-statements are strategies for finding safer substitutes.

Contingency management provides consequences for taking steps in a particular direction. Although contingency management can include the use of punishments, we found that self-changers rely on rewards much more than punishments. Therefore reinforcements are emphasized, because a philosophy of the stage model is to work in harmony with people's natural ways of changing. Contingency contracts, overt and covert reinforcements, and group recognition are procedures for increasing reinforcement and the probability that healthier responses will be repeated.

Stimulus control removes cues for unhealthy habits and adds prompts for healthier alternatives. Avoidance, environmental reengineering, and self-help groups can provide stimuli that support change and reduce risks for relapse.

Social liberation requires an increase in social opportunities or alternatives, especially for people who are relatively deprived or oppressed. Advocacy, empowerment procedures, and appropriate policies can produce increased opportunities for health promotion among minority, gay, and impoverished populations. These same procedures, such as smoke-free zones, salad bars in school lunchrooms, and easy access to condoms and other contraceptives, can also be used to help all people change.

Decisional Balance

Decisional balance reflects an individual's relative weighing of the pros and cons of changing. Originally, we relied on Janis and Mann's model (1977) of decision making, which included four categories of pros (instrumental gains for self and for others and approval for self and for others) and four categories of cons (instrumental costs to self and to others and disapproval from self and from others). In a long series of studies attempting to produce this structure of eight factors, we always found a much simpler structure—just the pros and cons of changing.

Self-Efficacy

Self-efficacy has two parts.

Confidence, the primary construct in self-efficacy, is the situation-specific confidence people have that they can cope with high-risk situations without relapsing to their unhealthy or high-risk habits. This construct was adapted from Bandura's self-efficacy theory (1977, 1982). (Self-efficacy is discussed in greater detail in Chapter Eight.)

Temptation describes the intensity of urges to engage in a specific habit when in the midst of difficult situations. The three most common types of tempting situations are negative affect or emotional distress, positive social occasions, and cravings.

Critical Assumptions

The Transtheoretical Model concentrates on five stages of change, ten processes of change, the pros and cons of changing, and self-efficacy and temptation. The model is also based on critical assumptions about the nature of behavioral change and about the interventions that can best facilitate such change.

The following set of assumptions drives both TTM research and TTM practice.

1. No single theory can account for all the complexities of behavioral change. Therefore, a more comprehensive model will most likely emerge from an integration across major theories.
2. Behavioral change is a process that unfolds over time through a sequence of stages.
3. Stages are both stable and open to change just as chronic behavioral risk factors are both stable and open to change.

4. Without planned interventions, populations will remain stuck in the early stages. There is no inherent motivation to progress through the stages of intentional change as there seems to be for stages of physical and psychological development.

5. The majority of at-risk populations are not prepared for action and will not be served by traditional action-oriented prevention programs. Health promotion can have much greater impact if it shifts from an action paradigm to a stage paradigm.

6. Specific processes and principles of change need to be applied at specific stages if progress through the stages is to occur. In the stage paradigm, intervention programs must be matched to each individual's stage of change.

7. Chronic behavioral patterns are under some combination of biological, social, and self-control. Stage-matched interventions have been designed primarily to enhance self-control.

Empirical Support: Basic Research

Each of the core constructs we describe here has been subjected to a wide variety of studies across a broad range of behaviors and populations. Only a sampling of these studies can be reviewed here. The review covers in most detail the investigations conducted by researchers at the University of Rhode Island.

Stage Distribution. If interventionists are to match the needs of entire populations, they need to know the stage distributions of specific high-risk behaviors. A series of studies on smoking has assessed smokers in the stages prior to action (see Table 4.2). The results demonstrated that less than 20 percent of smokers are in the preparation stage in most populations (see, for example, Velicer and others, 1995a). Approximately 40 percent of smokers are in the contemplation stage, and another 40 percent are in precontemplation. These results show that action-oriented cessation programs will not match the needs of the vast majority of smokers.

In a sample of 20,000 members of a health maintenance organization (HMO), stage distribution was assessed for fifteen health behaviors (Rossi, 1992b). Although there are variations in the distributions for these high-risk behaviors, the results support a general rule of thumb: 40 percent in precontemplation, 40 percent in contemplation, and 20 percent in preparation.

Pros and Cons Analyzed Across Twelve Behaviors. Across studies of twelve different behaviors (smoking cessation, quitting cocaine, weight control, dietary fat reduction, safer sex, condom use, exercise acquisition, sunscreen use, radon testing, delinquency reduction, mammography screening, and physicians practicing preventive medicine), the two-factor structure was remarkably stable.

TABLE 4.2. DISTRIBUTION OF FOUR SAMPLES OF SMOKERS BY STAGE.

Sample	Precontemplation (percent)	Contemplation (percent)	Preparation (percent)	Sample Size
Random digit dial	42.1	40.3	17.6	4,144
Four U.S. worksites	41.1	38.7	20.1	4,785
California	37.3	46.7	16.0	9,534
Rhode Island high schools	43.8	38.0	18.3	208

Note: These studies assess current smokers; therefore, no respondents are in action or maintenance.

Analysis of Stage Change in Pros and Cons. Stage is not a theory; it is a variable. Over the years, researchers at the University of Rhode Island have studied the stages of change for more than twelve behaviors. In twelve studies focusing on these different health behaviors, the pros of changing were higher than the cons for people in precontemplation (Prochaska and others, 1994a). Likewise, the pros increase between precontemplation and contemplation. There were no systematic differences in the cons between precontemplation and contemplation. But from contemplation to action, across all twelve behaviors, the cons of changing were lower in action than in contemplation. In eleven of the twelve studies, the pros of changing were higher than the cons for people in action.

These basic findings suggest principles for progressing through the stages (Prochaska, 1994b). To progress from precontemplation to contemplation, the pros of changing must increase. To progress from contemplation to action, the cons of changing must decrease. So with people in precontemplation, practitioners would target the pros for intervention and save the cons for people who have progressed to contemplation. Before an individual progresses to action, the pros and cons should cross over, with the pros becoming higher than the cons, as a sign that the person is well prepared for action.

Strong and weak principles of progress. Across these same twelve studies, mathematical relationships were found between the pros and cons of changing and progress across the stages. The Strong Principle is:

$$PC \rightarrow A \cong 1 \text{ SD} \uparrow \text{Pros}$$

Progress from contemplation to action involves approximately one standard deviation increase in the pros of changing. On intelligence tests, a one SD increase would be fifteen points, which is a substantial increase.

The Weak Principle is:

$$PC \rightarrow A \cong .5 \text{ SD} \downarrow \text{Cons}$$

Progress from precontemplation to action involves approximately an 0.5 SD decrease in the cons of changing.

The practical implications of these principles are that the pros of changing must increase twice as much as the cons must decrease. Perhaps twice as much emphasis should be placed on raising the benefits as on reducing the costs or barriers.

Processes of Change Across Behaviors. One assumption of The Transtheoretical Model is that there is a common set of change processes that people apply across a broad range of behaviors. The higher-order structure of the processes (experiential and behavioral) has been replicated across problem behaviors better than specific processes have (Rossi, 1992a). Typically, we have found support for our standard set of ten processes across such behaviors as smoking, choice of diet, using cocaine, exercising, using condoms, and receiving sun exposure. But the structure of the processes across studies has not been as consistent as the structure of the stages and the pros and cons of changing. It is also very possible that people may use fewer change processes with particular behaviors. For an infrequent behavior like a yearly mammogram, for example, fewer processes may be required to progress to long-term maintenance (Rakowski, Dube, and Goldstein, forthcoming; Rakowski and others, forthcoming).

Relationship Between Stages and Processes of Change. One of the earliest empirical integrations was the discovery of systematic relationships between the stage people were in and the processes they were applying. This discovery allowed an integration of processes from theories typically seen as incompatible and in conflict. Table 4.3 presents our current empirical integration (Prochaska, DiClemente, and Norcross, 1992). The integration suggests that in early stages, people apply cognitive, affective, and evaluative processes to progress through the stages. In later stages, people rely more on commitments, conditioning, contingencies, environmental controls, and support for progressing toward termination.

Table 4.3 has important practical implications. To help people progress from precontemplation to contemplation, practitioners need to apply such processes as consciousness raising and dramatic relief. Applying processes like contingency management, counterconditioning, and stimulus control to people in precontemplation represents a theoretical, empirical, and practical mistake. But for people in action, such strategies represent an optimal matching.

Like the structure of the processes, the integration of the processes and stages has not been as consistent as the integration of the stages and pros and cons of changing. Although part of the problem may be the greater complexity of integrating ten processes across five stages, the processes of change need more basic research.

TABLE 4.3. STAGES OF CHANGE IN WHICH CHANGE PROCESSES ARE MOST EMPHASIZED.

	Stages of Change				
	Precontemplation	Contemplation	Preparation	Action	Maintenance
Processes	Consciousness raising Dramatic relief Environmental reevaluation	Self-reevaluation	Self-liberation	Contingency management Helping relationships Counterconditioning Stimulus control	

Application: A Conceptual and Practical Review of Research on Smoking Cessation

Smoking is costly to individual smokers and to society. In the United States, approximately 47,000,000 Americans continue to smoke. Over 400,000 preventable deaths per year are attributable to smoking (U.S. Department of Health and Human Services, 1990). Of the people alive in the world today, 500,000,000 are expected to die from this single behavior, losing approximately five billion years of life to tobacco use (Peto and Lopez, 1990). If researchers and practitioners can make even modest gains in the science and practice of smoking cessation, they can prevent millions of premature deaths and help preserve billions of years of life.

Currently, smoking cessation clinics achieve only modest public health impact. When offered for free by HMOs in the United States, such clinics recruit only about 1 percent of HMO subscribers who smoke. Such behavioral health services simply cannot make much difference if they treat such a small percentage of the problem (Orleans and others, 1988). Likewise, the results of the heart health programs have been disappointing (Luepker and others, 1994; Glasgow and others, 1995; Lando and others, 1995; Schmid, Jeffrey, and Hellerstedt, 1989).

One alternative is to shift from an action paradigm to a stage paradigm, in order to increase reach and interact with a much higher percentage of populations at risk. The stage paradigm has been applied to four of the most important phases of planned interventions, as described in the following sections.

Recruitment

Action-oriented cessation programs often falter in this first phase of intervention and produce low participation rates. Across four different samples, Velicer and others (1995a) found that 20 percent or less of smokers were in the preparation stage. Thus, when action-oriented programs were advertised or announced, less than 20 percent of a population was explicitly or implicitly targeted. The other 80 percent–plus were left on their own (see Table 4.2).

In two home-based programs with approximately five thousand smokers in each study, we reached out either by telephone alone or by personal letters followed by telephone calls, if needed, and recruited smokers to stage-matched interventions. For each of the five stages, the interventions included at least one of the following: self-help manuals; individualized computer feedback reports based on assessments of the pros and cons, processes, and self-efficacy and temptations; and counselor protocols based on the computer reports. Using the two proactive recruitment methods and stage-matched interventions, we were able to recruit 82 percent to 85 percent, respectively (Prochaska, Velicer, Fava, and Laforge, 1996; Prochaska, Velicer, Fava, and Rossi, 1996). Such quantum increases in participation rates provide the potential for practitioners to generate unprecedented impacts with entire populations of smokers.

Population impact equals participation rate times the rate of efficacy or action. Historically, if a health promotion program produced 30 percent efficacy (such as long-term abstinence), it was judged to be better than a program that produced 25 percent abstinence. But a program that generates 30 percent efficacy but only 5 percent participation has an impact of only 1.5 percent (30 percent × 5 percent). A program that produces only 25 percent efficacy but 60 percent participation has an impact of 15 percent—a 1,000 percent greater impact on a high-risk population.

The stage paradigm would shift outcomes from efficacy alone to impact. To achieve such high impact, practitioners need to shift from reactive recruitment, where they advertise or announce their programs and react when people reach them, to proactive recruitments, where they reach out to interact with all potential participants. To optimize public health impact, they need to use proactive protocols to recruit participants to stage-matched programs. But it is not enough to recruit people; they also must be retained.

People with a precontemplation profile should not be treated as if they were ready for action interventions. Relapse prevention strategies are indicated for smokers who are taking action. But those in precontemplation are more likely to need drop-out prevention strategies.

Matching interventions to stage of change is the best strategy to promote retention. In four smoking cessation studies using such matching strategies, we were able to retain smokers in the precontemplation stage at the same high levels as those who started in the preparation stage (Prochaska, 1994a).

Progress

The amount of progress participants make as they follow health promotion programs is directly related to the stage they were in at the start of the interventions. This stage effect is illustrated in Figure 4.1. Smokers initially in precontemplation showed the smallest amount of abstinence over eighteen months and those in preparation progressed the most (Prochaska, DiClemente, and Norcross, 1992). Across sixty-six different predictions of progress, smokers starting in contemplation were about two-thirds more successful than those in precontemplation at six-, twelve-, and eighteen-month follow-ups. Similarly, at the same follow-ups, those in preparation were about two-thirds more successful than those in contemplation (Prochaska, Velicer, Fava, and Laforge, 1996; Prochaska, Velicer, Fava, and Rossi, 1996).

These results can be used clinically. A reasonable goal for each therapeutic intervention with smokers is to help them progress one stage. If over the course of brief therapy, they progress two stages, they will be about 2.66 times more successful at long-term follow-ups (Prochaska and others, 1996a).

Process

To help populations progress through the stages, practitioners need to understand the processes and principles of change. One of the fundamental principles for progress is that different processes of change need to be applied at different stages of change. Classic conditioning processes like counterconditioning, stimulus control, and contingency control can be highly successful for participants taking action but can produce resistance from individuals in precontemplation. With these individuals, more experiential processes, like consciousness raising and dramatic relief, can move them cognitively and affectively and help them shift to contemplation (Prochaska, Norcross, and DiClemente, 1994).

After fifteen years of research, we have identified fourteen variables on which to intervene in order to accelerate progress across the first five stages of change (Prochaska, Norcross, and DiClemente, 1994). At any particular stage, practitioners only need to intervene on a maximum of six variables. To guide individuals at each stage of change, we have developed computer-based expert systems that can deliver individualized and interactive interventions to entire populations

FIGURE 4.1. POINT-PREVALENT ABSTINENCE BY STAGE OF CHANGE.

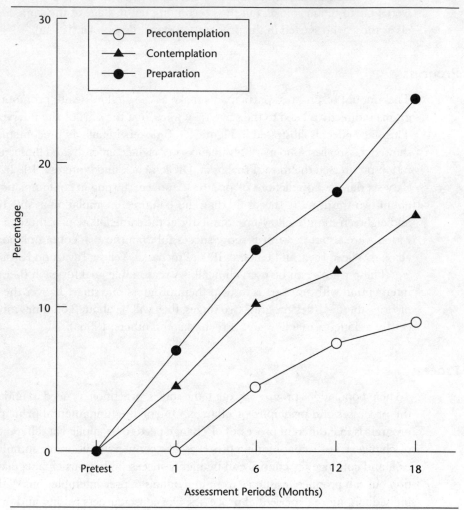

(Velicer and others, 1993). These computer programs can be used alone or in conjunction with counselors.

Outcomes

In the first large-scale clinical trial, we compared four treatments: (1) one of the best home-based action-oriented cessation programs (standardized), (2) stage-matched manuals (individualized), (3) expert system computer reports plus manuals (interactive), and (4) counselors plus expert system computer reports and manuals (personalized). We randomly assigned, by stage, each of 739 smokers to one of the four treatments (Prochaska, DiClemente, Velicer, and Rossi, 1993) (see Figure 4.2).

For the computer-aided treatments, participants completed forty questions by mail or telephone and the responses were entered in central computers. The feedback reports that were generated informed participants about their stage of change, their pros and cons of changing, and their use of change processes appropriate to their stages. At baseline, participants were given positive feedback on what they were doing correctly and guidance on which principles and processes they needed to apply more of in order to progress. In two progress reports delivered over the next six months, participants also received positive feedback on any improvement they made on any of the variables relevant to progressing. Thus, demoralized and defensive smokers could begin progressing without having to quit and without having to work too hard. Smokers in the contemplation stage could begin taking small steps, like delaying their first cigarette in the morning for an extra thirty minutes. They could choose small steps that would increase their self-efficacy and help them become better prepared for quitting.

In the personalized treatment, smokers received four proactive counselor calls over the six-month intervention period. Three of the calls were based on the computer reports. Counselors reported much more difficulty in interacting with participants when there were no progress data.

The two self-help manual treatment groups paralleled each other for twelve months. At eighteen months, the stage-matched manuals moved ahead. This is an example of a delayed-action effect, which is often observed with stage-matched programs specifically and which others have observed with self-help programs generally (Glynn, Anderson, and Schwarz, 1992). It takes time for participants in early stages to progress all the way to action. Therefore, some treatment effects, as measured by action, will be observed only after considerable delay. But it is encouraging to find treatments producing therapeutic effects months and even years after treatment ended.

The computer reports alone and the computer reports plus counselor treatments paralleled each other for twelve months. Then, the effects of the counselor

FIGURE 4.2. COMPARISON OF EFFECTIVENESS OF FOUR TREATMENTS.

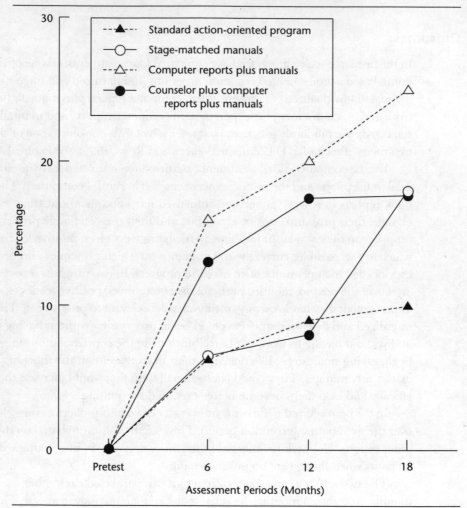

condition flattened out while the computer condition effects continued to increase. We can only speculate as to the delayed differences between these two conditions. Participants in the personalized condition may have become somewhat dependent on the social support and social control of the counselor calling. The last call was after the six-month assessment, and benefits would be observed at twelve months. The group whose counselors were terminated could make no further progress after the twelve months because of the loss of social support and control. The classic pattern in smoking cessation clinics is rapid relapse beginning as soon as the treatment is terminated. Some of this rapid relapse could well be due to the sudden loss of social support or social control provided by the counselors and other participants in the clinic.

A comparison of "reactive" smokers in one study (Prochaska, DiClemente, Velicer, and Rossi, 1993) to "proactive" smokers in another study (Prochaska, Velicer, Fava, and Laforge, 1996) yields remarkable results (see Figure 4.3). Both groups received the same home-based expert system computer reports delivered over a six-month period. Although the reactively recruited subjects were slightly more successful at each follow-up, what is striking is how similar are the results.

If these results continue to be replicated, health promotion programs will be able to produce unprecedented impacts on entire populations. Achieving such unprecedented impacts will require scientific and professional shifts

From an action paradigm to a stage paradigm

From reactive to proactive recruitment

From expecting participants to match program needs to having the programs match participant needs

From clinic-based to community-based behavioral health programs that still apply the field's most powerful individualized and interactive intervention strategies

With these shifts in health promotion strategies, this country may be better prepared to respond to the huge unmet needs and the great opportunities related to the prevention of chronic diseases and premature death.

Application: Development of a Stage-Matched Multiple-Risk Behavior Intervention for Minority Adolescent Females

A stage-matched intervention program for cervical cancer prevention recently developed and implemented in the Philadelphia metropolitan area serves as an

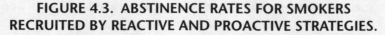

FIGURE 4.3. ABSTINENCE RATES FOR SMOKERS
RECRUITED BY REACTIVE AND PROACTIVE STRATEGIES.

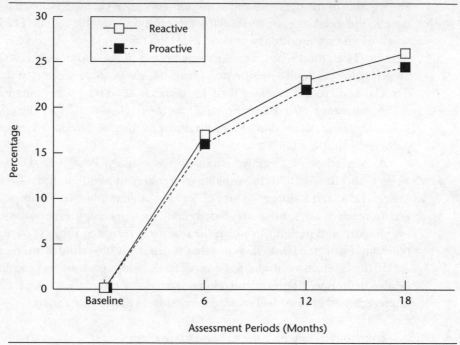

example of TTM intervention development. This collaborative multiple behavioral risk program for cervical cancer prevention implemented in several family planning clinics (Prochaska and others, 1993, 1996b; Redding and others, 1993) and funded by the National Cancer Institute is called Step By Step: Steppin' for Healthier Teens. A randomized trial of a stage-matched intervention package, it aims both to increase condom use and decrease cigarette smoking in sexually active female teens between the ages of fourteen and seventeen, as compared to the members of a usual care, information-only comparison group (Prochaska and others, 1993). The intervention package includes both computer-based, multimedia, individualized expert system feedback, and stage-matched counseling.

One strength of this research is its goal of primary outcomes relating directly to behavior rather than disease. Reducing smoking and increasing condom use have many more health benefits than preventing cervical cancer, including prevention of lung cancer, sexually transmitted diseases (STDs), heart disease, HIV, and unwanted pregnancy. By targeting these two behaviors, interventionists can use one integrated intervention package to reduce risks for multiple disease states.

It remains to be seen whether multiple-risk behavior interventions such as this one will demonstrate an interaction effect that will make them more effective than delivering each behavioral intervention separately.

This intervention package is delivered within family planning health care settings, which may be the sole or primary health care contact for many of these young women. Family planning clinics offer proactive counseling on various reproductive health options. This counseling has better prepared women for their health care visits and helped them make informed choices. It provided the basis for offering the stage-matched counseling proactively to the intervention group. This stage-matched intervention package in family planning clinics can serve as a model in many ways for other interventions in other health care settings: by intervening proactively with clients; by using the data-based Transtheoretical Model; by treating two risky teen behaviors together, as they are practiced and experienced, instead of focusing on only one behavior or one disease risk at a time; and by integrating complementary components (expert system feedback and counseling) into one stage-matched intervention package.

Expert system computer technology offers many advantages. It can systematically address multiple-risk behaviors. It is relevant for participants at all stages of change and not just for those prepared for action. Proactive recruitment and intervention strategies result in higher participation rates. This technology can incorporate visual and audio stimuli, enhancing a program's ability to reach and interact with lower literacy youth. It can be individualized to clients' needs. The technology is novel and can result in higher participation rates. Expert systems can maintain client confidentiality and provide potentially cost-effective expert feedback, without incurring the costs of bringing the experts to the health clinics. They consistently provide the same quality of intervention implementation. Expert systems can be easily updated to add new information, new response modalities, and other health promotion topic areas. Finally, they have the potential for adaptation and dissemination to multiple settings including other health clinics, schools, worksites, and so forth.

This project is tailored to inner-city African American teenage females. However, far less is known about these teens than about adult smokers. Two questions that should be addressed to develop and stage-match interventions are, first, What can current research teach us? and, second, What still needs to be known to help these participants progress toward healthier behaviors?

Research has demonstrated that a stage-matched smoking cessation program that works well with adults (Prochaska and others, 1993, 1996b; Velicer and others, 1993) has also been accepted by high school–aged adolescents, but outcome data are only preliminary (Pallonen and others, 1993, 1994, 1995). TTM constructs do apply equally well to male and female adolescents (Pallonen and others, 1994), and tailoring the expert system intervention to an adolescent audience should increase participants' levels of attention and enjoyment (Pallonen and others, 1995). The TTM's core constructs apply well to condom use and sexual behavior change across many different populations (Bowen and Trotter, 1995; Cabral and others, forthcoming; Evers and Harlow, 1995; Freeman, Cohn, Corby, and Wood, 1991; Galavotti and others, 1995; Grimley, Riley, Bellis, and Prochaska, 1993; Grimley, Prochaska, and Prochaska, 1993; Grimley, Prochaska, Velicer, and Prochaska, 1995; Grimley, DiClemente, Prochaska, and Prochaska, 1995; Grimley and others, forthcoming; Harlow, Quina, and Morokoff, 1992; Holtgrave and others, 1995; Prochaska and others, 1990, 1994a, 1994b; Redding and others, 1993; Redding and Rossi, 1993, forthcoming; Schnell, Galavotti, and O'Reilly, 1993). This descriptive and predictive model already has improved interventionists' understanding of how individuals change from risky to healthful sexual behaviors. For example, from many cross-sectional applications of the pros and cons of safer sex and condom use, it can be seen that increasing the pros of condom use is much more important and more feasible than decreasing the cons.

Validation of constructs was a necessary first step in this population. Pilot data collection and formative research conducted from 1994 to 1995 (Coviello and others, 1995; Redding and others, 1996a, 1996b) both supported the measures used in this intervention and provided reasonable estimates of normative reference points for participants at each stage in this population on these measures. Formative research guided the choice of language to express constructs. Pilot data also replicated relationships between core TTM constructs and stage of change and suggested that looking at alcohol use in addition to sexual behavior and smoking would be useful (Coviello and others, 1995; Redding, Laforge, and Armstrong, 1995). One challenge of conducting multiple-risk behavioral research is the sheer response burden for participants. Collecting data on stages, pros and cons, efficacy, and processes for two behaviors could add up to a prohibitively long survey. Using pilot data, attempts were also made to balance construct validity with response burden, but this forced reduction of the number of items per scale.

The expert system for smoking had different sections for stage of change, pros and cons of smoking, temptation to smoke, and processes of change (Pallonen and others, 1995; Velicer and others, 1993). The pilot data supported the development of a condom use expert system with parallel sections: stage of change, pros and cons of condom use, confidence in condom use, and processes of condom adoption. As in the smoking expert system, within each section, participants at each stage of change received feedback that compared them to others at the same stage who had made progress. This normative feedback is the only type of feedback possible at first contact. After that, ipsative feedback is also possible, comparing current responses to those that the participant gave previously. This makes the exact combination of feedback paragraphs anyone receives highly individualized, especially after the first contact. We believe that the more expert scientific knowledge we can program into our expert systems, the better our outcomes will be.

All intervention materials were designed with the goal of helping people at each stage to progress to the next stage. This breaks down the behavioral change process into fairly discrete, feasible steps for participants. For example, it may be easier for a precontemplater to hear a suggestion to think about something (prodding her or him toward contemplation) than to respond to the current standard intervention in the field, which is to ask the person to move to action in spite of the fact that she or he is clearly not ready yet. Some of a practitioner's more complex decisions include, for example, choosing which processes will be the subject of specific feedback for each stage and which specific subscales of confidence will also be the subject of feedback.

All the decisions and feedback in the expert system are based on statistical or scientific decision making, that is, they are based on data, not on clinical judgment alone. Statistical decision making about behavior outperforms clinical judgment. Now, all of us have the science and technology to build programs with each piece based on the best our current data have to offer.

Conclusion and Future Directions

Research on the TTM is vibrant. Researchers and practitioners around the world continue to extend the stages-of-change concepts to new problems, populations, and settings. Yet, there are many unanswered questions. Although expert system technology may be one of the waves of the future, adequate data sets are needed to develop the decision rules for each TTM variable, and computers are necessary to handle the complexity of stage-matching on these variables (although computers are not essential to generate stage-tailored health promotion materials).

What does research demonstrate regarding the efficacy of stage-tailored interventions? A series of studies across problem areas supports the efficacy of stage-tailored health education materials when compared to action-oriented materials or no treatment (Campbell and others, 1994; Greene and others, 1994; Marcus and others, 1992; Skinner, Strecher, and Hospers, 1994). In contrast, however, for smoking cessation, stage-tailored manuals did not outperform the "gold standard," American Lung Association (ALA) manuals, and the stage-matched expert system group clearly outperformed the action-oriented manuals (Prochaska, DiClemente, Velicer, and Rossi, 1993).

In the most recent smoking cessation studies, the stage-matched expert system intervention was compared to stage-tailored manuals in different groups that received series of one, two, three, or six doses. In this study, stage-matched expert systems clearly outperformed stage-tailored manuals (Prochaska, Velicer, Fava, and Laforge, 1996; Prochaska, Velicer, Fava, and Rossi, 1996; Prochaska and others, 1996a). Furthermore, the stage-tailored intervention group did not outperform the proactive assessment alone control group. Proactive assessment alone does produce some active effect, which may have negated any difference between stage-tailored and assessment alone.

Further research is needed to determine the relative efficacy, impact, and cost effectiveness of stage-matched interactive systems compared to noninteractive stage-tailored programs. Research results to date are encouraging, yet much still needs to be done to advance The Transtheoretical Model. Basic research needs to be done with other theoretical variables, such as perceived risk, subjective norms, and severity of the problem, to determine if such variables relate systematically to the stages and if they predict progress across particular stages. More research is needed on the structure of the processes and stages of change across a broad range of health behaviors. Can measurement be simplified in public health settings? How much tailoring is needed? What modifications are most needed for specific types of behavior, such as fewer processes, perhaps, for infrequent behaviors like annual mammograms? What additional behaviors, such as stress, gambling, depression, and social isolation, could be understood from a stage perspective? Does the model hold only for changing chronic behaviors like smoking or can it be useful with acute conditions like acute depression?

Can the stage model be useful in describing, explaining, and predicting changes beyond the individual level, such as changes in couples, families, organizations, and communities? What happens when two or more people are trying to change together and they are in different stages? Can social policies be made more effective by matching policies to a community's stage of readiness to change? Are there particular types of public health campaigns, such as media campaigns, that can best produce progress in communities in early stages of change?

How do diverse populations respond to stage-matched interventions and to high-tech systems? How might a program best be tailored to meet the needs of diverse populations?

At the individual level much more research needs to be done on the most cost-effective interventions for producing progress through the stages across a variety of health behaviors. What are the minimum interventions needed to accelerate progress at each stage?

The Transtheoretical Model is a dynamic theory of change and it must remain open to modification as more students, scientists, and practitioners apply the stage model to a growing number of theoretical and public health problems.

References

Bandura, A. "Self-Efficacy: Toward a Unifying Theory of Behavior Change." *Psychological Review*, 1977, *84*, 191–215.

Bandura, A. "Self-Efficacy Mechanism in Human Agency." *American Psychologist*, 1982, *37*, 122–147.

Bowen, A. M., and Trotter, R. "HIV Risk in IV Drug Users and Crack Smokers: Predicting Stage of Change for Condom Use." *Journal of Consulting and Clinical Psychology*, 1995, *63*, 238–248.

Cabral, R. J., and others. "Paraprofessional Delivery of a Theory-Based HIV Prevention Counseling Intervention for Women." *Public Health Reports*, forthcoming.

Campbell, M. K., and others. "Improving Dietary Behavior: The Effectiveness of Tailored Messages in Primary Care Settings." *American Journal of Public Health*, 1994, *84*, 783–787.

Coviello, D., and others. "Step by Step: A Cervical Cancer Prevention Project." Paper presented at the annual meeting of the American Public Health Association, San Diego, Oct. 1995.

DiClemente, C. C., and Prochaska, J. O. "Self Change and Therapy Change of Smoking Behavior. A Comparison of Processes of Change in Cessation and Maintenance." *Addictive Behavior*, 1982, *7*, 133–142.

Evers, K. E., and Harlow, L. L. "Longitudinal Prediction of Stage of Condom Use in Women in Psycho-Attitudinal Variables." Paper presented at the 103rd annual convention of the American Psychological Association, New York, Aug. 1995.

Freeman, A., Cohn, D., Corby, N., and Wood, R. "Patterns of Sexual Behavior Change Among Homosexual/Bisexual men: Selected U.S. Sites 1987–1990." *Morbidity and Mortality Weekly Report*, 1991, *40*(46), 792–794.

Galavotti, C., and others. "Validation of Measures of Condom and Other Contraceptive Use Among Women at High Risk for HIV Infection and Transmission: Stage of Change, Decisional Balance, and Self-Efficacy." *Health Psychology*, 1995, *14*, 570–578.

Glanz, K., and others. "Stages of Change in Adopting Healthy Diets: Fat, Fiber, and Correlates of Nutrient Intake." *Health Education Quarterly*, 1994, *21*, 499–519.

Glasgow, R. E., and others. "Take Heart: Results from the Initial Phase of a Work-Site Wellness Program." *American Journal of Public Health*, 1995, *85*(2), 209–216.

Glynn, T. J., Anderson, D. M., and Schwarz, L. "Tobacco Use Reduction Among High Risk Youth: Recommendations of a National Cancer Institute Expert Advisory Panel." *Preventive Medicine*, 1992, *24*, 354–362.

Greene, G. W., and others. "Stages of Change for Reducing Dietary Fat to 30 percent of Energy or Less." *Journal of the American Dietetic Association*, 1994, *94*, 1105–1110.

Grimley, D. M., DiClemente, R. J., Prochaska, J. O., and Prochaska, G. E. "Preventing Adolescent Pregnancy, STDs and HIV: A Promising New Approach." *Family Life Educator*, 1995, *13*, 7–15.

Grimley, D. M., Prochaska, G. E., and Prochaska, J. O. "Condom Use Assertiveness and the Stages of Change with Main and Other Partners." *Journal of Applied BioBehavioral Research*, 1993, *1*, 152–173.

Grimley, D. M., Prochaska, J. O., Velicer, W. F., and Prochaska, G. E. "Contraceptive and Condom Use Adoption and Maintenance: A Stage Paradigm Approach." *Health Education Quarterly*, 1995, *22*, 455–470.

Grimley, D. M., Riley, G. E., Bellis, J. M., and Prochaska, J. O. "Assessing the Stages of Change and Decision-Making for Contraceptive Use for the Prevention of Pregnancy, Sexually Transmitted Diseases, and Acquired Immunodeficiency Syndrome." *Health Education Quarterly,* 1993, *20,* 455–470.

Grimley, D. M., and others. "Cross-Validation of Measures Assessing Decision-Making and Self-Efficacy for Condom Use." *American Journal of Health Behavior, Education, and Promotion,* forthcoming.

Harlow, L. L., Quina, K., and Morokoff, P. *Predicting HIV-Risky Heterosexual Behavior in Women.* NIMH grant no. MH47233, 1992.

Holtgrave, D. R., and others. "An Overview of the Effectiveness and Efficiency of HIV Prevention Programs." *Public Health Reports,* 1995, *110,* 134–146.

Janis, I. L., and Mann, L. *Decision Making: A Psychological Analysis of Conflict, Chance and Commitment.* New York: Free Press, 1977.

Lando, H. A., and others. "Changes in Adult Cigarette Smoking in the Minnesota Heart Health Program." *American Journal of Public Health,* 1995, *85,* 201–208.

Luepker, R. V., and others. "Community Education for Cardiovascular Disease Prevention: Risk Factor Changes in the Minnesota Heart Health Program." *American Journal of Public Health,* 1994, *84,* 1383–1393.

Marcus, B. H., and others. "Using the Stages of Change Model to Increase the Adoption of Physical Activity Among Community Participants." *American Journal of Health Promotion,* 1992, *6,* 424–429.

Orleans, C. T., and others. "Effectiveness of Self-Help Quit Smoking Strategies." Presented at the symposium *Four National Cancer Institute-Funded Self-Help Smoking Cessation Trials: Interim Results and Emerging Patterns* (T. Glynn, chair) at the annual meeting of the Association for the Advancement of Behavior Therapy, New York, Nov. 1988.

Pallonen, U. E., and others. "Applying the Stages of Change and Processes of Change Concepts to Adolescent Smoking Cessation." *Annals of Behavioral Medicine,* 1993, *15* (supp.), 131.

Pallonen, U. E., and others. "A 2-Year Self-Help Smoking Cessation Manual Intervention Among Middle-Aged Finnish Men: An Application of The Transtheoretical Model." *Preventive Medicine,* 1994, *23,* 507–514.

Pallonen, U. E., and others. "Computer-Based Smoking Cessation Interventions Among Adolescents: 12 Month Follow-Up Results." *Annals of Behavioral Medicine* 1995, *17* (supp.), 68.

Peto, R., and Lopez, A. "World-Wide Mortality from Current Smoking Patterns." In B. Durstone and K. Jamrogik (eds.), *The Global War: Proceedings of the Seventh World Conference on Tobacco and Health.* East Perth, Western Australia: Organizing Committee of Seventh World Conference on Tobacco and Health, 1990.

Prochaska, J. O. *Systems of Psychotherapy: A Transtheoretical Analysis.* (2nd ed.) Pacific Grove, Calif.: Brooks-Cole, 1984. (Originally published 1979.)

Prochaska, J. O. "Staging: A Revolution in Health Promotion." Master science lecture at the annual meeting of the Society for Behavioral Medicine, Boston, April 1994a.

Prochaska, J. O. "Strong and Weak Principles for Progressing from Precontemplation to Action Based on Twelve Problem Behaviors." *Health Psychology,* 1994b, *13,* 47–51.

Prochaska, J. O., and DiClemente, C. C. "Stages and Processes of Self-Change of Smoking: Toward an Integrative Model of Change." *Journal of Consulting and Clinical Psychology,* 1983, *51,* 390–395.

Prochaska, J. O., DiClemente, C. C., and Norcross, J. C. "In Search of How People Change: Applications to the Addictive Behaviors." *American Psychologist,* 1992, *47*(9), 1102–1114.

Prochaska, J. O., DiClemente, C. C., Velicer, W. F., and Rossi, J. S. "Standardized, Individualized, Interactive, and Personalized Self-Help Programs for Smoking Cessation." *Health Psychology,* 1993, *12*(5), 399–405.

Prochaska, J. O., Norcross, J. C., and DiClemente, C. C. *Changing for Good.* New York: Morrow, 1994.

Prochaska, J. O., Velicer, W. F., Fava, J., and Laforge, R. "Toward Disease State Management for Smoking: Stage Matched Expert Systems for a Total Managed Care Population of Smokers." Unpublished manuscript, 1996.

Prochaska, J. O., Velicer, W. F., Fava, J., and Rossi, J. "A Stage Matched Expert System Intervention with a Total Population of Smokers." Unpublished manuscript, 1996.

Prochaska, J. O., and others. *Stages of Change, Self Efficacy, and Decisional Balance of Condom Use in a High HIV Risk Sample.* Technical report to the Centers for Disease Control, contract grant #0–4115–002. Kingston, R.I.: Cancer Prevention Research Center, 1990.

Prochaska, J. O., and others. *Changing Teen Behaviors: Cervical Cancer Prevention.* National Cancer Institute grant RO1 CA63745, 1993.

Prochaska, J. O., and others. "Stages of Change and Decisional Balance for Twelve Problem Behaviors." *Health Psychology,* 1994a, *13,* 39–46.

Prochaska, J. O., and others. "The Transtheoretical Model and Human Immunodeficiency Virus Prevention: A Review." *Health Education Quarterly,* 1994b, *4,* 471–486.

Prochaska, J. O., and others. "Stage, Interactive, Dose Response, Counseling and Stimulus Control Computer Effects in a Total Managed Care Population of Smokers." Unpublished manuscript, 1996a.

Prochaska, J. O., and others. "A Stage-Matched Multiple Risk Behavior Program Targeting Urban Teenagers." Unpublished manuscript, 1996b.

Rakowski, W., Dube, C. E., and Goldstein, M. G. "Considerations for Extending The Transtheoretical Model of Behavior Change to Screening Mammography." *Health Education Research,* forthcoming.

Rakowski, W., and others. "Screening Mammography and Constructs from The Transtheoretical Model: Associations Using Two Definitions of the Stages-of-Adoption." *Annals of Behavioral Medicine,* forthcoming.

Redding, C. A., Laforge, R., and Armstrong, K. *Impact of Alcohol Use on Women's Condom Use and Smoking.* Office of Research on Women's Health Administrative Supplement to National Cancer Institute grant RO1 CA63745, 1995.

Redding, C. A., and Rossi, J. S. "The Processes of Safer Sex Adoption." *Annals of Behavioral Medicine,* 1993, *15* (supp.), 106.

Redding, C. A., and Rossi, J. S. "Testing a Model of Situational Self-Efficacy for Safer Sex Among College Students: Stage and Gender-Based Differences." *Psychology & Health,* forthcoming.

Redding, C. A., and others. "The Transtheoretical Model and Cervical Cancer Prevention Among Minority Female Adolescents." In *Proceedings of PsychoOncology V: Psychosocial Factors in Cancer Risk and Survival.* New York: Memorial Sloan-Kettering Cancer Center, 1993.

Redding, C. A., and others. "Pros, Cons, and Efficacy for Condom Use in At-Risk Adolescent Females." Paper presented at the 17th annual meeting of the Society of Behavioral Medicine, Washington, D.C., Mar. 1996a.

Redding, C.A., and others. "Stages and Processes of Condom Use Adoption in At-Risk Female Teens." Paper presented at the 17th annual meeting of the Society of Behavioral Medicine, Washington, D.C., Mar. 1996b.

Rossi, J. S. "Common Processes of Change Across Nine Problem Behaviors." Paper presented at the 100th meeting of the American Psychological Association, Washington, D.C., 1992a.

Rossi, J. S. "Stages of Change for 15 Health Risk Behaviors in an HMO Population." Paper presented at 13th annual meeting of the Society for Behavioral Medicine, New York, 1992b.

Rossi, J. S., Blais, L. M., Redding, C. A., and Weinstock, M. A. "Preventing Skin Cancer Through Behavior Change: Implications for Interventions." *Dermatologic Clinics,* 1995, *13,* 613–622.

Schmid, T. L., Jeffrey, R. W., and Hellerstedt, W. L. "Direct Mail Recruitment to House-Based Smoking and Weight Control Programs: A Comparison of Strengths." *Preventive Medicine,* 1989, *18,* 503–517.

Schnell, D. J., Galavotti, C., and O'Reilly, K. R. "An Evaluation of Sexual Behavior Change Using Statistical and Cognitive Models." *Statistics in Medicine,* 1993, *12,* 219–228.

Skinner, C. S., Strecher, V. J., and Hospers, H. J. "Physician Recommendations for Mammography: Do Tailored Messages Make a Difference?" *American Journal of Public Health,* 1994, *84,* 43–49.

Snow, M. G., Prochaska, J. O., and Rossi, J. S. "Stages of Change for Smoking Cessation Among Former Problem Drinkers: A Cross-Sectional Analysis." *Journal of Substance Abuse,* 1992, *4,* 107–116.

U.S. Department of Health and Human Services. *The Health Benefits of Smoking Cessation: A Report of the Surgeon General.* DHHS publication no. CDC 90–8416. Washington, D.C.: U.S. Government Printing Office, 1990.

Velicer, W. F., and others, "An Expert System Intervention for Smoking Cessation." *Addictive Behaviors,* 1993, *18,* 269–290.

Velicer, W. F., and others. "Distribution of Smokers by Stage in Three Representative Samples." *Preventive Medicine,* 1995a, *24,* 401–411.

Velicer, W. F., and others. "An Empirical Typology of Subjects Within Stages of Change." *Addictive Behaviors,* 1995b, *20,* 299–230.

CHAPTER FIVE

THE THEORY OF REASONED ACTION AND THE THEORY OF PLANNED BEHAVIOR

Daniel E. Montaño
Danuta Kasprzyk
Stephen H. Taplin

This chapter presents the Theory of Reasoned Action and the Theory of Planned Behavior. Both theories focus on theoretical constructs concerned with individual motivational factors as determinants of the likelihood of performing a specific behavior. Theory constructs are shown graphically in Figures 5.1 and 5.2 and are defined in Table 5.1. The theory of reasoned action (TRA) includes measures of attitude and social normative perceptions that determine behavioral intention. Behavioral intention in turn affects behavior. The theory of planned behavior (TPB) is an extension of the TRA rather than an independent theory. The TPB adds a construct concerned with perceived control over performance of the behavior. Both theories assume that all other factors including demographics and environment operate through the model constructs and do not independently contribute to explaining the likelihood of a person's performing a behavior. The TRA has been used extensively in recent years to understand health behaviors and to develop interventions (Jemmott, Jemmott, and Fong, 1992; Montaño, 1986; Montaño and Taplin, 1991; Lierman, Young, Kasprzyk, and Benoliel, 1990; Gillmore, Morrison, Lowery, and Baker, 1994). The TPB is a more recent evolution of the TRA and has not been as extensively tested or applied to explain health behaviors.

The Theory of Reasoned Action, first introduced in 1967, is concerned with the relations between beliefs (behavioral and normative), attitudes, intentions, and behavior. Fishbein (1967) developed the TRA through an effort to understand the relationship between attitudes and behavior. Many previous studies of this relationship found relatively low correspondence between attitudes and behavior, and some theorists moved toward eliminating attitude as a factor underlying behavior (Fishbein, 1993; see, for example, Abelson, 1972; Wicker, 1969). In his work that led to development of the TRA, Fishbein distinguished between attitude toward an object and attitude toward a behavior with respect to that object. A health-related example of this is the *object* of breast cancer versus the *behavior* of seeking mammography screening for breast cancer. Most prior studies attempted to test the correspondence between attitude toward an object and behavior with respect to the object. Fishbein found that attitude toward a behavior is a much better predictor of that behavior than attitude toward the target at which the behavior is directed (Fishbein and Ajzen, 1975). Thus, in the breast cancer screening example, attitude toward breast cancer is expected to be a poor predictor while attitude toward seeking mammography screening is expected to be a good predictor of mammography screening behavior.

Fishbein draws clear distinctions in the definitions and measurement of beliefs, attitudes, intentions, and behavior. He argues that it is critical to have a high degree of correspondence between measures of attitude, intention, and behavior in terms of action, target, context, and time. Operationalization of the TRA constructs was developed from a long history of attitude measurement theory, rooted in the concept that an attitude (toward an object or an action) is determined by expectations or beliefs concerning the attributes of the object or action and by evaluations of those attributes. This expectancy value conceptualization has been applied extensively in psychology in many areas, including learning theory, attitude theory, and decision making (for example, see Rotter, 1954; Rosenberg, 1956; Edwards, 1954).

The main constructs of the Theory of Reasoned Action and the Theory of Planned Behavior are described in more detail in the remainder of this chapter along with a description of measurement of the constructs and empirical support for the theories. We also describe the similarity between these theories' key constructs and constructs from other behavioral theories. Too much attention has been paid to differences between theories while their similarities have often been ignored (Weinstein, 1993). Finally, we describe two applications of the theories to understand health behaviors.

The Theory of Reasoned Action

The Theory of Reasoned Action (Figure 5.1), asserts that the most important determinant of *behavior* is a person's *behavioral intention*. The direct determinants of an individual's behavioral intention are his *attitude* toward performing the behavior and his *subjective norm* associated with the behavior. Attitude is determined by the individual's beliefs about outcomes or attributes of performing the behavior (*behavioral beliefs*), weighted by evaluations of those outcomes or attributes. Thus, a person who holds strong beliefs that mostly positively valued outcomes will result from performing a behavior will have a positive attitude toward that behavior. Conversely, a person who holds strong beliefs that negatively valued outcomes will result from a behavior will have a negative attitude toward that behavior. Similarly, a person's subjective norm is determined by his *normative beliefs*—whether important referent individuals approve or disapprove of performing the behavior, weighted by his motivation to comply with those referents. Thus, a person who believes that certain referents think he should perform a behavior, and who is motivated to meet the expectations of those referents, will hold a positive subjective norm. Conversely, a person who believes certain referents think he should not perform the behavior will have a negative subjective norm, and a person who is less motivated to comply with the referents will have a relatively neutral subjective norm.

FIGURE 5.1. THEORY OF REASONED ACTION.

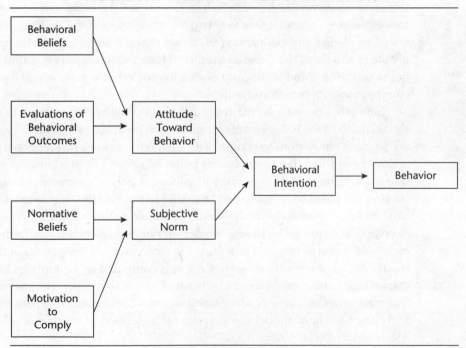

Source: Based on Ajzen and Fishbein, 1980, p. 8.

The TRA assumes a causal chain: behavioral beliefs and normative beliefs are linked to behavioral intention and behavior via attitude and subjective norm. The measurement of model components and causal relationships among the components are clearly specified (Ajzen and Fishbein, 1980). A person's behavioral beliefs about the likelihood that performance of the behavior will result in certain outcomes are measured on bipolar "unlikely"-"likely" or "disagree"-"agree" scales. Evaluations of each outcome are measured on bipolar "good"-"bad" scales. For example, one perceived outcome of "my quitting smoking" might be that this "will cause me to gain weight." A person's behavioral belief about this outcome is measured by having her rate the likelihood that "my quitting smoking will cause me to gain weight." The person's evaluation of this outcome is measured when she rates the degree to which "my gaining weight" is good or bad. These behavioral belief and evaluation ratings are usually scored from −3 to +3, thus capturing the psychology of double negatives, that is, a belief that a behavior will *not* result in a negative outcome contributes positively to the person's attitude.

A person's attitude toward performing the behavior is computed by first multiplying her behavioral belief concerning each outcome by her corresponding outcome evaluation ratings and then summing these product scores across all outcomes of the behavior. In the previous example, a person may believe that quitting smoking is very unlikely to result in gaining weight (belief scored as −3) and may evaluate gaining weight as very bad (evaluation scored as −3). Thus, the product of this belief and evaluation (+9) shows that the belief and evaluation contribute positively to this person's attitude. However, this is only one outcome of quitting smoking, and beliefs and evaluations of other outcomes will enter into computation of a person's attitude.

Similarly, a person's normative beliefs about whether each referent thinks she should perform the behavior are measured on bipolar scales scored −3 to +3, and the person's motivations to comply with each referent are measured on unipolar scales scored 1 to 7. For example, one potential referent for the behavior of quitting smoking might be the person's physician. A person's normative belief concerning her physician is measured by asking her to rate the degree to which she believes her physician thinks she should or should not quit smoking. Motivation to comply is measured by having the person rate her agreement versus disagreement with the statement: "Generally, I want to do what my physician thinks I should do." The person's subjective norm is computed by multiplying her normative belief about each referent by her motivation to comply with that referent and then summing these product scores across all referents. (The measurement and computation of model components are described in much more detail by Ajzen and Fishbein, 1980.)

A prospective study design is recommended to discern the relationships between the constructs, with attitude, subjective norm, and intention measured at one time point and behavior measured during a following interval. A cross-sectional study may provide poor prediction and understanding of previous behavior if study respondents' motivations change subsequent to the behavior. Multiple regression is usually used to test the relationships in the TRA, assessing the effect of attitude and subjective norm in explaining intention at that time and in predicting subsequent behavior. The relative weights of attitude and subjective norm depend upon the behavior and the population under investigation. Some behaviors are entirely under attitudinal control, and others are under normative control. The same behavior has been found to be under attitudinal control in one population but under normative control in another population (Fishbein, 1990). The relative weights are determined empirically for the particular behavior and population under investigation, and this information suggests whether attitude or subjective norm is the best focus for behavioral change efforts. Correlation and analysis of variance can be used to determine which specific behavioral beliefs or normative beliefs are most strongly associated with intention and behavior, thus providing empirically identified targets for intervention efforts.

The name of this theory has sometimes led to the misperception that it is a model of *rational behavior*. This is far from correct. The assumption of the TRA is that individuals are *rational actors*. That is, all individuals process information and are motivated to act on it. The TRA assumes that there are underlying reasons that determine an individual's motivation to perform a behavior. These reasons, made up of a person's behavioral and normative beliefs, determine that person's attitude and subjective norm, regardless of whether those beliefs are rational, logical, or correct by some objective standard. The strength of the TRA is that it provides a framework for discerning those underlying reasons, a means to decipher actions by identifying, measuring, and combining beliefs that are relevant to individuals or groups, allowing practitioners and researchers to understand the specific reasons of specific individuals or groups, the reasons that motivate the behavior of interest. The TRA does not specify the particular beliefs about behavioral outcomes or normative referents that should be measured. The relevant behavioral outcomes and referents will be different for different behaviors. Likewise, they may be different for the same behavior among different populations. For example, the outcomes affecting mammography use appear to be quite different for low-income and for middle-income women (Thompson and others, forthcoming).

A critical step in applying the TRA involves conducting open-ended elicitation interviews to identify the relevant behavioral outcomes and referents for each particular behavior and population under investigation. Elicitation interviews are conducted with a sample of at least fifteen to twenty individuals from the population under investigation, about half of whom have performed or intend to perform the behavior under investigation and half of whom have not performed the behavior. These individuals are asked to provide two types of information. First, they are asked to describe any positive or negative reasons for performing the behavior, and second, they are asked to describe any individuals or groups to whom they might listen who are either in favor of or opposed to their performing the behavior. The elicitation interviews are then content analyzed to identify the relevant attributes or outcomes of the behavior and the relevant social referents. This information then provides the questionnaire content, and the TRA measures are developed. A poorly conducted elicitation phase will likely result in inadequate identification of the underlying outcomes and referents, resulting in poor TRA measures and poor behavioral prediction and thus yielding inadequate information for the development of effective interventions.

The TRA builds a framework for identifying key behavioral and normative beliefs affecting behavior. Interventions can then be designed to target and change these beliefs or the value placed upon them, thereby affecting attitude and subjective norm and leading to a change in intention and behavior. The TRA has been used successfully to predict and explain a wide range of health behaviors including smoking, drinking, contraceptive use, clinical breast exam and mammography use, flu vaccine use, exercising, seat belt use, and safety helmet use (Fishbein, 1993). The primary purpose of the TRA is to explain *behavioral intention* regardless of whether the behavior is under volitional control. However, the success of the theory in explaining *actual behavior* is dependent upon the degree to which the behavior is under volitional control (that is, occurring in situations where individuals can exercise a large degree of control over the behavior). Under conditions of high volitional control, motivation as measured by intention and its attitudinal and normative determinants is expected to be the main determinant of behavior. However, it is not clear that the TRA components are sufficient for predicting behaviors in which volitional control is reduced. For example, a person who has high motivation to perform a behavior may not actually perform that behavior due to intervening environmental conditions. Thus, Ajzen and colleagues developed the Theory of Planned Behavior (TPB) to predict behaviors over which people have incomplete volitional control. (Table 5.1 summarizes the key concepts just discussed.)

The Theory of Planned Behavior

The Theory of Planned Behavior (TPB) is an extension of the TRA and is summarized in Figure 5.2. Ajzen and colleagues (Ajzen, 1991; Ajzen and Driver, 1991;

TABLE 5.1. TRA AND TPB CONSTRUCTS AND DEFINITIONS.

Concept	Definition	Measure
Behavioral intention	Perceived likelihood of performing the behavior	Bipolar unlikely-likely scale; scored −3 to +3
Attitude		
Behavioral belief	Belief that behavioral performance is associated with certain attributes or outcomes	Bipolar unlikely-likely scale; scored −3 to +3
Evaluation	Value attached to a behavioral outcome or attribute	Bipolar bad-good scale; scored −3 to +3
Subjective norm		
Normative belief	Belief about whether each referent approves or disapproves of the behavior	Bipolar disagree-agree scale; scored −3 to +3
Motivation to comply	Motivation to do what each referent thinks	Unipolar unlikely-likely scale; scored 1 to 7
Perceived behavioral control		
Control belief	Perceived likelihood of occurrence of each facilitating or constraining condition	Unlikely-likely scale; scored −3 to +3 or 1 to 7
Perceived power	Perceived effect of each condition in making behavioral performance difficult or easy	Bipolar difficult-easy scale; scored −3 to +3

Ajzen and Madden, 1986) added *perceived behavioral control* to the TRA in an effort to account for factors outside the individual's control that may affect his intention and behavior. This extension was based in part on the idea that behavioral performance is determined jointly by motivation (intention) and ability (behavioral control). Ajzen argues that a person will expend more effort to perform a behavior when his perception of behavioral control is high. A person's perception of control over behavioral performance, together with intention, is expected to have a direct effect on behavior, particularly when his perceived control is an accurate assessment of actual control over the behavior and when volitional control is not high. The effect of perceived control declines and intention is a sufficient behavioral predictor in situations in which volitional control over the behavior is high (Madden, Ellen, and Ajzen, 1992).

Additionally, the theory postulates that perceived control is an independent determinant of behavioral intention along with attitude toward the behavior and subjective norm. Holding attitude and subjective norm constant, a person's perception

FIGURE 5.2. THEORY OF PLANNED BEHAVIOR.

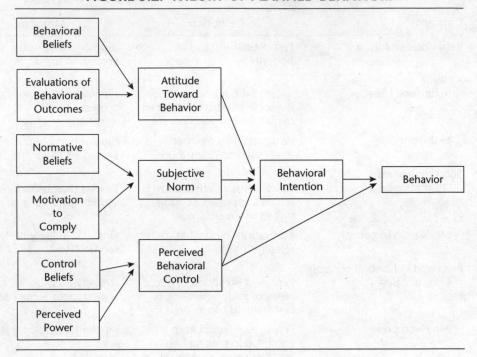

of the ease or difficulty of behavioral performance will affect his behavioral intention. The relative weights of these three factors in determining intention are expected to vary for different behaviors and populations.

According to the TPB, perceived control is determined by *control beliefs* concerning the presence or absence of resources for and impediments to behavioral performance, weighted by the *perceived power* or impact of each resource and impediment to facilitate or inhibit the behavior. Thus, a person who holds strong control beliefs about the existence of factors that facilitate the behavior will have high perceived control over the behavior. Conversely, a person who holds strong control beliefs about the existence of factors that impede the behavior will have low perceived control over the behavior. Few studies have operationalized perceived control using the underlying measures of control beliefs and perceived power.

As in the TRA, the particular resources and impediments that are to be measured are not specified by the theory but are identified through elicitation interviews for the particular population and behavior under investigation. Once these factors are identified, a person's control beliefs and perceived power regarding each factor are measured. Although Ajzen has not completely specified how control beliefs are to be measured, applications of the TPB suggest that control beliefs regarding each factor should be measured on a bipolar likelihood-of-occurrence scale scored −3 to +3. Perceived power of each factor is measured on a bipolar "easy"-"difficult" scale (Terry, Gallois, and McCamish, 1993; Ajzen, 1991). For example, elicitation interviews might identify "restaurant smoking policies" as a factor that affects a person's perceived behavioral control over quitting smoking. A person's control belief regarding this factor is measured by having him rate his likelihood of encountering a restaurant smoking policy, and perceived power is measured by having him rate his perception of the effect of restaurant smoking policies in making it either easier or more difficult to quit smoking. These measures are obtained for all factors identified as facilitating or impeding the behavior. The person's perceived behavioral control is then computed by multiplying each control belief by the corresponding perceived power (impact) rating, and then summing these product scores across all control factors (Ajzen and Driver, 1991).

Ajzen's construct of perceived behavioral control is very similar to Bandura's construct of self-efficacy (1991), an individual's judgment of how well he can perform a behavior under various inhibiting conditions. However, operationalization of the constructs is somewhat different in TPB.

Perceived control is also very similar to Triandis's concept (1980) of *facilitating conditions*, which is concerned with the characteristics of an individual (for example, knowledge or ability) or of the environment that make it easier or more difficult to perform the behavior, independent of an individual's behavioral intention. Facilitating conditions are considered to moderate the effect of intention on behavior. However, Triandis has not described methods for measuring facilitating conditions as has been done for perceived control. Each of these theorists is describing different dimensions of the same construct, one concerned with the factors that influence whether intention is translated into behavior. Both Triandis and Ajzen view this construct as moderating the effect of intention on behavior. Intention will have a greater effect on behavioral performance if perceived behavioral control is high, and perceived behavioral control will have a greater effect on performance if intention is high. However, this interaction hypothesis has received very little empirical support (Ajzen, 1991).

Relatively few studies have used TPB to examine health behaviors. Of those few, most have looked at exercise behavior (Blue, 1995). Applications of TPB generally have found support for perceived control as a direct predictor of both intention and behavior (Ajzen, 1991). However, most of these studies have used a single overall measure of perceived control rather than computing perceived control from measures of control beliefs and perceived power concerning specific facilitators and constraints. A couple of studies have measured control beliefs and found them to be important predictors of behavior (Ajzen and Driver, 1991). Clearly, if perceived behavioral control is an important determinant of intention or behavior, knowledge of the effects of control beliefs on each facilitator or constraint would be useful when developing interventions. Such findings can designate a focus, helping practitioners target those specific environmental factors where control beliefs are most strongly associated with intention or behavior.

In this chapter, we provide two examples of research applying the models. The first study primarily focused on the TRA but also examined facilitating conditions (similar to perceived control in the TPB). The second study measured perceived behavioral control as described by Ajzen (1991). These examples describe the phases in application of the models, including the critical elicitation phase, descriptions of model component measurement, and descriptions of analyses to predict behavior.

Application: Prediction of Mammography Use

Mammography use in the early 1980s appeared disappointingly low despite the long history of evidence that it afforded a benefit (Howard, 1987). Evidence suggested that fewer than 15 to 20 percent of women had ever had mammograms at that time (Fink, Shapiro, and Lewison, 1986). Work had begun in the United Kingdom and the United States to explain why use was low, but evidence was sparse and largely based on cross-sectional retrospective surveys that were descriptive, generally documenting demographic differences in usage rates (Reeder, Berkanovic, and Marcus, 1980; Maclean, Sinfield, Klein, and Harnden, 1984; Lane and Fine, 1983; French and others, 1982). These descriptive studies suggested that younger married women from higher sociodemographic groups were more likely to get mammograms (Reeder, Berkanovic, and Marcus, 1980; Hobbs, Smith, George, and Sellwood, 1980).

Calnan's prospective study (1984) based on the Health Belief Model was an exception to this collection of cross-sectional surveys. He concluded that some components of the Health Belief Model could discriminate among women who did and did not get mammograms but that the model explained a relatively modest proportion of the variance. The variables that contributed to the discriminant model included health motivation (that is, use of a dentist, prior cervical cancer screening, and an index of personal health behavior) and the value of illness threat reduction (perceived vulnerability, concern about breast cancer, and perceived costs and benefits).

We concluded that there was a need to explore alternative behavioral models to explain mammography use rates, with an emphasis on identification of factors that would lend themselves to health education efforts to increase those rates. Clearly, little could be done to influence an individual's demographic characteristics. At the same time, developing a health education approach based upon an incomplete understanding of the factors that affect a woman's mammogram-seeking behavior might have unintended consequences. For example, there is some evidence that increasing women's sense of susceptibility to breast cancer might result in levels of fear that discourage getting mammograms (Leventhal, 1989; Janis and Mann, 1977; Weinstein, 1987). These concerns led to the study described here, in which we tried to ascertain the factors associated with mammography use, especially focusing on those that could be influenced through subsequent health education interventions.

Methods

During the mid- to late 1980s, we worked with colleagues at Group Health Cooperative of Puget Sound (GHC) to conduct a prospective study and develop intervention trials. GHC is a predominantly staff model health maintenance organization (HMO) in the Northwest, established in 1946 and governed by a consumer board. The HMO has an active breast cancer screening program that mails letters prompting women to schedule mammograms when they are due for screening (Thompson, Taplin, Carter, and Schnitzer, 1989). The program involves more than 50,000 women ages forty and above.

We used the Theory of Reasoned Action as the framework for our first study (Montaño and Taplin, 1991). An important feature of the study was that participants had completed a prior breast cancer risk factor questionnaire. Response to this risk factor questionnaire was high (85 percent), and the information allowed stratification of the sample by risk levels (Taplin, Anderman, and Grothaus, 1989). Questionnaires based on the TRA were mailed to women within two weeks after they received a letter prompting them to schedule a screening mammogram. From GHC's automated records, we then determined whether women scheduled a mammogram within six months of receiving their letter. The prospective design allowed us to test the associations between measured variables and subsequent participation in the mammography program (Montaño and Taplin, 1991; Taplin and Montaño, 1993).

A critical step in applying the TRA was conducting elicitation interviews with women who were GHC enrollees in order to identify the content of each of the TRA constructs to be measured. Semistructured open-ended elicitation interviews were conducted with twenty-two women who previously had been invited by GHC to obtain a mammogram, eight of whom had not scheduled to get one. These women were asked to describe positive and negative outcomes or attributes associated with having a mammogram, people or groups they would listen to about getting a mammogram, factors that made it easy or difficult to get a mammogram, and their feelings about the idea of getting a mammogram. Content analysis of these elicitation interviews identified behavioral outcomes and normative referents, and this information was used to develop TRA measures of attitude and subjective norm. The content analysis also revealed that women mentioned environmental factors that make it easier or more difficult to get a mammogram, so these were used to develop measures of a facilitating conditions construct, as theorized by Triandis (1980). Women also described emotional reactions to the idea of getting a mammogram, and this information was used to develop a measure of affect, described by Triandis as being independent of the belief-based measure of attitude. Final construct scores were based on sets of items that showed high internal consistency (Cronbach's alpha > .65).

Model component measures and computation were as follows:

Behavior. Mammography participation was obtained from medical records during the six months after each woman's invitation to obtain a mammogram.

Intention. Intention to obtain a mammogram was measured on a 7-point bipolar scale with endpoints "extremely unlikely" and "extremely likely."

Attitude. Eight outcomes or attributes of mammography were identified in the content analysis (see Table 5.4 later in this chapter), and behavioral belief and evaluation measures were developed for each. Behavioral beliefs were measured for each behavioral outcome using 7-point scales with endpoints "extremely unlikely" and "extremely likely." These measures included items such as, "My having a mammogram this year would involve physical discomfort." Evaluations of each behavioral outcome were rated on 7-point bipolar scales with endpoints "extremely bad" and "extremely good." Evaluation ratings were coded −3 to +3, and belief ratings were coded 1 to 7. There is some support for this unipolar scoring of beliefs to measure probability. However, more recent analyses indicate that bipolar scoring (−3 to +3) for both belief and evaluation measures provides optimal scaling (Ajzen, 1991). Attitude scores were computed by multiplying each outcome belief and corresponding evaluation, and summing these products. Internal consistency of this attitude scale was Cronbach's alpha = .79.

Subjective norm. Eight sources of influence (referents) were identified from the elicitation interviews: physician, husband, women friends, daughters, sisters, nurse, prominent women, and GHC. Participants' normative beliefs about whether each source of influence thought the participant should get a mammogram were made on 7-point bipolar scales with endpoints "extremely unlikely" and "extremely likely," coded −3 to +3. Ratings of their motivation to comply with each source of influence were made on 7-point scales with endpoints "disagree" and "agree," coded 1 to 7. Subjective norm scores were calculated for each study participant by computing the mean of her normative belief times motivation to comply products. A mean was used because several influence sources were not applicable to all participants. The internal consistency of this scale was Cronbach's alpha = .91.

Affect. Four semantic differential items were used to measure affect associated with getting a mammogram. These were 7-point bipolar scales with opposite adjective pairs at each end representing affective reactions to the idea of getting a mammogram: "good"-"bad," "beneficial"-"harmful," "pleasant"-"unpleasant," "frightening"-"reassuring." These were summed to provide a measure of affect for each study participant. The internal consistency of the scale was Cronbach's alpha = .67.

Facilitating conditions. Facilitating conditions were measured by having participants rate the degree to which three environmental factors (schedule, time of year, and transportation) made it easy or difficult to get a mammogram. These ratings were made on 7-point scales with endpoints "easy" and "difficult." These items were summed to compute a facilitating condition score for each study participant. Internal consistency was Cronbach's alpha = .68.

Other measures. The questionnaire also included measures of demographic characteristics, health-related behaviors, and items measuring the Health Belief Model components of susceptibility, severity, and efficacy.

Analysis

Analysis of the data from this study involved model testing and conducting an exploration of the effect of behavioral beliefs and normative beliefs reported by women. To test the model, the analysis proceeded in three steps: (1) testing the correlations between model constructs (attitude, subjective norm, behavioral intention, affect, and facilitating conditions); (2) using multiple regression to test the model's prediction of mammography behavior; and (3) evaluating the contribution of other variables assessed (that is, demographic characteristics and other preventive health behaviors—for example, from the Health Belief Model) as compared to the TRA model constructs in the prediction of mammography behavior. We next assessed the effect of behavioral beliefs and normative beliefs on mammography participation. Finally, we tested whether the effects of model constructs and behavioral beliefs were different for older and younger women (Taplin and Montaño, 1993).

Results

Seventy-two percent of the study sample (683 out of 939) returned the study survey, and participation in mammography screening was 52 percent. Attitude, subjective norm, affect, and facilitating conditions each correlated significantly with behavioral intention and behavior. Results from regression analyses to test the model in explaining intention and behavior are presented in Table 5.2. The TRA components (attitude and subjective norm) were entered first, followed by the addition of affect for predicting intention, and both affect and facilitating conditions for predicting behavior. The analysis demonstrates that the TRA model constructs predicted behavior and that the addition of the constructs of affect and facilitating conditions significantly improved the explanatory power of the basic model. Although subjective norm did not have a significant weight in the multivariate model's predicting behavior in two of the prediction equations due to multicollinearity with other model constructs, it was correlated significantly with intention and behavior. Within measures of subjective norm, physician had the strongest influence. A surprising finding was that facilitating conditions had the strongest weight in the model.

The improvement of the model's prediction of behavior was also tested using hierarchical stepwise regression, by entering demographic and Health Belief Model measures after TRA measures. As shown in Table 5.3, the expanded TRA constructs accounted for most of the variance explained, although education, age, and marital status did improve the model's explanatory power. Health Belief Model components, women's beliefs about how much breast cancer would affect their lives (severity), and women's susceptibility to breast cancer had very low correlations with behavior and did not improve the multiple correlation after the TRA constructs were entered into the model.

When specific beliefs about mammography were examined, it was not surprising to see that women who got mammograms compared to those who did not had higher attitude scores, indicating a more positive attitude toward getting a mammogram. Table 5.4 illustrates that all eight behavioral beliefs used to compute

TABLE 5.2. MODEL PREDICTIONS OF MAMMOGRAPHY INTENTION AND BEHAVIOR.

	R
Intention = 0.34 A_{act} + 0.27 SN	0.52
Intention = 0.18 A_{act} + 0.12 SN + 0.43 AF	0.62
Behavior = 0.27 A_{act} + 0.12 SN	0.34
Behavior = 0.19 A_{act} + 0.06 SN[a] + 0.20 AF	0.38
Behavior = 0.16 A_{act} − 0.01 SN[a] + 0.15 AF + 0.27 F	0.45

Note: A_{act} = attitude; SN = subjective norm; AF = affect; F = facilitating conditions. All beta weights significant at $p < 0.01$, except [a] = not significant.

Source: Adapted from Montaño and Taplin, 1991, p. 737.

TABLE 5.3. HIERARCHICAL STEPWISE REGRESSION TESTING THE TRA AND OTHER VARIABLE PREDICTION OF MAMMOGRAPHY USE.

	R^2	R^2 Change	Significance
Expanded TRA measures			
Attitude	0.10	0.10	0.01
Facilitating conditions	0.17	0.07	0.01
Subjective norm	0.17	0.002	n.s.
Affect	0.19	0.02	0.01
Other variables entering stepwise			
Education	0.23	0.04	0.01
Age dummy (60–75 vs. remainder)	0.24	0.01	0.01
Marital status dummy (never married vs. remainder)	0.26	0.01	0.01
Variables not entering			
Seat belt use	—	—	—
Number pap smears	—	—	—
Exercise	—	—	—
Income	—	—	—
Susceptibility	—	—	—
Severity	—	—	—
Efficacy	—	—	—
Risk status (high vs. moderate or borderline)	—	—	—

Source: Adapted from Montaño and Taplin, 1991, p. 738.

attitude were significantly associated with mammography use, suggesting that each belief could be targeted with intervention efforts to change women's attitudes toward getting a mammogram. A comparison of these associations by age found that the TRA model explained a larger proportion of the variance among women aged sixty-five and older compared to women aged forty to sixty-four ($R = 0.57$ versus $R = 0.40$, respectively). Additionally, the correlations between all eight beliefs and behavior were higher for older women (sixty-five and older) than for younger women (forty to sixty-four). This suggests that interventions targeting these behavioral beliefs may be more effective among older than younger women. It may also suggest that more needs to be done to understand the beliefs of women less than sixty-five years of age.

Based in part on this study, two interventions targeting women were developed, both using a randomized trial study design. The first intervention, conducted in the late 1980s, was designed using a simple low-cost approach with methods easily implemented in GHC's screening program (Taplin and others, 1994). The above results demonstrated that subjective norm was significantly correlated with women's mammography intentions and behavior. Normative perceptions concerning the

TABLE 5.4. MEAN ATTITUDE SCORES (BELIEF X VALUE) FOR EIGHT BEHAVIORAL BELIEFS AMONG MAMMOGRAPHY PARTICIPANTS AND NONPARTICIPANTS.

Behavioral Belief	Women Obtaining a Mammogram	Women Not Obtaining a Mammogram	t Test
1. Test for breast cancer when no symptoms exist	14.33	8.96	7.61[a]
2. Detects breast cancer I cannot find myself	18.61	14.54	6.18[a]
3. Is inconvenient	5.86	3.55	3.50[a]
4. Is unfamiliar	7.27	4.82	3.65[a]
5. Can detect a breast cancer my MD cannot find	18.04	14.25	5.67[a]
6. Exposes me to excessive radiation	2.69	0.15	4.44[a]
7. Involves physical discomfort	6.00	3.48	4.59[a]
8. Detects breast cancer in early stage	18.96	16.63	4.47[a]

Note: Difference in scores is significant: $p < 0.01$.

Source: Adapted from Taplin and Montaño, 1993, p. 18.

woman's physician and GHC were significant. Thus, physician normative influence was targeted by the intervention because we felt it might be modifiable through simple communications from GHC. Because the GHC mammography program uses a centralized correspondence system, we hypothesized that a personalized letter signed by the woman's physician, as compared to the usual practice of correspondence from the screening program, might increase physician normative influence and thereby increase women's likelihood of getting a mammogram. We also decided to test the effect of a reminder postcard sent subsequent to the initial mammography invitation. This low-cost intervention, found to be effective with other behaviors (Larson and others, 1982), might act as a facilitating factor. In fact, reminder postcards nearly doubled a woman's odds of getting a mammogram, but having the correspondence signed by the woman's physician did not add to the impact.

The lack of an effect for the physician's signature may have been due to the success of the usual screening program correspondence in convincing women that their provider supported mammography screening. We did not measure TRA constructs, so it is not clear whether the reminder postcard worked as a facilitating condition or simply reinforced the normative belief concerning GHC providers. These post hoc explanations cannot be tested because the relevant measures were not obtained after the interventions.

In order to improve the intervention, we developed a second intervention trial, which built directly on the results of the prospective study. This randomized trial was designed to target beliefs and affect as well as social norm and facilitating factors. Our earlier work found significant effects of facilitating conditions, subjective norm, affect, and attitude in determining intention and mammography participation. The current intervention is testing whether motivational telephone counseling will increase the use of mammography beyond that achieved by reminders alone. In this trial, we are comparing the motivational interview against a simple reminder telephone call or postcard. The motivational call first identifies a woman's concerns through open-ended questions, then tailors the discussion to respond to affect, beliefs, values, and facilitating conditions. The callers respond primarily to the concerns expressed, but they can encourage expression by modeling other women's concerns. For example, the caller might say, "Some women say that the thought of a mammogram is frightening." We believe that affect is a factor that lends itself to influence during the personalized interactive conversation afforded by a telephone call.

Discussion and Implications

The application of the Theory of Reasoned Action to the problem of how to increase mammography participation helped organize the basic research and influenced the development of interventions now being implemented in GHC's breast cancer screening program. The TRA served to increase our understanding of the factors that influence women's mammography-seeking behavior. In addition, elicitation interviews helped define the measures of the TRA constructs (attitude and subjective norm) and alerted us to potential additional theoretical constructs (affect and facilitating conditions) that might influence women's behavior. The research and methods were important in assessing factors that predict behavior and in designing intervention messages likely to increase mammography behavior among women. We applied the data gathered using the TRA framework and methods when we went on to the development of the messages to be used in the motivational telephone call.

Our research showed that there was a need to expand the theory in order to better understand and potentially influence women's behavior (McBride and others, 1993; Curry and others, 1993). The basic tenets of the model are intuitive and appealing. Our research found additional factors that are amenable to manipulation through an intervention. In the development of interventions, we thought about how to influence each construct of the model that predicted behavior and where to place the emphasis for intervention. We also are conducting similar work using the TRA as a framework to understand mammography behavior and to develop a behavioral change intervention among low-income women at an inner-city adult care clinic (Thompson and others, forthcoming).

Application: Prediction of Condom Use Among High STI Risk Groups

The transmission of sexually transmitted infections (STIs), including HIV, can be prevented through consistent use of latex condoms. Unfortunately, rates of condom use among some groups at risk for STIs remain low enough to sustain the STI epidemics. Thus, a great deal of recent research has been designed to understand the factors associated with condom use and to develop interventions to increase condom use among individuals at risk for STIs.

Epidemiological and sociological approaches focus on macro factors such as age, gender, and socioeconomic status to describe behavior and can be useful for identifying groups to target with scarce intervention resources. However, these studies have limited utility in driving the design of intervention messages. To succeed in designing interventions that influence behavior, studies must uncover such changeable factors as attitudes or perceptions of norms. These findings can then drive the design of intervention and health education messages. Demographic factors may then be useful for segmenting audiences if descriptive analyses indicate that mutable factors are different among different groups.

Focusing on behavioral models important to intervention development is key if practitioners want to affect health behavior. Some studies focusing on condom use and sexual behavior have used behavioral models, but most have been descriptive, presenting condom use rates and types of sexual behavior (Tanfer, Grady, Klepinger, and Billy, 1993; Lauman, Gagnon, Michael, and Michaels, 1994; Catania and others, 1992).

Almost all studies that have examined factors affecting condom use among individuals at risk for STIs are either retrospective or cross-sectional. These study designs make it difficult to identify the *predictors* of behavior. Factors predicting future behavior may be different from factors that are correlates of behavior measured cross-sectionally. Thus, there was a need to conduct a theory-driven prospective study to identify and understand the factors affecting the likelihood of condom use among people who are at higher risk than the general population for contracting or transmitting HIV. We expected that such a study would provide useful insights into the development of more effective HIV prevention intervention programs. Between 1990 and 1994, we conducted such a study, applying an integrated behavioral model that included components from several behavioral theories. That model is described elsewhere (Fishbein and others, 1992; Montaño, Kasprzyk, and Fishbein, 1996). Here we describe the findings from the application of the TRA and the TPB components.

Methods

The study was conducted in Seattle and targeted four groups at risk for HIV infection: injecting drug users (IDUs), men who have sex with men (MSMs), female commercial sex workers (CSWs), and multipartnered heterosexuals (MPHs). Purposive sampling was used to recruit approximately equal numbers of each risk group and to stratify the groups to include about equal numbers of whites, blacks, and Hispanics. The IDU and MPH groups were also stratified to include equal numbers by gender. Community-based recruitment was conducted by a multiracial multi-ethnic team recruiting study participants from locations identified through prior ethnographic research. The recruitment effort included support and coordination from other community-based HIV prevention projects.

A prospective design was used with participants recruited for two interviews. They were interviewed at intake with a questionnaire that measured all model components including self-reported condom use. Participants were interviewed again, three months later, to measure all model components and self-reported condom use during the previous three months. A total of 935 participants completed Time 1 interviews and were asked to return for follow-up interviews, with 686 returning for Time 2 interviews (73 percent return).

The questionnaire used in this study was developed through an extensive ethnographic elicitation phase. Semistructured open-ended interviews were conducted with 171 individuals from the four target groups. Participants were asked open-ended questions about factors that might affect their use of condoms with different types of partners (regular, casual, customers) and for different types of sex (vaginal, anal, oral). The interview included questions to elicit information concerning beliefs about outcomes or attributes of using condoms, people or groups the participants listened to about condom use, and factors that made it easier or more difficult to use condoms. Participants also were asked whether they thought there were any other factors that might affect their condom use behavior with sexual partners. Content analysis of responses to these questions developed the measures for attitude, subjective norm, and perceived control, respectively. Separate measures of model constructs were developed for condom use with each type of partner for each type of sex. It was clear from the ethnographic interviews that these different types are distinct behaviors, and participants described different factors affecting each behavior.

Model component measures and computation were as follows.

Behavior. At Time 2, participants rated on a 10-point scale how often they had each type of sex with each type of partner during the previous three months.

For each type of partner and type of sex, they rated how often they used a condom. They used a 7-point scale with endpoints "never" and "all the time." The validity of this measure was assessed by testing its correlation with rates obtained using a thirty-day-calendar recall measure. Correlations were between .81 and .94.

Intention. Intention to use condoms for each type of sex with each type of partner was measured on a 7-point bipolar scale with endpoints "extremely unlikely" and "extremely likely."

Attitude. Attitude toward condom use for each type of sex with each type of partner was constructed from belief and evaluation items. The elicitation interview content analysis identified between thirty and thirty-two outcomes and attributes of each condom use behavior. Behavioral belief measures were developed for each behavior using 7-point bipolar scales with endpoints "extremely unlikely" and "extremely likely." These measures included such items as "using a condom every time you have vaginal sex during the next three months with your regular partner will decrease your sexual sensation" or "using a condom implies you don't trust your partner." Evaluations of each behavioral outcome were rated on 7-point bipolar scales with endpoints "extremely bad" and "extremely good." Belief and evaluation ratings were coded from −3 to +3 and attitude scores were computed by summing the products of beliefs and evaluations. Internal consistency of these scales, measured by Cronbach's alpha, ranged from .83 to .89.

Subjective norm. Subjective norm scores were obtained by having participants rate their normative beliefs about whether fifteen different referents thought they should use condoms and about their motivation to comply with those referents. Referents identified from the elicitation interviews included such people as friends, mothers, counselors, and sexual partners. Normative beliefs for each source of influence were rated on 7-point bipolar scales with endpoints "extremely unlikely" and "extremely likely," and coded −3 to +3. Ratings of motivation to comply with each source of influence were made on 7-point scales with endpoints "disagree" and "agree," coded 1 to 7. Subjective norm scores were calculated by computing the mean of normative belief times motivation to comply products. A mean was used because several influence sources were not applicable to all participants. The internal consistency of these scales, measured by Cronbach's alpha, ranged from .90 to .93.

Perceived behavioral control. The content analysis of elicitation interviews identified ten circumstances and conditions that facilitate or impede condom use. Facilitators include having sex in a usual place and having a partner who is open to the idea of using condoms. Barriers include being high on drugs and being in a hurry to have sex. Measures of perceived control were obtained by asking participants to rate how often each of the ten conditions occurred when they had sex with each type of partner (control beliefs) and the degree to which each condition made it easy or difficult to use a condom (perceived power). Control beliefs were rated on a 10-point scale ranging from "0 of 10 times" to "10 of 10 times." Perceived power of each condition was rated on 7-point bipolar scales with endpoints "difficult" and "easy," coded −3 to +3. Perceived control scores were computed by summing the products of control belief and perceived power ratings. We used the label "facilitators/constraints" to describe this construct. Internal consistency of these scales, measured by Cronbach's alpha, ranged from .69 to .71.

Results

The measures obtained in this study allowed us to conduct separate analyses to predict condom use for different types of sex with different types of partners. Additionally, the design allowed us to compare findings for various sample subgroups by risk group, gender, and race or ethnicity. To simplify the description of findings from this study, this chapter presents only the findings for prediction of condom use for vaginal sex with regular and casual partners and for the overall study sample not broken down by subgroups.

Correlation and multiple regression analyses were conducted to test the effects of attitude, subjective norm, and perceived control in explaining condom use intention and behavior. The top two rows in Table 5.5 present the contributions of attitude, subjective norm, and perceived control measured at Time 1 to explain behavioral intention. All three components had significant correlations with intentions, with attitude having consistently the strongest correlation, followed by perceived control. All three also provided significant independent contributions to the prediction of intention using multiple regression. The regression weights suggest that attitude is relatively more important in predicting intention to use condoms with a regular partner and perceived control is more important in predicting intention to use condoms with a casual partner.

The bottom two rows of Table 5.5 show the findings from analyses to predict behavior at Time 2, using attitude, subjective norm, and perceived control measured at Time 1. All three components correlated significantly with behavior, with attitude again having the highest correlations. Multiple regression analyses found that attitude contributed the most to predicting condom use with both regular and casual partners. Perceived control also had significant regression coefficients for both regular and casual partners, but subjective norm was significant only for condom use with a regular partner. These findings provide support for the importance of environmental facilitators and constraints, as measured by perceived control, in improving the prediction of behavior from attitude and subjective norm alone.

As in the mammography research, we looked at the correlations between behavior and the belief items making up each of the TPB components because this

TABLE 5.5. PREDICTION OF CONDOM USE INTENTION AND BEHAVIOR FROM ATTITUDE, SUBJECTIVE NORM, AND PERCEIVED BEHAVIORAL CONTROL.

	Correlation			Regression Coefficient			
Dependent Variable	A	SN	PBC	A	SN	PBC	R
Condom use intention with							
Regular partner	.59	.40	.48	.40	.14	.21	.64
Casual partner	.42	.36	.36	.26	.22	.45	.51
Condom use behavior with							
Regular partner	.43	.30	.37	.28	.10	.19	.47
Casual partner	.37	.19	.31	.25	n.s.	.17	.41

Note: A = attitude; SN = subjective norm; PBC = perceived behavioral control. All correlations, regression coefficients, and multiple *Rs* listed were significant at $p < .05$ or less.

information can be used in the development of behavioral change intervention messages and strategies. Of the thirty-one behavioral beliefs measured and used to compute attitude, twenty-eight were significantly correlated with condom use with a regular partner and nineteen were significantly correlated with condom use with a casual partner. Table 5.6 presents a few of these beliefs to illustrate typical differences in patterns of correlations with condom use behavior with regular and casual partners. Beliefs about feeling relaxed, reduced sensation, intimacy, partner anger, and trust between partners (the top rows of Table 5.6) were more strongly correlated with condom use with regular than with casual partners. Beliefs concerning spontaneity and discomfort were more strongly correlated with condom use with casual than with regular partners. Several beliefs, including embarrassment and others not listed, were nearly equally correlated for regular and casual partner condom use.

The center rows of Table 5.6 show correlations between normative beliefs and condom use with regular and casual partners. Perceptions about normative support from family were equally important for both types of partner, although normative support from friends had a stronger influence on condom use with regular than with casual partners. Finally, the bottom rows of Table 5.6 show correlations between behavior and perceived control beliefs concerning environmental facilitators and constraints. Perceptions that the partner is open to the idea of condom use or has suggested condom use are more strongly correlated with condom use behavior with regular than casual partners, although being in a hurry to have sex is more strongly correlated with casual than regular partners. Clearly the correlations in Table 5.6 suggest that different interventions should be developed to in-

TABLE 5.6. CORRELATIONS OF BELIEFS WITH CONDOM USE BEHAVIOR.

	Regular Partner (Vaginal)	Casual Partner (Vaginal)
Behavioral beliefs		
Partner will feel relaxed	.40	.29
Will decrease your sensation	.18	.04[a]
Is less intimate	.26	.01[a]
Makes partner angry	.22	.06[a]
Implies you don't trust partner	.27	.15
Is less spontaneous	.04[a]	.20
Is embarrassing	.23	.24
Is too dry for you	.24	.34
Normative beliefs		
Counselor	.15	.01[a]
Mother	.16	.21
Other family	.24	.18
Best friend	.32	.12
Friends	.25	.01[a]
Regular partner	.44	.14
Control beliefs (facilitators and constraints)		
Have condoms available	.35	.32
Partner open to idea of using condoms	.44	.32
In a hurry to have sex	.03[a]	.12[a]
Partner suggests using condoms	.41	.30
Sex in a usual place	.24	.20

Note: All correlations listed were significant at $p < .05$ or less, except [a] = not significant.

fluence condom use with regular partners on the one hand and with casual partners on the other. These interventions would target different sets of beliefs in order to effect changes in attitude, subjective norm, and perceived control for these two behaviors and thereby change the respective intentions and behaviors.

We also conducted separate analyses for different demographic and risk subgroups from our study sample. We found that the regression coefficients for attitude, subjective norm, and perceived control varied by study subgroup as well as by partner type and type of sex. Additionally, we found that the specific behavioral beliefs predictive of behavior varied for different subgroups within the study sample. This variation in the significant behavioral predictors by subgroup in addition to partner type and type of sex suggests the need to tailor interventions differently for each subgroup (Kasprzyk and Montaño, 1993). For example, for one subgroup, the intervention might be focused on attitude, and for another, the intervention might be more effective if focused on perceived control or subjective norm.

Discussion and Implications

The application of the TRA components (attitude and subjective norm) and the addition of perceived control from the TPB resulted in an organizational framework for studying and explaining condom use. This framework provided a structure for the elicitation interviews, which identified beliefs underlying attitude, subjective norm, and perceived control that are relevant to the population and behaviors under investigation. All three components were important determinants of behavioral intention, and the prospective design found all three to be important predictors of subsequent behavior. This study confirmed the complexity of explaining and attempting to change condom use. We found that use of condoms for each type of sex and with each type of partner is a different behavior from use of condoms with other types of sex and types of partner. We also found that these different behaviors have different predictors and that these predictors varied by sample subgroups' demographic characteristics. The data from this study contain a wealth of information that can be used to design effective behavioral change interventions. Our analyses of the beliefs underlying each model component provide very specific information about the focus for intervention messages. The next phase of this research involves the development of interventions designed to change the appropriate sets of beliefs found to predict condom use behavior for certain subgroups.

Conclusion

Theoretical frameworks organize thought and planning of research, analysis, and intervention. The Theory of Reasoned Action and the Theory of Planned Behavior provide excellent frameworks for conceptualizing, measuring, and identifying factors that determine behavior. The TRA focuses on cognitive factors (beliefs and values) that determine motivation (behavioral intention), and the theory has been very useful in explaining behavior, particularly behavior under volitional control. The TRA provides a very precise rationale for identifying and measuring behavioral and normative beliefs and for testing their association with intention and behavior. In applying behavioral theories, it is important to reassess them continually and to consider other theory-driven constructs that may add to the explanatory power. The TPB extends the TRA by adding perceived behavioral control, which relates to facilitating or constraining conditions that affect intention and behavior. This is particularly important for dealing with behaviors over which a person has less volitional control. This component has not been as extensively tested as the TRA components, and Ajzen only recently specified control beliefs as the underlying determinants of behavioral control. Our studies on mammography use and condom use found strong support for construct of facilitators and constraints as behavioral determinants. The condom use study measured and found support for control beliefs.

We cannot stress enough the importance of conducting in-depth open-ended elicitation interviews to identify the behavioral outcomes, referents, and facilitators and constraints that are relevant to the particular behavior and population under investigation and that are to be measured. In addition to supplying specific information that can later be used in the process of designing specific intervention messages, the interview process allows researchers to ground the measures empirically.

If theory is to assist the interventions that researchers and practitioners conduct, it must focus attention on how to select the important factors that can be influenced from among the many factors that exist. The Theory of Reasoned Action and its extension in the Theory of Planned Behavior seem particularly useful in this regard. Application of these models to understand a particular behavior will identify underlying beliefs that determine an individual's attitude, subjective norm, and perceived behavioral control, and thereby affect that individual's likelihood of performing the behavior. Often the important beliefs affecting behavior are different for different related behaviors and for different populations, as was the case in the condom use study.

The TRA and TPB provide a framework for empirically identifying factors on which intervention efforts should focus. However, selection of the specific beliefs to change through health education interventions must be done carefully. Targeting a few beliefs may not be effective if they are a small proportion of the total set of beliefs affecting intention. Similarly, targeting beliefs that constitute a model component that does not have a strong regression coefficient may be ineffective. It is also important to consider the effect of intervention messages on the entire set of beliefs underlying behavior. An intervention communication may change one targeted belief in the desired direction while adversely affecting other important beliefs, thus negating the effect of changing the targeted belief. Additionally, intervention development must pay attention to all model components simultaneously. For example, attempting to modify control beliefs concerning factors that facilitate carrying out one's intention will not be effective if a person is not motivated to perform the behavior in the first place. Conversely, changing attitude and intention may not result in behavioral change if the person holds strong control beliefs about conditions that constrain the behavior.

It is therefore critical to assess the effect of interventions on the beliefs targeted and on other components of the model. The TRA and TPB form a basis for evaluating behavioral change interventions because they allow us to hypothesize how the intervention targeting a set of beliefs will affect the model component (attitude, for example) that those items compose and thereby will affect intention and behavior. It is important to use an evaluation design that includes the measurement of the TRA and TPB components, both at baseline and after the intervention has been implemented, to assess how they are affected by the intervention.

References

Abelson, R. P. "Are Attitudes Necessary?" In B. T. King and E. McGinnies (eds.), *Attitudes, Conflict, and Social Change.* Orlando, Fla.: Academic Press, 1972.

Ajzen, I. "The Theory of Planned Behavior." *Organizational Behavior and Human Decision Processes,* 1991, *50,* 179–211.

Ajzen, I., and Driver, B. L. "Prediction of Leisure Participation from Behavioral, Normative, and Control Beliefs: An Application of the Theory of Planned Behavior." *Leisure Sciences,* 1991, *13,* 185–204.

Ajzen, I., and Fishbein, M. *Understanding Attitudes and Predicting Social Behavior.* Englewood Cliffs, N.J.: Prentice Hall, 1980.

Ajzen I., and Madden, T. J. "Prediction of Goal-Directed Behavior: Attitudes, Intentions, and Perceived Behavioral Control." *Journal of Experimental Social Psychology,* 1986, *22,* 453–474.

Bandura, A. "Social Cognitive Theory of Self Regulation." *Organizational Behavior and Human Decision Processes,* 1991, *50,* 248–285.

Blue, C. L. "The Predictive Capacity of the Theory of Reasoned Action and the Theory of Planned Behavior in Exercise Research: An Integrated Literature Review." *Research in Nursing and Health,* 1995, *18*(2), 105–121.

Calnan, M. "The Health Belief Model and Participation in Programmes for the Early Detection of Breast Cancer: A Comparative Analysis." *Social Science and Medicine,* 1984, *19,* 823–830.

Catania, J. A., and others. "Prevalence of AIDS-Related Risk Factors and Condom Use in the United States." *Science,* 1992, *258,* 1101–1106.

Curry, S. J., and others. "A Randomized Trial of the Impact of Risk Assessment and Feedback on Participation in Mammography Screening." *Preventive Medicine,* 1993, *22,* 350–360.

Edwards, W. "The Theory of Decision Making." *Psychological Bulletin,* 1954, *51,* 380–417.

Fink, R., Shapiro, S., and Lewison, J. "The Reluctant Participant in a Breast Cancer Screening Program." *Public Health Reports,* 1986, *83,* 479–490.

Fishbein, M. (ed.). *Readings in Attitude Theory and Measurement.* New York: Wiley, 1967.

Fishbein, M. "AIDS and Behavior Change: An Analysis Based on the Theory of Reasoned Action." *Interamerican Journal of Psychology,* 1990, *24,* 37–56.

Fishbein, M. Introduction. In D. J. Terry, C. Gallois, and M. McCamish (eds.), *The Theory of Reasoned Action: Its Application to AIDS Preventive Behaviour.* Oxford, England: Pergamon Press, 1993.

Fishbein, M., and Ajzen, I. *Belief, Attitude, Intention and Behavior: An Introduction to Theory and Research.* Reading, Mass.: Addison-Wesley, 1975.

Fishbein, M., and others. *Factors Influencing Behavior and Behavior Change.* Final Report, Theorists Workshop. Bethesda, Md.: National Institute of Mental Health, 1992.

French, K., and others. "Attendance at a Breast Screening Clinic: A Problem of Administration or Attitudes?" *British Medical Journal,* 1982, *285,* 617–620.

Gillmore, M. R., Morrison, D. M., Lowery, C., and Baker, S. A. "Beliefs About Condoms and Their Association with Intentions to Use Condoms Among Youths in Detention." *Journal of Adolescent Health,* 1994, *15*(3), 228–237.

Hobbs, P., Smith, A., George, W. D., and Sellwood, R. A. "Acceptors and Rejectors of an Invitation to Undergo Breast Screening Compared with Those Who Referred Themselves." *Journal of Epidemiology and Community Health,* 1980, *34,* 19–22.

Howard, J. "Using Mammography for Cancer Control: An Unrealized Potential." *CA: A Cancer Journal for Clinicians,* 1987, *37,* 33–48.

Janis, I. L., and Mann, L. *Decision Making: A Psychological Analysis of Conflict, Chance and Commitment.* New York: Free Press, 1977.

Jemmott, J. B., Jemmott, L. S., and Fong, G. T. "Reductions in HIV Risk—Associated Sexual Behaviors Among Black Male Adolescents: Effects of an AIDS Prevention Intervention." *American Journal of Public Health,* 1992, *82*(3), 372–377.

Kasprzyk, D., and Montaño, D. E. "Theory Based Identification of Determinants of Condom Use." Poster presented at the IX International Conference on AIDS, Berlin, June 6–11, 1993.

Lane, D. S., and Fine, H. L. "Compliance with Mammography Referrals: Implications for Breast Cancer Screening." *New York State Journal of Medicine,* 1983, *83,* 173–176.

Larson, E. G., and others. "Do Postcard Reminders Improve Influenza Vaccination Compliance?" *Medical Care,* 1982, *20,* 639–648.

Lauman, E. O., Gagnon, J. H., Michael, R. T., and Michaels, S. *The Social Organization of Sexuality: Sexual Practices in the United States.* Chicago: University of Chicago Press, 1994.

Leventhal, H. "Emotional and Behavioral Processes." In J. Johnston and L. Wallace (eds.), *Stress and Medical Procedures.* Oxford, England: Oxford Science and Medical Publications, 1989.

Lierman, L., Young, H., Kasprzyk, D., and Benoliel, J. "Predicting Breast Self-Examination Using the Theory of Reasoned Action." *Nursing Research,* 1990, *39*(2), 97–101.

Maclean, U., Sinfield, D., Klein, S., and Harnden, B. "Women Who Decline Breast Screening." *Journal of Epidemiology and Community Health,* 1984, *38,* 278–283.

Madden, T. J., Ellen, P. S., and Ajzen, I. "A Comparison of the Theory of Planned Behavior and the Theory of Reasoned Action." *Personality and Social Psychology Bulletin,* 1992, *18*(1), 3–9.

McBride, C. M., and others. "Exploring Environmental Barriers to Participation in Mammography Screening in an HMO." *Cancer Epidemiology, Biomarkers and Prevention,* 1993, *2,* 599–605.

Montaño, D. E. "Predicting and Understanding Influenza Vaccination Behavior: Alternatives to the Health Belief Model." *Medical Care,* 1986, *24,* 438–453.

Montaño, D. E., Kasprzyk, D., and Fishbein, M. "Application of an Integrated Behavioral Model to Predict Condom Use: A Prospective Study Among High HIV Risk Groups." *Journal of Applied Social Psychology.* Unpublished manuscript, 1996.

Montaño, D. E., and Taplin, S. H. "A Test of an Expanded Theory of Reasoned Action to Predict Mammography Participation." *Social Science and Medicine,* 1991, *32,* 733–741.

Reeder, S., Berkanovic, E., and Marcus, A. C. "Breast Cancer Detection Behavior Among Urban Women." *Public Health Reports,* 1980, *95,* 276–281.

Rosenberg, M. J. "Cognitive Structure and Attitudinal Affect." *Journal of Abnormal and Social Psychology,* 1956, *53,* 367–372.

Rotter, J. B. *Social Learning and Clinical Psychology.* Englewood Cliffs, N.J.: Prentice Hall, 1954.

Tanfer, K., Grady, W. R., Klepinger, D. H., and Billy, J.O.G. "Condom Use Among U.S. Men, 1991." *Family Planning Perspectives,* 1993, *25*(2), 61–66.

Taplin, S. H., Anderman, C., and Grothaus, L. "Breast Cancer Risk and Participation in Mammographic Screening." *American Journal of Public Health,* 1989, *79,* 1494–1498.

Taplin, S. H., and Montaño, D. E. "Attitudes, Age and Participation in Mammographic Screening: A Prospective Analysis." *Journal of the American Board of Family Practice,* 1993, *6,* 3–23.

Taplin, S. H., and others. "Using Physician Correspondence and Postcard Reminders to Promote Mammography Use." *American Journal of Public Health,* 1994, *84,* 571–574.

Terry, D., Gallois, C., and McCamish, M. "The Theory of Reasoned Action and Health Care Behaviour." In D. J. Terry, C. Gallois, and M. McCamish (eds.), *The Theory of Reasoned Action: Its Application to AIDS Preventive Behaviour.* Oxford, England: Pergamon Press, 1993.

Thompson, B., and others. "The Use of Qualitative Methodology to Identify Attitudes and Beliefs Toward Mammography Among Women Utilizing an Urban Public Hospital." *Journal of Health Care for the Poor and Underserved,* forthcoming.

Thompson, R. S., Taplin, S. H., Carter, A. P., and Schnitzer, F. "Cost Effectiveness in Program Delivery." *Cancer,* 1989, *64,* 2682–2689.

Triandis, H. C. "Values, Attitudes and Interpersonal Behavior." In H. E. Howe, Jr. (ed.), *Nebraska Symposium on Motivation.* Vol. 27. Lincoln: University of Nebraska Press, 1980.

Weinstein, N. D. "Unrealistic Optimism About Susceptibility to Health Problems: Conclusions from a Community-Wide Sample." *Journal of Behavioral Medicine,* 1987, *10*(4), 481–500.

Weinstein, N. D. "Testing Four Competing Theories of Health-Protective Behavior." *Health Psychology,* 1993, *12*(4), 324–333.

Wicker, A. W. "Attitudes vs. Actions: The Relationship of Verbal and Overt Behavioral Responses to Attitude Objects." *Journal of Social Issues,* 1969, *25,* 41–78.

CHAPTER SIX

STRESS, COPING, AND HEALTH BEHAVIOR

Caryn Lerman
Karen Glanz

An understanding of stress and coping is essential to health education, health promotion, and disease prevention. Stress can contribute to illness through its direct physiological effects and through its indirect effects, via maladaptive health behaviors (for example, smoking and poor eating habits). However, stress does not affect all people equally; some individuals live through terribly threatening experiences yet manage to cope well and do not become susceptible to illness. Among individuals who are ill or at risk for illness, ways of coping can have important influences on psychological and physical health outcomes. Influences of friends, family, and health care providers in the face of stress can have profound effects on these outcomes as well.

The illness experience, medical treatment, a diagnosis of illness, and fear of developing an illness can all provoke stressful reactions. The way individuals experience and cope with stress affects whether and how they seek medical care and social support and how well they adhere to health professionals' advice. Reactions to stressors can promote or inhibit healthful practices and influence a person's self-efficacy and hence his or her motivation to practice positive health habits. In all these situations, the psychosocial aspects of the situation affect the determinants and consequences of health behaviors. A better understanding of theory and the empirical literature on stress and coping is thus essential if researchers and practitioners are to develop strategies and programs to help individuals cope better with stress and to enhance their psychological and physical well-being.

The purpose of this chapter is to review major theories, research, and applications related to stress, coping, and health. We first provide a brief summary of historical concepts of health, stress, and coping, and we outline the most influential cognitive-behavioral theoretical framework, The Transactional Model of Stress and Coping. Key variables, definitions, relationships among concepts, and a summary of findings relevant to health behavior are presented. The second part of the chapter describes applications of the model to the design of health behavior interventions.

Historical Concepts of Health, Stress, and Coping

Conceptualizations of health, stress, and coping are derived from numerous branches of research, with the earliest work conducted by scientists in the fields of biology and psychophysiology. In addition, diverse health and behavioral science disciplines—including epidemiology, personality psychology, and cognitive and social psychology—have been influential in developing an understanding of stress and health.

Stressors are demands made by the internal or external environment that upset individuals' homeostasis, thus affecting their physical and psychological well-being and requiring action to restore that balance or equilibrium (Lazarus and Cohen, 1977). Early work on stress focused on physiological reactions to stressful stimuli. Cannon (1932) is credited with first describing the *fight-or-flight* reaction to stress. Hans Selye, considered the father of modern stress research, extended Cannon's studies with clinical observations and laboratory research. He hypothesized that living organisms, particularly rats and people, exhibited nonspecific changes in response to stressors, and he labeled this response a three-stage General Adaptation Syndrome (GAS). This syndrome consists of an alarm reaction, resistance, and exhaustion (Selye, 1956). Each stage evokes both physiological and behavioral responses, and if "curative" measures are not taken, physical and psychological deterioration is expected to occur.

Another major stream of stress research in the 1960s and 1970s focused on identifying and quantifying potential stressors, or *stressful life events*. Holmes and Rahe (1967) developed the Social Readjustment Rating Scale (SRRS), a tool to measure both positive and negative life events that were considered stressful by virtue of the need for adjustment. Studies showed that people with high scores on the SRRS had more illness episodes than those with low scores. This scale stimulated a substantial body of research (Dohrenwend and Dohrenwend, 1981), despite numerous methodological limitations. For example, the scales did not consider whether respondents regarded events as desirable or undesirable. In addition, some scale items were not independent of the outcomes being examined and retrospective designs were frequently used. Subsequent research examined life experiences using ratings of the subjective impact of the events (Sarason, Johnson, and Siegel, 1978). Other studies focused on the effects of minor day-to-day stressful events identified as daily hassles and uplifts (Kanner, Coyne, Schaefer, and Lazarus, 1981).

In the 1960s and 1970s, stress was considered to be a transactional phenomenon dependent on the meaning of the stimulus to the perceiver (Lazarus, 1966; Antonovsky, 1979). The central concept in these models is that a given event or situation may be perceived in different ways by various individuals. Moreover, these subjective perceptions—rather than the objective stressors—are seen to be the main determinants of effects on subsequent behaviors and on health status. Some researchers in the field of occupational stress and health used this concept as a foundation for an "interaction" model that viewed occupational stress as a result of the interaction between individual workers' characteristics and the work environment, or the "person-environment fit" (French and Kahn, 1962; House, 1974). These lines of theory and research also gave rise to examination of possible buffering, or moderating, factors and, in particular, to a focus on the role of social support (Cohen and Wills, 1985).

A large body of biological and epidemiological research has grown at the same time that social psychological research on stress and coping has evolved. Accumulating research supports the contention that some personality dispositions and psychological states (for example, fatalism, hostility, and emotional suppression) are linked to disease endpoints (Scheier and Bridges, 1995). There is evidence that chronic stressors and responses to them affect the sympathetic nervous system and endocrine functions, thus influencing the occurrence and progression of health problems including cancer, infectious diseases, and HIV/AIDS (Kiecolt-Glaser and Glaser, 1995). The difficulty of separating psychological and biological causal factors in health status and health behavior is underscored by the apparent complexity of mechanisms proposed for these associations (Borysenko, 1984).

Clearly, there are numerous and important areas of research and theory on stress and health. In this chapter, we emphasize cognitive-behavioral theory and research due to its direct relevance to health education and health behavior change.

Transactional Model of Stress and Coping: Overview, Key Constructs, and Empirical Support

The Transactional Model of Stress and Coping provides a framework for evaluating the processes of coping with stressful events. Stressful experiences are construed as person-environment *transactions* wherein the impact of an external stressor, or demand, is mediated by the person's appraisal of the stressor and the psychological, social, and cultural resources at his or her disposal (Lazarus and Cohen, 1977; Antonovsky and Kats, 1967; Cohen, 1984). When faced with a stressor, a person evaluates the potential threat or harm (*primary appraisal*), as well as his or her ability to alter the situation and manage negative emotional reactions (*secondary appraisal*). Actual *coping efforts,* aimed at problem management and emotional regulation, give rise to the *outcomes* of the coping process (for example, psychological well-being, functional status, adherence). Table 6.1 summarizes the key concepts, definitions, and applications of the Transactional Model of Stress and Coping. Figure 6.1 illustrates the interrelationships among these concepts. For an extensive discussion of theoretical underpinnings, readers should refer to the work of Lazarus and Folkman (Lazarus and Folkman, 1984; Lazarus, 1991a).

Primary Appraisal

Primary appraisal is a person's judgment about the significance of an event as stressful, positive, controllable, challenging, benign, or irrelevant. Health problems

FIGURE 6.1. DIAGRAM OF TRANSACTIONAL MODEL OF STRESS AND COPING.

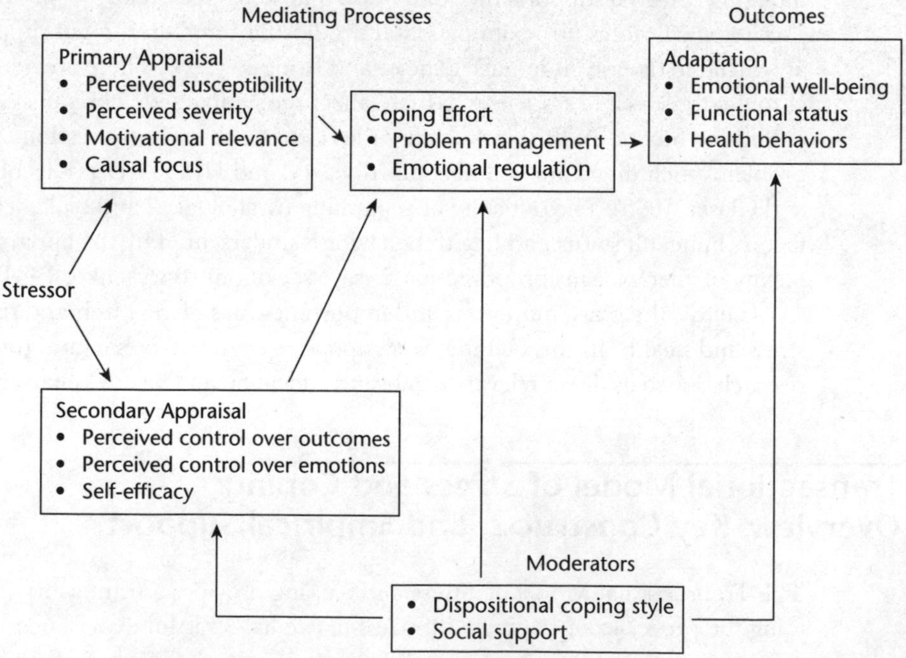

TABLE 6.1. TRANSACTIONAL MODEL OF STRESS AND COPING.

Concept	Definition	Application
Primary appraisal	Evaluation of the significance of a stressor or threatening event	Perceptions of an event as threatening can cause distress. If an event is perceived as positive, benign, or irrelevant, little negative threat is felt.
Secondary appraisal	Evaluation of the controllability of the stressor and a person's coping resources	Perception of one's ability to change the situation, manage one's emotional reaction, or cope effectively can lead to successful coping and adaptation.
Coping efforts	Actual strategies used to mediate primary and secondary appraisals	
Problem management	Strategies directed at changing a stressful situation	Active coping, problem solving, and information seeking can be used.
Emotional regulation	Strategies aimed at changing the way one thinks or feels about a stressful situation	Venting feelings, avoidance, denial, and seeking social support may be used.
Outcomes of coping (adaptation)	Emotional well-being, functional status, health behaviors	Coping strategies may result in short- and long-term positive or negative adaptation.
Dispositional coping styles	Generalized ways of behaving that can affect a person's emotional or functional reaction to a stressor; relatively stable across time and situations.	
Optimism	Tendency to have generalized positive expectancies for outcomes	Optimists may experience fewer symptoms or faster recovery from illness.
Information seeking	Attentional styles that are vigilant (monitoring) versus those that involve avoidance (blunting)	Monitoring may increase distress and arousal; it may also increase active coping. Blunting may mute excessive worry, but may reduce adherence.
Locus of control	Generalized belief about one's ability to control events	Internal locus of control can lead to more active coping and increased adherence.

are usually evaluated initially as threatening, that is, as negative stressors. Two basic primary appraisals are perceptions of *susceptibility* to the threat and perceptions of *severity* of the threat. According to the Transactional Model of Stress and Coping, appraisals of personal risk and threat severity prompt efforts to cope with the stressor. For example, a woman who perceives herself at risk for breast cancer may be motivated to obtain mammograms (problem-focused coping) and may seek social support to cope with her concerns about this threat (emotion-focused coping). However, heightened perceptions of risk can also generate distress. For example, among women with a family history of ovarian cancer, those who perceive themselves as highly susceptible are more prone to experience intrusive ideation and psychological distress (Schwartz and others, 1995). Appraisals of high threat can also prompt escape-avoidance behaviors (Folkman and others, 1986), which can have the paradoxical effect of reducing adherence to health-promoting practices (Lerman and Schwartz, 1993). For example, heightened distress about personal risk of breast cancer has been associated with decreased adherence to recommended breast cancer screening guidelines (Lerman and others, 1993; Kash, Holland, Halper, and Miller, 1992).

Primary appraisals can also serve to minimize the significance of the threat, particularly when a health threat is ambiguous or uncertain. This *appraisal bias* was demonstrated in a series of well-designed studies by Croyle and colleagues (Ditto and Croyle, 1995; Croyle and Sandman, 1988). Employing a test for a fictitious enzyme disorder, they showed that persons who were informed of "abnormal" test results rated the disorder as less serious and the test itself as less valid than did those who received "normal" test results. Such minimizing appraisals have also been shown to reduce distress associated with real health threats. For example, breast cancer patients who perceived themselves as "invulnerable" to a recurrence experienced less distress and had better overall adjustment than other patients (Timko and Janoff-Bulman, 1985). Among HIV-positive men, beliefs of invulnerability enhanced perceived control and active coping and reduced distress, without compromising performance of safe sexual behaviors (Taylor and others, 1992). However, other studies suggest that minimizing appraisals may also diminish motivation to adopt recommended preventive health behaviors such as cholesterol screening and dietary restriction (Weinstein, 1989; Croyle, 1992). This minimization effect may be particularly pronounced among smokers. For example, Chapman, Wong, and Smith (1993) found that smokers were significantly more likely than nonsmokers to perceive themselves as less personally susceptible to the health effects of smoking.

Other primary appraisals involve the *motivational relevance* and *causal focus* of the stressor. When a stressor is appraised as having a major impact on a person's goals or concerns (high motivational relevance), that person is likely to experience anxiety and situation-specific distress (Smith and Lazarus, 1993). This may be especially true when the relevance is to the person's own physical health or well-being (Folkman and others, 1986). Perceiving oneself as responsible for the stressor (self-causal focus) may be more likely to generate guilt and depression than anxiety (Smith, Haynes, Lazarus, and Pope, 1993; Lewis and Daltroy, 1990). When coping with illness, the congruence of the appraisal with the appraisal of a significant other may be more important than the individual's focus of causality (Manne and Taylor, 1993). Alternatively, the most important aspect of causal appraisals of illness may be whether or nor they are generated at all (Lowery, Jacobsen, and DuCette, 1993).

Secondary Appraisal

Secondary appraisal is an assessment of a person's coping resources and options (Cohen, 1984). In contrast to primary appraisals that focus on the features of the stressful situation, secondary appraisals address what one can do about the situation. Key examples of secondary appraisals are *perceived ability to change the situation* (for example, perceived control over the threat), *perceived ability to manage one's emotional reactions* to the threat (for example, perceived control over feelings), and *expectations about the effectiveness of one's coping resources* (for example, coping self-efficacy).

Positive associations between perceptions of control over illness and psychological adjustment have been demonstrated across a wide variety of diseases, including cancer (Marks, Richardson, Graham, and Levine, 1986), coronary heart disease (Taylor, Helgeson, Reed, and Skokan, 1991), and HIV/AIDS (Taylor and others, 1992). Moreover, perceived control over illness may improve physical well-being by increasing the likelihood that a person will adopt recommended health behaviors (Thompson and Spacapan, 1991). For example, perceived control over health outcomes has been shown to relate positively to breast cancer screening behaviors (Hallal, 1982) and to safe sexual behavior (Taylor and others, 1992). However, in situations that cannot be altered (for example, severe or fatal disease), high levels of perceived control may actually increase distress and dysfunction (Affleck, Tennen, Pfeiffer, and Fifield, 1987; Thompson and others, 1993). Thus, beliefs about personal control are likely to be adaptive only to the extent that they fit with reality (Brownell, 1991).

Beliefs about one's ability to perform the behaviors necessary to exert control (that is, self-efficacy) have been shown to play a central role in the performance of a variety of health behaviors (Strecher, DeVellis, Becker, and Rosenstock, 1986). For example, self-efficacy beliefs predict success with smoking cessation attempts (Strecher, DeVellis, Becker, and Rosenstock, 1986) and maintenance of exercise and diet regimens (Ewart, Taylor, Reese, and Debusk, 1983; Jeffrey and others, 1984). Self-efficacy, a central construct of Social Cognitive Theory (Bandura, 1989;

see Chapter Eight), is specific to a given behavior and is not a global personality trait. For example, a sedentary nonsmoker may have high self-efficacy for avoiding tobacco use but low self-efficacy for exercising regularly.

Coping Efforts

According to the Transactional Model, the emotional and functional effects of primary and secondary appraisals are mediated by actual *coping strategies* (Lazarus and Folkman, 1984; Lazarus, 1991a). Original formulations of the model conceptualized coping efforts along two overarching dimensions: problem management and emotional regulation. Also referred to as problem-focused coping, problem management strategies are directed at changing the stressful situation. Examples of problem-focused coping include active coping, planning problem solving, and information seeking. By contrast, emotion-focused coping efforts aim not to alter the situation but to change the way one thinks or feels about it. These strategies include seeking social support, venting of feelings, avoidance, and denial. The model predicts that problem-focused coping strategies will be most adaptive for stressors that are changeable, while emotion-focused strategies are most adaptive when the stressor is unchangeable or when all problem-focused coping attempts have been made. However, some strategies, such as denial, are considered to be maladaptive in both types of situations.

There are some interesting parallels between the coping strategies in the Transactional Model and the change processes in The Transtheoretical Model, also known as the Stages of Change Model (Prochaska, DiClemente, and Norcross, 1992; see Chapter Four). For example, "self-reevaluation" is a change process shown to facilitate progression from the contemplation stage of behavioral change to the preparation stage. Similar to emotion-focused coping strategies such as reappraisal, self-reevaluation involves assessing and, in some cases, altering how one feels about a problem. Likewise, change processes such as stimulus control and counterconditioning (that is, substitution of alternatives for problem behaviors) could be considered problem-focused coping strategies.

Recent empirical studies of coping have focused on the extent to which an individual engages versus disengages with the stressor (Carver and others, 1993). When a stressor is perceived as highly threatening and uncontrollable, a person may be more likely to use disengaging coping strategies (Taylor and others, 1992). Examples of disengaging coping strategies include distancing, cognitive avoidance, behavioral avoidance, distraction, and denial. By avoiding thoughts and feelings about the stressor, individuals may minimize their initial distress (Suls and Fletcher, 1985). Ultimately, however, avoidance or denial may lead to intrusive thoughts that can generate increased distress (Schwartz and others, 1995). By contrast, when a stressor is appraised as controllable and a person has favorable beliefs about self-efficacy, he or she is more likely to use engaging coping strategies (Aspinwall and Taylor, 1992). Examples of engaging coping strategies include active coping, planning problem solving, information seeking, and using social support. These are also considered problem-focused strategies, as noted above. Other common coping responses to health threats include positive reinterpretation, acceptance, and use of religion and spirituality (Carver and others, 1993; Reed and others, 1994).

Several theoretically driven questionnaires have been developed to assess coping efforts. Typically, respondents are asked to describe a stressful situation they have experienced and to answer questions about how they would evaluate and respond to the situation. The most widely used subscales address problem-focused coping and emotion-focused coping (Stone, Greenberg, Kennedy-Moore, and Newman, 1991). Examples of available tools include the Ways of Coping Inventory (WOC) (Folkman and Lazarus, 1980), the Multidimensional Coping Inventory (Endler and Parker, 1990), and the Coping Orientations to Problems Experienced (COPE) scale (Carver, Scheier, and Weintraub, 1989). The COPE questionnaire, one of the more recent inventories, uses twelve subscales for types of coping strategies: active coping, suppression of competing activities, planning, restraint, social support, positive reframing, religion, acceptance, denial, disengagement, humor, and self-distraction (Carver and others, 1993). There are also scales to measure daily use of coping strategies (Stone and Neale, 1984); these scales may provide more precise assessments of coping transactions (Stone, Kennedy-Moore, and Neale, forthcoming).

The Transactional Model has generated an extensive body of literature on coping strategies, adjustment to illness, and health behavior. In general, these studies provide evidence for the psychological benefits of active coping strategies and acceptance and reappraisal over avoidant or disengaging strategies (for example, Carver and others, 1993; Taylor and others, 1992). In addition to its adverse effects on psychological well-being, avoidant coping may increase the likelihood of negative health behaviors, such as IV drug use in people with AIDS (Fleishman and Vogel, 1994). By contrast, using spirituality and seeking social support may reduce the chances that a person will engage in risky behaviors, such as unprotected sexual intercourse (Folkman, Chesney, Pollack, and Phillips, 1992). The extent to which specific coping strategies result in desirable or undesirable outcomes may depend on whether short- or long-term outcomes are considered more important (Cohen, 1984). In addition, coping flexibility (the ability to employ a variety of different strategies) has been found to be important in health promotion, particularly in prevention of relapse in smokers (Bliss, Garvey, and Heinold, 1989). Moreover, cognitive-behavioral interventions that enhance coping flexibility can improve maintenance of health behavior changes such as smoking cessation (Brandon, Copeland, and Saper, 1995).

Most research on coping strategies evaluates efforts to cope with a particular situation as distinct from generalized coping styles (Stone and Porter, 1995). However, as discussed in the next section, the effects of specific coping strategies on the emotional and functional outcomes of a health threat and the accompanying stress may depend on a person's dispositional coping style and his or her perceptions of support in the environment.

Coping Outcomes

Coping outcomes represent individuals' adaptations to stressors, following from their appraisal of the situation (primary appraisal) and resources (secondary appraisal) and influenced by coping efforts. Because a problem or stressor may change over time, outcomes may occur in differing time frames. Three main categories of outcomes are emotional well-being, functional status (or health status, disease progression, and so forth), and health behaviors. These outcomes may interact with one another. For example, emotional reactions may affect functional or health status through physiological processes of the endocrine, immune, and nervous systems (Kiecolt-Glaser and Glaser, 1995; Scheier and Bridges, 1995). Health behaviors such as seeking care, communication with health providers, and adherence to treatment recommendations may be influenced by physical limitations (functional status) and by emotional reactions such as worry, depression, and denial.

Theoretical Extensions

Further factors with theoretical relevance to stress and coping are dispositional coping styles, the role of social support, and practical stress management techniques.

Dispositional Coping Styles

In contrast to coping efforts, coping styles are conceptualized as dispositional or stable characteristics of the individual. Another important distinction between coping efforts and coping styles is that the former are situation specific while the latter are generalized (Lazarus, 1993). Coping efforts change as a function of primary and secondary appraisals, and these processes influence how a person will react emotionally and functionally to the stressor. Thus, coping efforts can be considered *mediators* of the effects of stress and appraisals on emotional and functional outcomes—in other words, mediators of the mechanism by which these effects are exerted (Baron and Kenny, 1986). By contrast, coping styles are enduring traits believed to drive appraisal and coping efforts (Lazarus, 1993). Individual differences in coping styles can be considered *moderators* of the impact of stress on coping processes and outcomes (Baron and Kenny, 1986). That is, the specific effect of a stressful event or a specific coping behavior on adjustment may depend, in part, on the person's coping style, which may produce a modifying interaction. Coping styles can also have direct effects on the emotional and physical outcomes of a stressful event.

Early conceptualizations and research on dispositional coping styles focused on characterizing persons who remained relatively healthy while undergoing stressful life experiences. Hinkle (1974) observed that such people tended to be emotionally insulated and less involved with other people. In contrast, Antonovsky (1979) and Kobasa (1979) suggested that people who exhibited healthful adaptation to internal and environmental stressors had strong resistance resources and a sense of meaningfulness in their lives. Antonovsky (1979) described a "sense of coherence" that involves a strong sense of confidence that the world is predictable and that things will work out "as well as reasonably can be expected." He further proposed that sense of coherence could be found not only in well-adapted individuals but in groups and cultures as well. Kobasa (1979) identified a constellation of features she called "hardiness," marked by a strong sense of meaningfulness and commitment to self, a vigorous attitude toward life, and an internal locus of control (discussed later in this chapter). She found that "hardy" professionals were less likely to report illness after experiencing many stressful events (Kobasa, 1979), but the findings did not hold in a second, prospective study of lawyers (Kobasa, Maddi, and Kahn, 1982). This work was a forerunner of more recent research on dispositional optimism.

Optimism. Perhaps the most widely researched coping style is dispositional optimism—the tendency to have positive (optimistic) rather than negative (pessimistic) generalized expectancies for outcomes. These expectancies have been shown to be relatively stable over time and across situations (Scheier and Carver, 1992). The direct beneficial effects of optimism on psychological adjustment have been demonstrated in prospective studies of cancer patients (Carver and others, 1993), coronary patients (Scheier and others, 1989), and HIV-positive men (Taylor and others, 1992). Optimists also have been shown to experience fewer physical symptoms during life stresses (Scheier and Carver, 1985) and faster recovery following myocardial infarction (Scheier and others, 1989).

Studies exploring the effects of optimism on coping responses and adaptation to illness are relevant to the Transactional Model. For example, Carver and colleagues (1993) conducted a one-year prospective study of the effects of optimism and coping strategies on psychological well-being among early stage breast cancer patients. Dispositional optimism was found to predict psychological adjustment at each time point. Moreover, this beneficial effect of optimism was mediated by the use of active coping, planning, problem solving, and acceptance. Optimism was related inversely to avoidance, a coping strategy that generated distress in this sample. Among gay men at risk for AIDS, dispositional optimism was associated with perceived lower risk of AIDS (primary appraisal), higher perceived control over AIDS (secondary appraisal), more active coping strategies, less distress, and more risk-reducing health behaviors in men at risk for AIDS (Taylor and others, 1992). Dispositional optimism also has been related to performance of exercise following coronary bypass surgery (Scheier and Carver, 1987). Thus, dispositional optimism appears to exert effects on each of the key processes of the Transactional Model. These effects, in turn, influence how optimists and pessimists respond emotionally and physically to health threats and illness.

Information Seeking. In addition to optimism, there is a wealth of support for the influence of attentional styles: *monitoring,* or seeking relevant information, and *blunting,* or avoiding such information (Miller, 1987). Several studies have shown that the vigilant style of individuals who are monitors contributes to their heightened perceived risk and excessive worry about health threats (Phipps and Zinn, 1986; Wardle and others, 1993). In a recent study of women at increased risk for ovarian cancer, monitoring was associated with heightened perceived risk of disease, intrusive thoughts, and distress (Schwartz and others, 1995). In this study, perceived risk, an appraisal variable, acted as a mediator of the effects of monitoring on psychological distress.

Effects of monitoring on physical outcomes of stressful events have also been demonstrated. For example, among cancer patients undergoing chemotherapy, monitoring has been associated with more severe nausea and vomiting (Lerman and others, 1990). Monitors have also been shown to experience more physical distress and arousal during an invasive medical procedure than blunters (Miller and Mangan, 1983). In a randomized trial comparing alternate methods of cancer risk counseling in women at high risk for breast cancer, monitors showed increases in distress in both counseling conditions (Lerman and others, 1996). However, when stressors are short term and when monitors' needs for information are satisfied (for example, by preparation for stressful medical procedures), active coping is enhanced and emotional, and physical distress is minimized (Miller and Mangan, 1983).

Although the foregoing studies suggest that monitoring may be a less adaptive coping style than blunting, there are situations where this may not be the case. For example, monitors may be more inclined to seek health information that could have significant medical benefits, as was shown in a study of genetic testing for cancer susceptibility (Lerman, Daly, Masny, and Balshem, 1994). In addition, because monitors are more attentive to health threats, they may also adhere better to recommended health practices than blunters (Steptoe and Sullivan, 1986).

Locus of Control. Locus of control is a generalized belief about one's ability to control events by virtue of one's own efforts (Rotter, 1966). Persons with internal locus of control are more likely to initiate change on their own, while those with external locus of control are more likely to be influenced by others. Also, individuals with an internal locus of control are more likely to use vigilant coping strategies than avoidant coping strategies; for example, they would more likely want to know what is occurring during surgery than to receive general anesthesia (Cohen, 1984). The perception that the environment is controllable is likely to lead to more active coping or greater efforts to influence the outcome or more action directed at coping. The concept of locus of control has been extended to beliefs about health-related events and threats (Wallston and Wallston, 1978). For example, a person with an external locus of control might believe that injuries from an automobile accident were due to chance or fate and might not invest great effort in rehabilitation or future preventive actions. In contrast, someone with an internal locus of control might try vigorously to recover quickly and become a staunch advocate of seat belt use. It should be noted that locus of control, unlike self-efficacy, is considered a generalized belief rather than situation or behavior specific.

Social Support

Social support has been conceptualized in a variety of ways (Israel and Schurman, 1990). Some definitions focus on the quantitative and tangible dimensions (for example, number of friendships), and others focus on qualitative and nontangible dimensions (for example, feelings of interconnectedness and subjective appraisals of adequacy of support networks) (Heitzmann and Kaplan, 1988). Although conceptualizations and forms of measurement may vary, substantial evidence exists that social support has beneficial effects on psychological and physical well-being (Israel and Schurman, 1990).

Social support appears to have both direct effects and "stress-buffering" effects on well-being (Cohen and Wills, 1985). The stress-buffering hypothesis predicts that social support will strengthen in its positive effects on adjustment and physical well-being as a stressor becomes more intense or persistent. Evidence for the buffering model has been found in studies that measure the perceived availability of social support (Cohen and Hoberman, 1983; Littlefield, Rodin, Murray, and Craven,

1990). The direct effects of social support have been observed primarily in studies assessing the extent of social support networks (Schonfeld, 1991; Gill and others, 1991).

By influencing the key processes posited in the Transactional Model of Stress and Coping, social support can influence how people adapt psychologically to a stressful event such as a significant health threat or illness. For example, the availability of friends to talk to could affect a person's perceptions of personal risk or of the severity of illness (primary appraisal). Social interactions can bolster beliefs about one's ability to cope with the situation and manage difficult emotions (secondary appraisal) (Cohen and McKay, 1984). Social support can serve as a mechanism for downward comparison—that is, a comparison between oneself and someone who is worse off (Cohen and Wills, 1985). Resultant increases in self-esteem and self-efficacy, in turn, can increase the likelihood of active coping strategies rather than avoidance (Holahan and Moos, 1986). A supportive environment can also protect against stress by providing opportunities for individuals to explore different coping options and to evaluate their efficacy (Holahan and Moos, 1986). In addition, disclosure of feelings has been shown to decrease avoidant coping and minimize negative emotional reactions to a stressor (Pennebaker and O'Heeron, 1984).

Social support also can influence health outcomes (Reifman, 1995). In a study of men with coronary artery disease, both quantitative and qualitative dimensions of social support predicted survival, even after controlling for medical variables (Williams and others, 1992). The results of studies of social support and cancer outcomes have been mixed, however (Reifman, 1995). A mechanism by which social support may benefit physical well-being is the promotion of active coping behaviors such as adherence to recommended health behaviors (Heitzmann and Kaplan, 1988). For example, among African Americans, social support has been associated with increased use of mammography and stool blood tests for cancer screening (Kang and Bloom, 1993). Alternatively, by enhancing the expression of negative feelings, social support may have direct physiological and immunological benefits (Pennebaker, 1990). (Social support is also discussed in Chapter Nine.)

Stress Management Interventions

A variety of techniques to manage stress, improve coping, and reduce the deleterious effects of stressors on physical and psychological well-being have been developed and tested in recent years. The limitations of this chapter preclude a full discussion of intervention strategies; however, we will briefly describe a sampling of methods based on both psychophysiological and cognitive-behavioral models.

Biofeedback and deep relaxation strategies focus on the interplay between biological and psychological responses to stressors (Kaplan, Sallis, and Patterson,

1993). Biofeedback systems aim to develop awareness and control of maladaptive responses to stressors and to reduce stress and tension in response to everyday situations. Use of relaxation techniques assumes that individuals possess alternative responses to fight-or-flight, responses that counteract the effects of stress. The basic elements of the relaxation response, which can be achieved through progressive relaxation training, hypnosis, yoga, and other techniques, are use of a constant mental stimulus, passive attitude, decreased muscle tone, and a quiet environment (Benson, 1984).

Cognitive-behavioral approaches to coping with stress are usually based on five key modes of coping: information seeking, direct action, inhibition of action, intrapsychic processes, and turning to others for support (Cohen and Lazarus, 1979). These approaches, most closely derived from the Transactional Model, focus on teaching individuals to evaluate their primary appraisals of stressful situations, to achieve accurate (rather than distorted) primary appraisals, and to evaluate their coping resources and enhance them as necessary (Kaplan, Sallis, and Patterson, 1993). Psychoeducational approaches, such as information in preparation for surgery, may play a central role in these interventions. Strategies to mobilize individuals to modify their objective sources of stress (that is, to change their environment) and to enhance social support are also important health promotion approaches (Israel and Schurman, 1990).

Applications to Specific Health Behavior Research

Examples of cognitive-behavioral intervention strategies to improve coping and adaptation are given in the applications that follow. These applications relate to breast cancer and HIV/AIDS.

Application: Problem-Solving Training for First-Degree Relatives of Newly Diagnosed Breast Cancer Patients

Women with a first-degree relative with breast cancer have a two- to fourfold increased risk of developing this disease (Claus, Risch, and Thompson, 1990). Yet research shows that many high-risk women do not adhere to breast cancer screening (Vogel and others, 1990). In addition, a substantial proportion of these women experience problems in psychological adjustment (Kash, Holland, Halper, and Miller, 1992; Lerman and Schwartz, 1993). Anxiety and distress in high-risk women can interfere with adherence to recommended breast cancer screening (Lerman and others, 1993). For first-degree relatives of newly diagnosed breast cancer patients, psychological adjustment and adherence issues may be especially challenging, as they must cope with concerns about both their own breast cancer risk and the welfare of loved ones.

The Transactional Model of Stress and Coping is being used as the theoretical foundation for the development and evaluation of a cognitive-behavioral intervention to promote adjustment and adherence among first-degree relatives of newly diagnosed breast cancer patients (Lerman and others, 1993–1997). This intervention uses the Problem-Solving Training (PST) approach (D'Zurilla, 1986; Haaga and Davison, 1991) to facilitate adaptive appraisals and to promote effective problem-focused and emotion-focused coping with stresses resulting from the relative's breast cancer diagnosis.

The PST intervention is delivered to the relatives of newly diagnosed breast cancer patients during an extended individual visit with a health educator or nurse. The approach has five steps. The first step is to assess the participant's appraisal of the situation, focusing on her attributions, perceptions of control, and perceptions of coping resources. Attention is paid to attributions of causability and control, as these beliefs are key determinants of adjustment (Taylor, Lichtman, and Wood, 1984). An adaptive appraisal is fostered by emphasizing that a relative's breast cancer diagnosis can be viewed as a opportunity to protect one's own health and that negative emotions can be used as a "cue" for problem-solving activity. In addition, participants are presented with an overview of the stress and coping model and the problem-solving techniques. Second, specific problem statements are generated; for example, "What can I do to minimize my anxiety about my risk?" and, "What can I do to help my sister adjust better to her treatment?" The objective of this stage is to set realistic and attainable short-term goals. The third step is to generate alternative solutions to the problem, focusing on both problem-focused coping strategies and emotion-focused coping strategies. Participants are taught a brainstorming approach to generate a wide range of strategies. The fourth step is to examine the value of these solutions by considering the impact on the participant's well-being, the impact on the well-being of the affected relative, the time and effort required, and the potential for problem resolution. Standardized prompts are used to elicit the participant's expectations about the consequences and to apply a cost-benefit strategy to select the best alternative. Finally, evaluation of the success of the specific coping strategies is performed during follow-up telephone booster sessions.

The PST intervention is being evaluated in the context of a randomized trial conducted at six cancer centers across the United States. The evaluation focuses on the impact of PST, relative to general health counseling (control), on the following elements of the Transactional Model: (1) primary appraisals, including perceptions of risk and of threat to oneself and to the affected relative; (2) secondary appraisals, including perceived ability to control the situation and manage negative mood reactions and perceived coping resources; (3) coping behaviors, including active coping, avoidant coping, and spiritual acceptance of coping; (4) quality of life outcomes, including cancer worries, mood, stress impact, and functional health status; and (5) adherence behaviors, including use of mammography, clinical breast examination, and breast self-examination.

Although outcome data from this trial are not yet available, there is reason to expect a positive impact. Self-appraised effective problem solvers report greater self-efficacy, exhibit fewer dysfunctional coping efforts, experience less anxiety, and have better physical health than ineffective problem solvers (Heppner, Reeder, and Larson, 1983). In randomized trials, PST has had beneficial effects on psychological well-being and adherence (D'Zurilla, 1986). For example, Nezu (1986) found that among persons diagnosed with unipolar depression, those randomized to PST reported increases in self-appraised problem-solving effectiveness and reductions in depressive symptoms. In a follow-up dismantling study, the problem orientation step (the first step described earlier in this section) was found to be critical to PST efficacy (Nezu and Perri, 1989). Interventions that include problem-solving skills have also been shown to improve adjustment and adherence to self-care regimens in cancer patients (Glanz and Lerman, 1992; Fawzy and others, 1990; Andersen, 1992).

Application: Interventions to Improve Coping with HIV/AIDS

Persons who receive a diagnosis of HIV disease or AIDS often react with a mixture of emotions, including shock, depression, hopelessness, grief, anger, and fear. Later, disease progression is accompanied by diminished social and physical functioning, financial resources and corresponding financial well-being, and quality of life (Chesney and Folkman, 1994). In HIV-infected individuals, psychosocial and behavioral factors may explain some of the variation in disease progression that is not predicted by biological (for example, immunological and serological) factors. Behavioral factors of interest include referral to medical care, initiation of that care, and adherence to treatment. Psychosocial factors such as coping and social support may affect both disease progression and quality of life. For example, one study of 736 people with AIDS found that they practiced a variety of coping behaviors categorized as positive coping, social support seeking, and avoidance coping. These coping behaviors were associated with health behaviors (for example, history of injected drug use), affect (for example, depressive symptoms), and disease progression (as indicated by symptoms) in both cross-sectional and longitudinal analyses (Fleishman and Vogel, 1994). A second study also found that positive psychological well-being of both symptomatic and asymptomatic men with AIDS-related conditions was associated with higher perceived social support and less frequent use of avoidant coping strategies (Kurdek and Siesky, 1990).

Because coping can influence outcomes of both disease progression and quality of life, stress management interventions hold promise for improving adaptation. Several types of interventions have been successful in enhancing adaptive coping and reducing distress. These include structured group interventions (Fawzy, Namir, and Wolcott, 1989), a group cognitive-behavioral stress management program for HIV-positive men (Antoni and others, 1991), and exercise training (LaPerriere, Fletcher, and Klimas, 1991).

Coping Effectiveness Training (CET) intervention, a group-based program based on the Transactional Model (Lazarus and Folkman, 1984), was developed and evaluated by the Center for AIDS Prevention Studies at the University of California. A detailed description of CET and its evaluation can be found in Chesney and Folkman (1994). The intervention is based on the view of stress as a person-environment transaction mediated by processes of cognitive appraisal and coping. The *metastrategy* taught in CET emphasizes building participants' skills to tailor coping strategies to specific stressful situations. This approach distinguishes CET from earlier cognitive-behavioral interventions for HIV/AIDS because previous strategies have developed individuals' skills for using only a few coping processes and sometimes only one (Fawzy, Namir, and Wolcott, 1989; Antoni and others, 1991).

CET involves two phases: training and maintenance. The training phase consists of weekly two-hour sessions and a daylong retreat. The maintenance phase includes bimonthly group meetings for one year. Skills taught in CET include appraising stressful situations, employing various approaches to problem- and emotion-focused coping, matching coping strategies to appraised stressors, using social support for coping assistance, and using cognitive-behavioral strategies to enhance self-efficacy and maintenance.

The CET program was evaluated in a controlled pilot study with twenty HIV-positive and twenty HIV-negative homosexual men. Subjects knew they were HIV-positive, had not been diagnosed with AIDS, and had depressed mood but were not under psychiatric care. The randomized design included four groups: one CET group and one waiting-list control group each for HIV-positive and HIV-negative participants. Results of the pilot study showed that CET could improve coping and positive morale and ease depression among both HIV-positive and HIV-negative men. The effect was associated with reduction in self-blame coping and shifts in coping profiles that reflected increased use of adaptive coping strategies (for example, problem solving and positive reappraisal) and reduced use of maladaptive coping strategies (for example, avoidance and self-blame) (Chesney and Folkman,

1994). Based on the findings of the pilot study, a larger clinical trial is under way. It will examine the effects of CET on immune function as well as mood and morale among HIV-positive men (Chesney and Folkman, 1994).

The CET intervention is unique in its derivation from the Transactional Model and its attention to developing skills to *match* coping strategies to stressful situations. Even though it is a rather intensive intervention, it may nonetheless be a cost-effective approach to slow or halt the progression of HIV/AIDS and to improve functioning and quality of life. Although the CET pilot study did not address the intervention's impact (if any) on other health care behaviors, this type of intervention might also affect referral success, adherence, and continuity of care. Other, more narrow interventions may also be beneficial with AIDS patients and those with other serious chronic diseases. It would ultimately be useful to compare the relative advantages of different intervention approaches.

Conclusion

The theory and research presented in this chapter illustrate the complexities of stress and the effects of coping on psychological well-being, health behavior, and health. This work suggests that the outcomes of the stress and coping process are determined by an interplay of situational factors, individual appraisals of the situation, and the coping strategies employed. No particular pattern of relationships among these factors has been related consistently to positive outcomes of the coping process. Rather, the effects of stress and coping processes depend on context (for example, controllability of the stressor), timing (short- versus long-term adaptation), and individual characteristics (for example, information-processing styles).

Although it is difficult to offer simple generalizations about the adaptiveness of specific coping processes or the efficacy of interventions, the extensive research conducted in this area has several implications for the practice of health promotion and health education. First, because individuals' emotional and health behavior responses to health threats are influenced to a large degree by their subjective interpretations, these appraisals must be assessed. For example, in a study of the determinants of lifestyle practices of cancer patients following treatment, the interventionist should assess primary appraisals (for example, perceptions of risk of recurrence), secondary appraisals (for example, self-efficacy in adopting health behavior recommendations), and specific coping strategies (for example, both problem-focused and emotion-focused coping). The inclusion of appraisal assessments is expected to increase the predictive validity of the model for lifestyle practices and to provide useful information about appraisals that facilitate versus those that hinder such practices. Such information can be useful for designing motivational messages and coping skills training techniques to be incorporated into standardized health promotion interventions for the population at issue.

A second implication of research on stress and coping relates to dispositional coping styles. As described in this chapter, coping strategies are likely to be beneficial to the extent that they fit with the features of the stressful situation and with the individual's own needs for information, control, and level of optimism versus pessimism. Incorporation of coping styles assessments into health promotion and psychoeducational interventions will facilitate the tailoring of these strategies to individual needs. As yet, there are no published studies of the efficacy of interventions tailored to these dispositional coping styles. However, in the smoking cessation area, interventions tailored to individuals' smoking behaviors and readiness to quit appear very promising (Curry, 1993; Velicer and others, 1993). Research on stress, coping, and health behavior suggests that interventions tailored to individual appraisals and coping behaviors are likely to be most effective in terms of enhancing coping, reducing stress, and improving health behavior and physical well-being.

References

Affleck, G., Tennen, H., Pfeiffer, C., and Fifield, H. "Appraisals of Control and Predictability in Adapting to a Chronic Stress." *Journal of Personality and Social Psychology*, 1987, *53*, 273–279.

Andersen, B. L. "Psychological Interventions for Cancer Patients to Enhance the Quality of Life." *Journal of Consulting and Clinical Psychology*, 1992, *60*(4), 552–568.

Antoni, M. H., and others. "Cognitive Behavioral Stress Management Intervention Buffers, Distress Responses, and Immunologic Changes Following Notification of HIV-1 Seropositivity." *Journal of Consulting and Clinical Psychology*, 1991, *59*, 906–913.

Antonovsky, A. *Health, Stress, and Coping.* San Francisco: Jossey-Bass, 1979.

Antonovsky, A., and Kats, R. "The Life Crisis History as a Tool in Epidemiologic Research." *Journal of Health and Social Behavior*, 1967, *8*, 15–20.

Aspinwall, L. G., and Taylor, S. E. "Modeling Cognitive Adaptation: A Longitudinal Investigation of the Impact of Individual Differences and Coping on College Adjustment and Performance." *Journal of Personality and Social Psychology*, 1992, *63*(6), 989–1003.

Bandura, A. "Human Agency in Social Cognitive Theory." *American Psychologist*, 1989, *44*, 1175–1184.

Baron, R. M., and Kenny, D. A. "The Moderator-Mediator Variable Distinction in Social Psychological Research: Conceptual, Strategic, and Statistical Considerations." *Journal of Personality and Social Psychology*, 1986, *51*(6), 1173–1182.

Benson, H. "The Relaxation Response and Stress." In J. D. Matarazzo and others (eds.), *Behavioral Health: A Handbook of Health Enhancement and Disease Prevention.* New York: Wiley, 1984.

Bliss, R. E., Garvey, A. J., and Heinold, J. W. "The Influence of Situation and Coping on Relapse Crisis Outcomes After Smoking Cessation." *Journal of Consulting and Clinical Psychology*, 1989, *57*(3), 443–449.

Borysenko, J. "Stress, Coping, and the Immune System." In J. D. Matarazzo and others (eds.), *Behavioral Health: A Handbook of Health Enhancement and Disease Prevention.* New York: Wiley, 1984.

Brandon, T. H., Copeland, A. L., and Saper, Z. L. "Programmed Therapeutic Messages as a Smoking Treatment Adjunct: Reducing the Impact of Negative Affect." *Health Psychology*, 1995, *14*(1), 41–47.

Brownell, K. D. "Personal Responsibility and Control Over Our Bodies: When Expectation Exceeds Reality." *Health Psychology*, 1991, *10*(5), 303–310.

Cannon, W. B. *The Wisdom of the Body.* New York: Norton, 1932.

Carver, C. S., Scheier, M. F., and Weintraub, J. K. "Assessing Coping Strategies: A Theoretically Based Approach." *Journal of Personality and Social Psychology*, 1989, *56*, 267–283.

Carver, C. S., and others. "How Coping Mediates the Effect of Optimism on Distress: A Study of Women with Early Stage Breast Cancer." *Journal of Personality and Social Psychology*, 1993, *65*(2), 375–390.

Chapman, S., Wong, W. L., and Smith, W. "Self-Exempting Beliefs About Smoking and Health: Differences Between Smokers and Ex-Smokers." *American Journal of Public Health*, 1993, *83*, 215–219.

Chesney, M. A., and Folkman, S. "Psychological Impact of HIV Disease and Implications for Intervention." *Psychiatric Clinics of North America*, 1994, *17*, 163–182.

Claus, E. B., Risch, N. J., and Thompson, W. D. "Age at Onset as an Indicator of Familial Risk of Breast Cancer." *American Journal of Epidemiology*, 1990, *131*(6), 961–972.

Cohen, F. "Coping." In J. D. Matarazzo and others (eds.), *Behavioral Health: A Handbook of Health Enhancement and Disease Prevention.* New York: Wiley, 1984.

Cohen, F., and Lazarus, R. S. "Coping with the Stress of Illness." In G. C. Stone, F. Cohen, and N. E. Adler (eds.), *Health Psychology: A Handbook.* San Francisco: Jossey-Bass, 1979.

Cohen, S., and Hoberman, H. M. "Positive Events and Social Supports as Buffers of Life Change Stress." *Journal of Applied Social Psychology*, 1983, *13*(2), 99–125.

Cohen, S., and McKay, G. "Social Support, Stress and the Buffering Hypothesis: A Theoretical Analysis." In A. Baum, J. E. Singer, and S. E. Taylor (eds.), *Handbook of Psychology and Health.* Vol. 4. Hillsdale, N.J.: Erlbaum, 1984.

Cohen, S., and Wills, T. A. "Stress, Social Support, and the Buffering Hypothesis." *Psychological Bulletin*, 1985, *98*(2), 310–357.

Croyle, R. T. "Appraisal of Health Threats: Cognition, Motivation, and Social Comparison." *Cognitive Therapy and Research*, 1992, *16*(2), 165–182.

Croyle, R. T., and Sandman, G. N. "Denial and Confirmatory Search: Paradoxical Consequences of Medical Diagnosis." *Journal of Applied Social Psychology*, 1988, *18*, 473–490.

Curry, S. J. "Self-Help Interventions for Smoking Cessation." *Journal of Consulting and Clinical Psychology*, 1993, *61*(5), 790–803.

Ditto, P. H., and Croyle, R. T. "Understanding the Impact of Risk Factor Test Results: Insights from a Basic Research Program." In R. T. Croyle (ed.), *Psychosocial Effects of Screening for Disease Prevention and Detection.* New York: Oxford University Press, 1995.

Dohrenwend, B. S., and Dohrenwend, B. P. *Stressful Life Events and Their Contexts.* New York: Prodist, 1981.

D'Zurilla, T. J. *Problem-Solving Therapy: A Social Competence Approach to Clinical Intervention.* New York: Springer, 1986.

Endler, N., and Parker, J. "Multidimensional Assessment of Coping: A Critical Evaluation." *Journal of Personality and Social Psychology,* 1990, *58,* 844–854.

Ewart, C. K., Taylor, C. B., Reese, L. B., and Debusk, R. F. "Effects of Early Postmyocardial Infarction Exercise Testing on Self-Perception and Subsequent Physical Activity." *American Journal of Cardiology,* 1983, *51,* 1076–1080.

Fawzy, F. I., and others. "A Structured Psychiatric Intervention of Cancer Patients: 1. Changes over Time in Methods of Coping and Affective Disturbance." *Archives of General Psychiatry,* 1990, *47,* 720–725.

Fawzy, I., Namir, S., and Wolcott, D. "Group Intervention with Newly Diagnosed AIDS Patients." *Psychiatric Medicine,* 1989, *7,* 35–46.

Fleishman J. A., and Vogel, B. Coping and Depressive Symptoms Among People with AIDS. *Health Psychology,* 1994, *13*(2), 156–169.

Folkman, S., Chesney, M. A., Pollack, L., and Phillips, C. "Stress, Coping, and High-Risk Sexual Behavior." *Health Psychology,* 1992, *11*(4), 218–222.

Folkman, S., and Lazarus, R. S. "An Analysis of Coping in a Middle-Aged Community Sample." *Journal of Health and Social Behavior,* 1980, *21,* 219–239.

Folkman, S., and others. "Dynamics of a Stressful Encounter: Cognitive Appraisal, Coping, and Encounter Outcomes." *Personality and Social Psychology,* 1986, *50*(5), 992–1003.

Folkman, S., and others. "Translating Coping Theory into an Intervention." In J. Eckenrode (ed.), *The Social Context of Coping.* New York: Plenum, 1991.

French, J.R.P., and Kahn, R. L. "A Programmatic Approach to Studying the Industrial Environment and Mental Health." *Journal of Social Issues,* 1962, *18,* 1–47.

Gill, M. J., and Harris, S. L. "Hardiness and Social Support as Predictors of Psychological Discomfort in Mothers of Children with Autism." *Journal of Autism and Developmental Disorders,* 1991, *21*(4), 407–416.

Glanz, K., and Lerman, C. "Psychosocial Impact of Breast Cancer: A Critical Review." *Annals of Behavioral Medicine,* 1992, *14*(3), 204–212.

Haaga, D. A., and Davison, G. C. "Cognitive Changes Methods." In F. H. Kanfer and A. P. Goldstein, *Helping People Change.* New York: Pergamon Press, 1991.

Hallal, J. C. "The Relationship of Health Beliefs, Health Locus of Control, and Self-Concept to the Practice of Breast Self-Examination in Adult Women." *Nursing Research,* 1982, *31*(3), 137–142.

Heitzmann, C. A., and Kaplan, R. M. "Assessment of Methods for Measuring Social Support." *Health Psychology,* 1988, *7*(1), 75–109.

Heppner, P. P., Reeder, B. L., and Larson, L. M. "Cognitive Variables Associated with Personal Problem-Solving Appraisal: Implications for Counseling." *Journal of Counseling and Psychology,* 1983, *30,* 537–545.

Hinkle, L. E. "The Effect of Exposure to Cultural Change, Social Change, and Changes in Interpersonal Relationships on Health." In B. S. Dohrenwend and B. P. Dohrenwend (eds.), *Stressful Life Events: Their Nature and Effects.* New York: Wiley, 1974.

Holahan, C. J., and Moos, R. H. "Personality, Coping, and Family Resources in Stress Resistance: A Longitudinal Analysis." *Journal of Personality and Social Psychology,* 1986, *51*(2), 389–395.

Holmes, T. H., and Rahe, R. H. "The Social Readjustment Rating Scale." *Journal of Psychosomatic Research,* 1967, *11,* 213–218.

House, J. S. "Occupational Stress and Coronary Heart Disease: A Review and Theoretical Integration." *Journal of Health and Social Behavior,* 1974, *15,* 12–27.

Israel, B. A., and Schurman, S. J. "Social Support, Control, and the Stress Process." In
  K. Glanz, F. M. Lewis, and B. K. Rimer (eds.), *Health Behavior and Health Education: Theory,
  Research, and Practice.* San Francisco: Jossey-Bass, 1990.

Jeffrey, R. W., and others. "Correlates of Weight Loss and Its Maintenance over Two Years of
  Follow-Up Among Middle-Aged Men." *Preventive Medicine,* 1984, *13,* 155–168.

Kang, S. H., and Bloom, J. R. "Social Support and Cancer Screening Among Older Black
  Americans." *Journal of the National Cancer Institute,* 1993, *85*(9), 737–742.

Kanner, A. D., Coyne, J. C., Schaefer, C., and Lazarus, R. S. "Comparison of Two Modes
  of Stress Measurement: Daily Hassles and Uplifts Versus Major Life Events." *Journal of
  Behavioral Medicine,* 1981, *4,* 1–39.

Kaplan, R. M., Sallis, J. F., and Patterson, T. L. "Stress and Coping." In R. M. Kaplan,
  J. F. Sallis, and T. L. Patterson (eds.), *Health and Human Behavior.* New York: McGraw-Hill,
  1993.

Kash, K. M., Holland, J. C., Halper, M. S., and Miller, D. G. "Psychological Distress and
  Surveillance Behaviors of Women with a Family History of Breast Cancer." *Journal of the
  National Cancer Institute,* 1992, *84,* 24–30.

Kiecolt-Glaser, J. K., and Glaser, R. "Psychoneuroimmunology and Health Consequences:
  Data and Shared Mechanisms." *Psychosomatic Medicine,* 1995, *57,* 269–274.

Kobasa, S. C. "Stressful Life Events, Personality, and Health: An Inquiry into Hardiness."
  Journal of Personality and Social Psychology, 1979, *37,* 1–11.

Kobasa, S. C., Maddi, S. R., and Kahn, S. "Hardiness and Health: A Prospective Study."
  Journal of Personality and Social Psychology, 1982, *42,* 168–177.

Kurdek, L. A., and Siesky, G. "The Nature and Correlates of Psychological Adjustment in
  Gay Men with AIDS-Related Conditions." *Journal of Applied Social Psychology,* 1990, *20,*
  846–860.

LaPerriere, A., Fletcher, M., and Klimas, N. "Aerobic Training in an AIDS Risk Group."
  International Journal of Sports Medicine, 1991, *12,* S53–S57.

Lazarus, R. S. *Psychological Stress and the Coping Process.* New York: McGraw-Hill, 1966.

Lazarus, R. S. *Emotion and Adaptation.* New York: Oxford University Press, 1991a.

Lazarus, R. S. "Progress on a Cognitive-Motivational-Relational Theory of Emotion." *American Psychologist,* 1991b, *46*(8), 819–834.

Lazarus, R. S. "Coping Theory and Research: Past, Present, and Future." *Psychosomatic Medicine,* 1993, *55,* 234–247.

Lazarus, R. S., and Cohen, J. B. "Environmental Stress." In I. Altman and J. F. Wohlwill
  (eds.), *Human Behavior and Environment.* Vol. 2. New York: Plenum, 1977.

Lazarus, R. S., and Folkman, S. *Stress, Appraisal, and Coping.* New York: Springer, 1984.

Lerman, C., Daly, M., Masny, A., and Balshem, A. "Attitudes About Genetic Testing for
  Breast-Ovarian Cancer Susceptibility." *Journal of Clinical Oncology,* 1994, *12*(4), 843–850.

Lerman, C., and Schwartz, M. "Adherence and Psychological Adjustment Among Women at
  High Risk for Breast Cancer." *Breast Cancer Research and Treatment,* 1993, *28,* 145–155.

Lerman, C., and others. "Effects of Coping Style and Relaxation on Cancer Chemotherapy
  Side Effects and Emotional Responses." *Cancer Nursing,* 1990, *13*(5), 308–315.

Lerman, C., and others. "Mammography Adherence and Psychological Distress Among
  Women at Risk for Breast Cancer." *Journal of the National Cancer Institute,* 1993, *85*(13),
  1074–1080.

Lerman, C., and others. "Counseling Women at Increased Risk for Breast Cancer." National
  Cancer Institute Grant no. RO1 CA63605, 1993–1997.

Lerman, C., and others. "A Randomized Trial of Breast Cancer Risk Counseling: Interacting Effects of Counseling, Education Level and Coping Style." *Health Psychology*, 1996, *15*, 75–83.

Lewis, F. M., and Daltroy, L. "How Causal Explanations Influence Health Behavior: Attribution Theory." In K. Glanz, F. M. Lewis, and B. K. Rimer (eds.), *Health Behavior and Health Education: Theory, Research, and Practice.* San Francisco: Jossey-Bass, 1990.

Littlefield, C. H., Rodin, G. M., Murray, M. A., and Craven, J. L. "Influence of Functional Impairment and Social Support on Depressive Symptoms in Persons with Diabetes." *Health Psychology*, 1990, *9*(6), 737–749.

Lowery, B. J., Jacobsen, B. S., and DuCette, J. "Causal Attribution, Control, and Adjustment to Breast Cancer." *Journal of Psychosocial Oncology*, 1993, *10*(4), 37–53.

Manne, S., and Taylor, K. "Support-Related Interactions Between Women with Cancer and Their Healthy Partners." Presented at the annual meeting of the American Psychological Association, Toronto, Aug. 1993.

Marks, G., Richardson, J. L., Graham, J. W., and Levine, A. "Role of Health Locus on Control Beliefs and Expectations of Treatment Efficacy in Adjustment to Cancer." *Journal of Personality and Social Psychology*, 1986, *51*(2), 443–450.

Miller, S. M. "Monitoring and Blunting: Validation of a Questionnaire to Assess Styles of Information Seeking Under Threat." *Journal of Personality and Social Psychology*, 1987, *52*, 345–353.

Miller, S. M., and Mangan, C. E. "The Interacting Effects of Information and Coping Style in Adapting to Gynecological Stress: Should the Doctor Tell All?" *Journal of Personality and Social Psychology*, 1983, *45*, 223–236.

Nezu, A. M. "Efficacy of a Social Problem-Solving Therapy Approach for Unipolar Depression." *Journal of Consulting and Clinical Psychology*, 1986, *54*(2), 196–202.

Nezu, A. M., and Perri, M. G. "Social Problem-Solving Therapy of Unipolar Depression: An Initial Dismantling Investigation." *Journal of Consulting and Clinical Psychology*, 1989, *57*(3), 408–413.

Pennebaker, J. W. *Opening Up: The Healing Power of Confiding in Others.* New York: Morrow, 1990.

Pennebaker, J. W., and O'Heeron, R. C. "Confiding in Others and Illness Rate Among Spouses of Suicide and Accidental Death Victims." *Journal of Abnormal Psychology*, 1984, *93*, 473–476.

Phipps, S., and Zinn, A. B. "Psychological Response to Amniocentesis: II. Effects of Coping Style." *American Journal of Medical Genetics*, 1986, *25*, 143–148.

Prochaska, J. O., DiClemente, C. C., and Norcross, J. C. "In Search of How People Change: Applications to the Addictive Behaviors." *American Psychologist*, 1992, *47*(9), 1102–1114.

Reed, G. M., and others. "Realistic Acceptance as a Predictor of Decreased Survival Time in Gay Men with AIDS." *Health Psychology*, 1994, *13*(4), 299–307.

Reifman, A. "Social Relationships, Recovery from Illness, and Survival: A Literature Review." *Annals of Behavioral Medicine*, 1995, *17*(2), 124–131.

Rotter, J. B. "Generalized Expectancies for Internal Versus External Control of Reinforcement." *Psychological Monographs*, 1966, *80*(1), 1–28.

Sarason, I. G., Johnson, J. H., and Siegel, J. M. "Assessing the Impact of Life Changes: Development of the Life Experiences Survey." *Journal of Consulting and Clinical Psychology*, 1978, *46*, 932–946.

Scheier, M. F., and Bridges, M. W. "Person Variables and Health: Personality and Predispositions and Acute Psychological States as Shared Determinants for Disease." *Psychosomatic Medicine*, 1995, *57*, 255–268.

Scheier, M. F., and Carver, C. S. "Optimism, Coping, and Health: Assessment and Implications of Generalized Outcome Expectancies." *Health Psychology*, 1985, *4*(3), 219–247.

Scheier, M. F., and Carver, C. S. "Dispositional Optimism and Physical Well-Being: The Influence of Generalized Outcome Expectancies on Health." *Journal of Personality*, 1987, *55*(2), 169–210.

Scheier, M. F., and Carver, C. S. "Effects of Optimism on Psychological and Physical Well-Being: Theoretical Overview and Empirical Update." *Cognitive Therapy and Research*, 1992, *16*(2), 201–228.

Scheier, M. F., and others. "Dispositional Optimism and Recovery from Coronary Artery Bypass Surgery: The Beneficial Effects on Physical and Psychological Well-Being." *Journal of Personality and Social Psychology*, 1989, *57*, 1024–1040.

Schonfeld, I. S. "Dimensions of Functional Social Support and Psychological Symptoms." *Psychological Medicine*, 1991, *21*(4), 1051–1060.

Schwartz, M. D., and others. "Coping Disposition, Perceived Risk, and Psychological Distress Among Women at Increased Risk for Ovarian Cancer." *Health Psychology*, 1995, *14*(3), 232–235.

Selye, H. *The Stress of Life*. New York: McGraw-Hill, 1956.

Smith, C. A., Haynes, K. N., Lazarus, R. S., and Pope, L. K. "In Search of the 'Hot' Cognitions: Attributions, Appraisals, and Their Relation to Emotion." *Journal of Personality and Social Psychology*, 1993, *65*(5), 916–929.

Smith, C. A., and Lazarus, R. S. "Appraisal Components, Core Relational Themes, and the Emotions." *Cognition and Emotion*, 1993, *7*(3–4), 233–269.

Steptoe, A., and Sullivan, J. "Monitoring and Blunting Coping Styles in Women Prior to Surgery." *British Journal of Clinical Psychology*, 1986, *24*, 143–144.

Stone, A., Greenberg, M., Kennedy-Moore, E., and Newman, M. "Self Report, Situation-Specific Coping Questionnaires: What Are They Measuring?" *Journal of Personality and Social Psychology*, 1991, *61*, 648–658.

Stone, A., Kennedy-Moore, E., and Neale, J. "Coping with Daily Problems." *Health Psychology*, forthcoming.

Stone, A., and Neale, J. "A New Measure of Daily Coping: Development and Preliminary Results." *Journal of Personality and Social Psychology*, 1984, *46*, 892–906.

Stone, A. A., and Porter, L. S. "Psychological Coping: Its Importance for Treating Medical Problems." *Mind/Body Medicine*, 1995, *1*, 46–54.

Strecher, V. J., DeVellis, B. M., Becker, M. H., and Rosenstock, I. M. "The Role of Self-Efficacy in Achieving Health Behavior Change." *Health Education Quarterly*, 1986, *13*(1), 73–91.

Suls, J., and Fletcher, B. "The Relative Efficacy of Avoidant and Nonavoidance Coping Strategies: A Meta-Analysis." *Health Psychology*, 1985, *4*(3), 249–288.

Taylor, S. E., Helgeson, V. S., Reed, G. M., and Skokan, L. A. "Self-Generated Feelings of Control and Adjustment to Physical Illness." *Journal of Social Issues*, 1991, *47*, 91–109.

Taylor, S. E., Lichtman, R. R., and Wood, J. V. "Attributions, Beliefs About Control and Adjustment to Breast Cancer." *Journal of Personality and Social Psychology*, 1984, *46*(3), 489–502.

Taylor, S. E., and others. "Optimism, Coping, Psychological Distress, and High-Risk Sexual Behavior Among Men at Risk for Acquired Immunodeficiency Syndrome (AIDS)." *Journal of Personality and Social Psychology*, 1992, *63*(3), 460–473.

Thompson, S. C., and Spacapan, S. "Perceptions of Control in Vulnerable Populations." *Journal of Social Issues*, 1991, *47*(4), 1–21.

Thompson, S. C., and others. "Maintaining Perceptions of Control: Finding Perceived Control in Low-Control Circumstances." *Journal of Personality and Social Psychology*, 1993, *64*(2), 293–304.

Timko, C., and Janoff-Bulman, R. "Attributions, Vulnerability, and Psychological Adjustment: The Case of Breast Cancer." *Health Psychology*, 1985, *4*(6), 521–544.

Velicer, W. F., and others. "An Expert System Intervention for Smoking Cessation." *Addictive Behaviors*, 1993, *18*, 269–290.

Vogel, V. G., and others. "Mammographic Screening of Women with Increased Risk of Breast Cancer." *Cancer*, 1990, *66*, 1613–1620.

Wallston, K. A., and Wallston, B. S. "Locus of Control and Health: A Review of the Literature." *Health Education Monographs*, 1978, *6*(2), 107–117.

Wardle, F. J., and others. "Psychological Impact of Screening for Familial Ovarian Cancer." *Journal of the National Cancer Institute*, 1993, *85*, 653–657.

Weinstein, N. D. "Optimistic Biases About Personal Risks." *Science*, Dec. 8, 1989, pp. 1232–1233.

Williams, R. B., and others. "Prognostic Importance of Social and Economic Resources Among Medically Treated Patients with Angiographically Documented Coronary Artery Disease." *Journal of the American Medical Association*, 1992, *267*, 520–524.

CHAPTER SEVEN

PERSPECTIVES ON INTRAPERSONAL THEORIES OF HEALTH BEHAVIOR

Barbara K. Rimer

We must understand theories that focus on the behavior of individuals if we are to change or explain individual health behavior. Part Two of this book describes four well-developed theories and models of health behavior: the Health Belief Model, the Theory of Reasoned Action and its companion, the Theory of Planned Behavior, The Transtheoretical Model, and theories of stress and coping. The theories and models included in this section were among the most widely cited in a literature search that uncovered 104 different theories of health behavior.

The Health Belief Model is one of the oldest and most resilient models of health behavior, and it has remained remarkably useful over time. The Theory of Reasoned Action and its later extension, the Theory of Planned Behavior, also have been robust models, used to study a wide range of health behaviors. The TRA and the HBM were discussed in the first edition of this book, also. The present edition incorporates two new theories. In the first edition, The Transtheoretical Model (TTM) was presented as a developing model. Now widely used in the study of health behavior, it deserves to stand on its own in a separate chapter in this edition. The other new theory presented in this edition is the Transactional Model of Stress and Coping. Models of stress and coping are especially appropriate in understanding the health behavior of high-risk populations and patients.

To conclude Part Two and the discussion of theory, this chapter considers some further perspectives on each of the four theories that have been presented and offers some thoughts on new theoretical directions.

The Health Belief Model

As Strecher and Rosenstock write in Chapter Three, the Health Belief Model (HBM) has been used "both to explain change and maintenance of health behavior and as a guiding framework for health behavior interventions."

The HBM is one of the few sociopsychological models to be developed expressly to understand health behavior. Health professionals have gained long experience with the model in a variety of health contexts, beginning with efforts to explain people's tuberculosis screening behaviors. A critical dimension of the HBM, the failure to believe in the possibility of having pathology in the absence of symptoms, is as relevant today in studying cancer, AIDS, and other diseases as it was in helping to explain tuberculosis screening behavior in the 1950s. Degree of belief in asymptomatology is probably a critical variable in explaining participation in cancer screening. We have learned, for example, that women are often reluctant to obtain mammograms when they are feeling healthy, even when they "know" that a mammogram can detect something too small to be found by a woman or her physician in any other way. It appears that it may take a belief in asymptomatology, almost an act of faith, to perform the behavior.

One of the most appealing aspects of the Health Belief Model is its acceptance not only by health educators but by psychologists, physicians, dentists, nurses, and other professionals. It has a sort of intuitive logic, the central tenets are clearly stated, and beliefs can be measured by a variety of techniques ranging from clinical interviews to population-based surveys. Mullen, Hersey, and Iverson (1987) have shown that the HBM is an economical model in terms of the number of questions needed to assess the key variables.

The Health Belief Model has been evaluated, and its limitations, too, have become evident. Critics might argue that according to the strictest definitions of theory, the HBM is not a theory at all. Certainly, it never has had the kind of rigorous quantification that Fishbein and Ajzen (1975) have achieved with the Theory of Reasoned Action. However, as Janz and Becker (1984) have shown, most of the concepts in the model have received some empirical support.

Some components of the Health Belief Model still are not well understood, and others, such as severity, have low predictive value. The concept of cue to action deserves further study and experimental manipulation. Chapter Three authors Strecher and Rosenstock also point out that we need to know more about the role of fear and how it may foster cognitive and behavioral changes. Other theoretical models, such as Protection Motivation Theory (Prentice-Dunn and Rogers, 1986), the Precaution Adoption Model (Weinstein, 1988), and Self-

Regulation Theory (Leventhal and Cameron, 1987), used in combination with the Health Belief Model, may be helpful in gaining this knowledge.

Strecher and Rosenstock have cautioned researchers and practitioners alike to be mindful of how the HBM is measured and analyzed. That is good advice. It is tempting to choose some components of the HBM on which to focus, but when a theory is taken out of context, the results may be both disappointing and difficult to explain.

In a particularly useful discussion, the authors of Chapter Three show that the HBM may be applicable to addictive behaviors. As they point out, people's beliefs have been understudied, and perceptions of threat and risk may play a central role in a smoker's readiness to quit. A combination of the HBM and the TTM might be appropriate for this purpose. The HBM can elucidate the personal beliefs that serve as barriers to quitting, and the TTM can characterize a person's stage and suggest interventions based on processes of change (Rimer, 1995).

The Health Belief Model is a thoroughly modern theory. Researchers and practitioners should be challenged to use the theory both to develop interventions and to evaluate them. One of the most significant HBM studies was conducted by Becker and Maiman (1980) in examining potential Tay-Sachs carriers. It may be especially timely to consider the HBM as a model for studying responses to genetic susceptibility testing.

The Theory of Reasoned Action and the Theory of Planned Behavior

The Theory of Reasoned Action (TRA) and the Theory of Planned Behavior (TPB), discussed in Chapter Five, share with the Health Belief Model roots in the tradition of value expectancy theories; however, the TRA and TPB are newer theories, dating to the late 1960s. As chapter authors Montaño, Kasprzyk, and Taplin discuss, these theories grew out of a need to understand the relationship between attitudes and behavior. The TRA and TPB assume a causal chain that links behavioral beliefs and normative beliefs to behavior through attitudes and subjective norms.

The Theory of Planned Behavior is a refinement of the Theory of Reasoned Action to include perceived behavioral control. This is an improvement and addresses concerns that the TRA is overly rational. The addition of perceived behavioral control means that all the theories discussed in Part Two include a variable akin to self-efficacy—a central variable in health education and health behavior research. But as the chapter authors note, one of the limitations of the TRA and TPB is that they are not behavioral change theories. They explain relationships between different types of beliefs, intentions, and behaviors. They might be used in conjunction with other theories described in this book when the goal is to develop interventions.

Fishbein and Ajzen (1975; Ajzen and Fishbein, 1980) have devoted much of their research effort to specifying the concepts within the Theory of Reasoned Action and, more recently, the Theory of Planned Behavior. The authors of Part Two have shown how each of the concepts, such as attitude toward the act, subjective norm, and behavioral intention, can be operationalized. Because their components have been so well codified, the TRA and TPB come closest of all the theories discussed here to meeting Kerlinger's strict definition of theory.

With increased precision of measurement has come improved precision of prediction. The theories are most predictive when the concepts are defined specifically and are measured in close temporal order. The TRA and TPB provide a method for systematically identifying those issues that are most important to a person's decisions about performing a specific behavior. The end product of these efforts is to identify important, mutable beliefs and attitudes for subsequent use in behavioral interventions. But the strategies for designing interventions must come from other theories.

One of the most important characteristics of the TRA and TPB is that they are grounded. In other words, preliminary work assures that they are grounded in issues relevant to the behavior and population of interest. It is easy to overlook important salient beliefs and attitudes when one does not use rigorous, comprehensive methods in collecting data prior to developing interventions.

Although very appealing, especially from a methodological point of view, the TRA and TPB do have limitations. Mullen, Hersey, and Iverson (1987) criticized the Theory of Reasoned Action as almost entirely rational and not recognizing emotional fear-arousal elements such as perceived susceptibility to illnesses. Thus, to explain behavior better, the TRA and TPB might need supplementation by the Health Belief Model or another theory, such as Protection Motivation Theory (Rogers and Mewborn, 1976) or Self-Regulation Theory (Leventhal and Cameron, 1987).

Further, the measurements required by the TRA and TPB models, even though powerful for prediction, may be cumbersome and time consuming in practice. They rely on extensive interviewer-administered personal interviews. Although ultimately useful, this can be a demanding, costly process. Collecting more than pilot data may be beyond the resources of most practitioners and can be laborious when programs must be developed quickly. Simplification of the theories for practice would make them more accessible to practitioners, who could then more easily use the constructs of the TRA and TPB to better understand, predict, and measure health behavior as well as to help people make better choices about health behavior.

The Transtheoretical Model

As mentioned earlier, The Transtheoretical Model, classified as a developing theory in the first edition of this book, has matured and been diffused so that it is now one of the most widely used models of health behavior, employed not just by health educators and psychologists but also by nurses, physicians, and other health providers. The Transtheoretical Model, discussed in Chapter Four, is directly applicable to practitioners' work, and this is one of the reasons it has become so widely accepted. Another reason for its widespread acceptance surely is its intuitive appeal. Treating people as though they are all the same will inevitably dilute the impact of interventions. The TTM allows practitioners to treat individuals as individuals. To make greater progress in some areas of behavioral science—for example, finding ways to further reduce the number of smokers and achieve greater public health impact—practitioners will have to learn to reach people in the precontemplation and contemplation stages (see Chapter Four). As Lerman, Orleans, and Engstrom (1993) and Abrams, Marlatt, and Sobell (1995) have observed, the vast majority (75 percent) of smokers are in these early stages.

Indeed, a paradigm shift has occurred, making The Transtheoretical Model one of the most popular models of health behavior. The TTM recognizes that people in the process of change should have access to interventions that start at their stage in the change process. For example, if a smoker has not started thinking about what smoking is doing to her, there is no point in providing detailed information about behavioral coping processes. It would be far better to raise her consciousness regarding the personal harms associated with smoking and the benefits to be achieved from quitting. This is not very different from the health education principle that Minkler discusses in Chapter Twelve in addressing community organization—start where the people are. Once the stage of change has been assessed, people can be provided with therapist-guided or self-initiated interventions that meet their needs.

Some important questions about the TTM remain. For example, must the processes of change always be measured? It certainly adds to the measurement burden. How many stages really exist? As the authors of Chapter Four discussed, that definition has changed over time. More attention also should be paid to extending the model to other populations, especially low-income and minority populations. For example, Tessaro and others (1996) found that Prochaska, DiClemente, Velicer, and Rossi's smoking pros and cons scale (1982) had little relevance to low-income African Americans in Durham, North Carolina. However, Rimer and others (forthcoming) found mammography pro-con scales developed by Rakowski and others (1993) to be very robust when applied to African Americans. As the TTM is extended to new health care settings and to screening behaviors, stage definitions will become more complex. For example, Rakowski and others (1993) found it necessary to add a relapse risk stage for mammography.

More research is also needed to determine what kinds of interventions are best for people in what stages. Although there has been some work in this area, far too little is known about how much and what kind of stage matching is needed. Early results (Prochaska and others, 1982) are encouraging. The TTM has an elegant simplicity, but both researchers and practitioners should be careful to use it wisely, carefully, comprehensively, and critically. Readers are encouraged to review a series of editorials about the TTM that appeared in the *British Journal of Addictions* (Davidson, 1992) for a discussion of some strengths and weaknesses of the TTM.

The Transactional Model of Stress and Coping

The focus now in theories of stress and coping is on the Transactional Model discussed in Chapter Six. The concepts of this model should be understood by those concerned with health education and health behavior. Who has not experienced stress? But one of the interesting things about stress is not only that it affects health (it does!) but that different people experience it differently. Moreover, people cope in individual ways, and some coping mechanisms are better than others. Why does one woman use her breast cancer as a stepping stone to personal growth while another remains locked in bitterness? How the women react to the stress is at least part of the answer.

These models may be especially relevant for the study of high-risk behaviors (for example, smoking and unprotected sex) and at-risk populations (for example, those with a family history of breast cancer and breast cancer patients). Stress and coping models share with the TTM, HBM, and TRA and TPB an emphasis on perceived control that can be defined broadly as self-efficacy.

It may be useful for those thinking about interventions to consider the two dimensions of coping discussed in Chapter Six: problem-focused coping (strategies to change a stressful situation) and emotion-focused coping (strategies to change the way one feels about a situation). Some of the coping methods sound remarkably like the processes of change in the TTM. And that makes sense—there tends to be a relatively finite set of coping behaviors.

Overall, health educators probably have paid too little attention to dispositional styles of coping (for example, information seeking and optimism), and as tailored interventions increasingly become possible, these dispositional styles should be considered.

An understanding of stress and coping can help researchers and practitioners not only to gain a better understanding of health behavior but also to design more effective interventions.

Future Directions

One emerging theory is particularly worthy of attention, and that is Weinstein's Precaution Adoption Model (1988).

The Precaution Adoption Model (PAM) suggests that people go through five stages in modifying their behavior: (1) they deny having heard of the hazard in question; (2) they acknowledge that the hazard poses risk to others; (3) they acknowledge that the hazard poses personal risk; (4) they make the decision to act; and (5) they adopt the behavioral change. The major determinants of each stage vary, although there are commonalities across some stages (Weinstein, 1988). For example, across the first three stages, indirect and direct experience with the hazard and the communication of who is at risk serve to facilitate movement across stages. The stage 3 actions of accepting personal risk (that is, understanding that a serious consequence can occur), and recognizing that a precaution is effective are vital to initiating the decision to act (stage 4). Unfortunately, individuals typically deny personal risk (that is, they are optimistically biased: Weinstein, 1980, 1984, 1987; Perloff and Fetzer, 1986) and are consequently less likely to seek out or pay attention to communication about the hazard (Weinstein, 1988). There may also be cultural determinants of inaccurate risk perceptions; for example, individuals in the Netherlands frequently underestimate their intake of dietary fat, even when it exceeds recommended levels (Brug and others, 1994). Thus, major goals of health interventions that prescribe precautionary behaviors should communicate information about risk that is clear, credible, salient, and personalized, to overcome the biases that may affect receptivity to this communication (Weinstein and Klein, 1995).

The Precaution Adoption Model provides a dynamic *cognitive* framework of behavioral change that emphasizes the important role of risk perceptions. It highlights processes overlooked in other frameworks, such as consideration of costs and benefits over time and the competition between precautionary behaviors and other life demands. The PAM also provides a heuristic model relevant to categorizing people at different stages of behavioral change, and it includes mediating variables amenable to intervention programs. This model has been studied primarily by Weinstein and his collaborators, but given the importance of risk perception, it is one that should be used more widely. It would be appropriate to combine it with the TTM. Both share a stage focus, but the PAM has a stronger emphasis on how people process risks and communications related to risks.

Conclusion

The theories in this section have much in common. Self-efficacy, by some name, is embodied in each of the theories. The concept of readiness (Abrams, personal communication with the author, Jan. 1996) is a central component of both the Health Belief Model and The Transtheoretical Model. Barriers are seen as inhibiting behavioral change in both the HBM and the TTM.

Some of the theories are easier to use than others. Sherry Turkle (1995) wrote about the appeal of appropriable theories, those that can be manipulated and played with. Part of the appeal of the HBM and TTM is undoubtedly that they are appropriable theories.

Each of the authors in Part Two has made clear that measurement is not for the weak-willed or faint of heart. Measurement of the theoretical variables requires the serious attention of those who use these theories to understand behavior and create interventions. The measurement of the TRA and TPB is perhaps most complex because of the need to conduct elicitation interviews prior to developing questionnaires.

Finally, theory is not theology. Theory needs questioners more than loyal followers. The advancement of each of the theories discussed here will come from those who are willing to use these theories, test them, and subject them to rigorous evaluation.

References

Abrams, D. B., Marlatt, G. A., and Sobell, M. G. "Overview of Section II: Treatment, Early Intervention, and Policy." In J. Fertig and R. Allen (eds.), *Alcohol and Tobacco: From Basic Science to Policy.* NIAAA Research Monograph, no. 19. Washington, D.C.: National Institute of Alcoholism and Alcohol Abuse, 1995.

Ajzen, I., and Fishbein, M. *Understanding Attitudes and Predicting Social Behavior.* Englewood Cliffs, N.J.: Prentice Hall, 1980.

Becker, M. H., and Maiman, L. A. "Strategies for Enhancing Patient Compliance." *Journal of Community Health,* 1980, *6,* 113–135.

Brug, J., and others. "Self-Rated Dietary Fat Intake: Association with Objective Assessment of Fat, Psychosocial Factors and Intention to Change." *Journal of Nutrition Education,* 1994, *26,* 218–233.

Davidson, R. "Prochaska and DiClemente's Model of Change: A Case Study?" *British Journal of Addictions,* 1992, *87,* 821–822.

Fishbein, M., and Ajzen, I. *Belief, Attitude, Intention and Behavior: An Introduction to Theory and Research.* Reading, Mass.: Addison-Wesley, 1975.

Janz, N. K., and Becker, M. H. "The Health Belief Model: A Decade Later." *Health Education Quarterly,* 1984, *11,* 1–47.

Lerman, C., Orleans, C. T., and Engstrom, P. F. "Biological Markers in Smoking Cessation Treatment." *Seminars in Oncology,* 1993, *20*(4), 359–367.

Leventhal, H., and Cameron, L. "Behavioral Theories and the Problem of Compliance." *Patient Education and Counseling,* 1987, *10,* 117–138.

Mullen, P. D., Hersey, J. C., and Iverson, D. C. "Health Behavior Models Compared." *Social Science and Medicine,* 1987, *24*(11), 973–981.

Perloff, L., and Fetzer, B. K. "Self-Other Judgments and Perceived Vulnerability to Victimization." *Journal of Personality and Social Psychology,* 1986, *2,* 502–510.

Prentice-Dunn, S., and Rogers, R. W. "Protection Motivation Theory and Preventive Health: Beyond the Health Belief Model." *Health Education Research,* 1986, *1,* 153–161.

Prochaska, J. O., DiClemente, C. C., Velicer, W. F., and Rossi, J. S. "Standardized, Individualized, Interactive, and Personalized Self-Help Programs for Smoking Cessation." *Health Psychology,* 1993, *12*(5), 399–405.

Prochaska, J. O., and others. "Self-Change Processes, Self-Efficacy and Self-Concept in Relapse and Maintenance of Cessation of Smoking." *Psychological Reports,* 1982, *51,* 983–990.

Rakowski, W., and others. "Women's Decision-Making About Mammography: An Application of the Relationship Between Stages of Adoption and Decisional Balance." *Health Psychology,* 1993, *12,* 209–241.

Rimer, B. K. "Audiences and Messages for Breast and Cervical Cancer Screening." *Wellness Perspectives: Research, Theory and Practice,* 1995, *11*(2), 13–39.

Rimer, B. K., and others. "Cancer Screening Practices Among Women in a Community Health Center Population." *American Journal of Preventive Medicine,* forthcoming.

Rogers, R. W., and Mewborn, C. R. "Fear Appeals and Attitude Change: Effects of a Threat's Noxiousness, Probability of Occurrence, and the Efficacy of Coping Responses." *Journal of Personality and Social Psychology,* 1976, *34,* 54–61.

Tessaro, I., and others. "Readiness to Change Smoking Behavior in a Community Health Center Population." *Journal of Community Health,* forthcoming.

Turkle, S. *Life on the Screen.* New York: Simon & Schuster, 1995.

Weinstein, N. D. "Unrealistic Optimism About Future Life Events." *Journal of Personality and Social Change,* 1980, *39,* 806–820.

Weinstein, N. D. "'Why It Won't Happen to Me': Perceptions of Risk Factors and Susceptibility." *Health Psychology,* 1984, *3,* 431–457.

Weinstein, N. D. "Unrealistic Optimism About Susceptibility to Health Problems: Conclusions from a Community-Wide Sample." *Journal of Behavioral Medicine,* 1987, *10*(4), 481–500.

Weinstein, N. D. "The Precaution Adoption Process." *Health Psychology,* 1988, *7*(4), 355–386.

Weinstein, N. D., and Klein, W. M. "Resistance of Personal Risk Perceptions to Debiasing Interventions." *Health Psychology,* 1995, *14,* 132–140.

PART THREE

MODELS OF INTERPERSONAL HEALTH BEHAVIOR

Frances Marcus Lewis

Individuals are social beings who derive their sense of self and personal efficacy from others through interpersonal exchanges. This interpersonal environment provides the means, models, reinforcements, and resources with which persons can learn about themselves and can affect their health behavior and health outcomes. The basic assumption of the chapters in Part Three is that the interpersonal environment is critical in affecting and predicting the individual's health behavior and, in turn, health outcomes. One theory and two theoretical frameworks are analyzed: Social Cognitive Theory, social support and social networks, and provider-patient communication.

Chapter Eight, by Baranowski, Perry, and Parcel, examines Social Cognitive Theory, highlighting two branches of social learning theory: an operant conditioning branch and a cognitive branch. The operant conditioning branch emphasizes the effects of external reinforcements and expectancies on a person's performance and expectations for future performance outcomes. The cognitive branch emphasizes how a person's cognitions, including expectations and imparted meaning about an event or situation, affect his or her performance and expectations. The operant conditioning branch views the person as a doer or a responder. The cognitive branch views the person as a thinker and an analyst, not just a doer. Baranowski, Perry, and Parcel synthesize these two branches of Social Learning Theory.

This chapter has been substantially updated since the first edition and includes two new case applications of the theory. These cases demonstrate how the concepts from both branches have been used to mold the components of both a community-based and a school-based intervention program.

In Chapter Ten, Roter and Hall carve a new direction for research in provider-patient communication. In the first edition of this book, the chapter on patient-provider communication (Joos and Hickam, 1990) analyzed the state of the literature and the applications at that time, making a timely contribution to our understanding of patient-provider interaction and remaining of interest and relevance today. Joos and Hickam examined four perspectives: cognition and information processing, interpersonal interaction, conflict resolution and negotiation, and social influence. Each of these perspectives has its own research tradition and offers either specific targets for increasing the effectiveness of the patient-provider interaction or methods for positively affecting it. Applications included reviews of both observational and intervention studies on patient-provider interactions.

In this new edition, Roter and Hall offer a complementary analysis that moves readers away from a traditional power-dominated model of patient-provider interaction to a theoretical framework that characterizes this interaction as one of reciprocal causation and complementary interaction. We offer their framework as an important new direction in research and practice in this area.

Chapter Nine, by Heaney and Israel, provides a theoretical framework for understanding the impact of social support and social networks on health behavior and health outcomes. Although it draws on the first edition chapter by Israel and Schurman (1990), it examines only social support and social networks, whereas the first version discussed stress and coping as well. In this edition, we have assigned separate chapters to these two topics, giving focused attention to each. Like the chapter on Social Cognitive Theory, the new chapter on social support and social networks highlights the importance of reciprocal determinism, or dynamic, multicausal relationships, between individuals and their interpersonal environments.

Together, all three chapters offer a set of theoretical frameworks from which to view the individual within his or her interpersonal context, and targets and methods for creating interpersonal environments that are health enhancing. Finally, Chapter Eleven offers some concluding observations on the uses of the theories and applications presented in Part Three and the concerns that remain to be dealt with.

References

Israel, B. A., and Schurman, S. J. "Social Support, Control, and the Stress Process." In
    K. Glanz, F. M. Lewis, and B. K. Rimer (eds.), *Health Behavior and Health Education: Theory,
    Research, and Practice.* San Francisco: Jossey-Bass, 1990.

Joos, S. K., and Hickam, D. H. "How Health Professionals Influence Health Behavior: Patient-Provider Interaction and Health Care Outcomes." In K. Glanz, F. M. Lewis, and B. K. Rimer (eds.), *Health Behavior and Health Education, Theory, Research, and Practice*. San Francisco: Jossey-Bass, 1990.

CHAPTER EIGHT

HOW INDIVIDUALS, ENVIRONMENTS, AND HEALTH BEHAVIOR INTERACT

Social Cognitive Theory

Tom Baranowski
Cheryl L. Perry
Guy S. Parcel

Social Cognitive Theory (SCT) addresses both the psychosocial dynamics influencing health behavior and the methods of promoting behavioral change. It emphasizes that a person's behavior and cognitions affect future behavior. Human behavior is explained in SCT in terms of a triadic, dynamic, and reciprocal model in which behavior, personal factors (including cognitions), and environmental influences all interact. An individual's behavior is uniquely determined by these interactions. Among the crucial personal factors are the individual's capabilities to symbolize behavior, to anticipate the outcomes of behavior, to learn by observing others, to have confidence in performing a behavior (including overcoming any barriers to performing the behavior), to self-determine or self-regulate behavior, and to reflect and analyze experience (Bandura, 1986).

Health educators and behavioral scientists have used SCT ideas creatively to develop procedures or techniques that influence these underlying cognitive variables, thereby increasing the likelihood of behavioral change. In this way, Social Cognitive Theory not only explains how people acquire and maintain certain behavioral patterns but also provides the basis for intervention strategies. This chapter offers a brief history of the development of Social Cognitive Theory,

The writing of this chapter was supported in part by the following grants to the authors: HL 47618, CA 61596, AA08596, and HL 39927.

descriptions of key concepts, and two recent examples of SCT use in designing health education programs.

Brief History of Social Cognitive Theory

Social Cognitive Theory incorporates an extensive range of theoretical concepts and has been employed in many areas of practice. Table 8.1 lists the SCT publication milestones in the areas of understanding and changing health behaviors.

Miller and Dollard (1941) originally introduced what they called Social Learning Theory (SLT) to explain imitation of behavior among animals and humans. The original SLT concepts were based on the classic learning principles and motivational ideas of Hull (1943). Learning theory explains behavior mechanistically. The person is seen as a "black box" that emits behaviors called responses to which reinforcements are applied by other people. These reinforcements or rewards, in turn, increase the likelihood of those behaviors. Reinforcements link the performance of certain responses to particular stimuli and thereby increase the likelihood of those responses in the presence of those stimuli and not others. Hull explained why certain kinds of behavior were more likely to occur than others by considering internal states called drives, not cognitions. Hull believed that animals and humans acquired drives, that is, physiological processes that motivate behavior. For example, hunger motivates food search and food consumption. Hull also maintained that one organism's responses are stimuli for other organisms. Social learning thereby attends to others' responses when motivated by an acquired drive.

Two streams of health-related research flowed from Miller and Dollard's (1941) seminal ideas. Rotter first applied these early social learning principles to clinical psychology (1954), which in turn led to his development of the idea of "generalized expectancies" of "reinforcement" (1966). Rotter contended that a person learns or is conditioned operantly on the basis of his or her history of positive or negative reinforcement. As a result, the person develops a sense of internal or external locus of control over the events in his or her life. Individuals with an internal locus of control are more likely to self-initiate change, whereas those who are externally controlled are more likely to be influenced by others or wait for chance occurrences. Within a learning theory framework, Zifferblatt (1975) applied behavioral analysis procedures to understand compliance behavior with medical regimens. Wallston and Wallston (1978) formulated a scale for the assessment of health *locus of control*. They proposed that their measure was more useful in health research than was a general measure of locus of control because an individual's sense of control often varies by domains of experience and action. The locus of control literature evolved to postulate a need or drive for control, with evidence that giving people control over their lives improved their health outcomes.

TABLE 8.1. DEVELOPMENT OF SOCIAL COGNITIVE THEORY: PUBLICATION MILESTONES.

1941	Miller and Dollard	Social Learning and Imitation
1954	Rotter	Social Learning and Clinical Psychology
1962	Bandura	"Social Learning Through Imitation"
1963	Bandura and Walters	Social Learning and Personality Development
1966	Rotter	"Generalized Expectancies for Internal Versus External Control of Reinforcement," Psychological Monographs
1969	Bandura	Principles of Behavior Modification
1973	W. Mischel	"Toward a Cognitive Social Learning Reconceptualization of Personality," Psychological Review
1975	Stokols	"The Reduction of Cardiovascular Risk: An Application of Social Learning Perspectives," Applying Behavioral Science to Cardiovascular Risk
1975	Zifferblatt	"Increasing Patient Compliance Through the Applied Analysis of Behavior," Preventive Medicine
1977	Bandura	Social Learning Theory
1977	Bandura	"Self-Efficacy: Toward a Unifying Theory of Behavior Change," Psychological Review
1977	Farquhar and others	"Community Education for Cardiovascular Health," Lancet
1978	Bandura	"The Self System in Reciprocal Determinism," American Psychologist
1978	Wallston and Wallston	"Locus of Control and Health: A Review of the Literature," Health Education Monographs
1981	Parcel and Baranowski	"Social Cognitive Theory and Health Education," Health Education
1983	Abrams and Follick	"Behavioral Weight-Loss Intervention at the Worksite: Feasibility and Maintenance," Journal of Consulting and Clinical Psychology
1986	Bandura	Social Foundations of Thought and Action: A Social Cognitive Theory
1988	Abrams and others	"Social Learning Principles for Organizational Health Promotion: An Integrated Approach," Health and Industry: A Behavioral Medicine Perspective
1995	Bandura	Self-Efficacy in Changing Societies

Although this is an important and interesting line of SLT research applied to health, this chapter emphasizes the second stream that has progressed beyond the behavioral theory headwaters, the employment of cognitive concepts to explain behavioral phenomena.

In 1962, Albert Bandura published an article on social learning and imitation. In contrast to operant learning theory, which maintained that rewards had to be directly applied for learning to occur, Bandura and Walters (1963) proposed that children could watch other children to learn a new behavior and did not need to be rewarded directly. Thus, a child learns by observing the behavior of others (modeling) and the rewards these others receive (vicarious reinforcement). In 1969, Bandura described a conceptual foundation for behavioral modification that heavily emphasized traditional learning theory. Mischel (1973) first proposed several cognitive constructs that formed a cognitive basis for Social Cognitive Theory. Stokols (1975) applied the observational learning concept to the area of cardiovascular disease risk reduction. In 1977, Bandura published his refutation of the adequacy of traditional learning theory principles for understanding learning and provided the first theoretical treatment of his cognitive concept of self-efficacy (Bandura, 1977a). Farquhar and others (1977) reported the first communitywide intervention for heart disease prevention based on SCT. In 1978, Bandura proposed the organizing concept of reciprocal determinism, in which environment, person, and behavior are seen to be continually interacting. In 1981, Parcel and Baranowski applied SCT to health education and delineated the stages in the behavioral change process at which each concept was most relevant. Abrams and Follick (1983) first applied social learning concepts to the design of worksite interventions. In 1986, Bandura published a comprehensive framework for understanding human social behavior and renamed Social Learning Theory as Social Cognitive Theory. Abrams and others (1986) used Social Cognitive Theory as a framework for understanding and integrating organizational and individual approaches to health behavior change. Bandura (1995) proposed self-efficacy as the construct undergirding many aspects of social change. Many other contributions could be cited, but this list reflects the major historical roots and some dominant contributions to the public health education literature.

SCT is particularly relevant to health education programs for three reasons. First, the theory synthesizes previously disparate cognitive, emotional, and behavioral understandings of behavioral change. Second, as demonstrated in this chapter, the constructs and processes identified by SCT suggest many important avenues for new behavioral research and practice in health education. Third, SCT permits the application of theoretical ideas developed in other areas of psychology to health behaviors and to behavioral change, thereby benefiting from their insights and understanding.

Social Cognitive Theory Constructs

Mischel (1973) and Bandura (1977b, 1986) formulated a number of SCT constructs that are important in understanding and intervening in health behavior. Table 8.2 summarizes these constructs as well as their implications for potential intervention strategies.

TABLE 8.2. MAJOR CONCEPTS IN SOCIAL COGNITIVE THEORY AND IMPLICATIONS FOR INTERVENTION.

Concept	Definition	Implications
Environment	Factors physically external to the person	Provide opportunities and social support
Situation	Person's perception of the environment	Correct misperceptions and promote healthful norms
Behavioral capability	Knowledge and skill to perform a given behavior	Promote mastery learning through skills training
Expectations	Anticipatory outcomes of a behavior	Model positive outcomes of healthful behavior
Expectancies	The values that the person places on a given outcome, incentives	Present outcomes of change that have functional meaning
Self-control	Personal regulation of goal-directed behavior or performance	Provide opportunities for self-monitoring, goal setting, problem solving, and self-reward
Observational learning	Behavioral acquisition that occurs by watching the actions and outcomes of others' behavior	Include credible role models of the targeted behavior
Reinforcements	Responses to a person's behavior that increase or decrease the likelihood of reoccurrence	Promote self-initiated rewards and incentives
Self-efficacy	The person's confidence in performing a particular behavior	Approach behavioral change in small steps to ensure success; seek specificity about the change sought
Emotional coping responses	Strategies or tactics that are used by a person to deal with emotional stimuli	Provide training in problem solving and stress management; include opportunities to practice skills in emotionally arousing situations
Reciprocal determinism	The dynamic interaction of the person, the behavior, and the environment in which the behavior is performed	Consider multiple avenues to behavioral change including environmental, skill, and personal change

Handwritten margin notes:
- Δ environment ⊕
- education knowledge
- training (teach do)
- modeling
- things important + relevant
- records reflections merits
- ⊕ models
- rewards
- small steps; can do!
- training + skills to deal = all arousing situations
- look @ dynamics

Reciprocal Determinism

In Social Cognitive Theory, behavior is dynamic, depending on aspects of the environment and the person, all of which influence each other simultaneously. This continuing interaction among the characteristics of a person, the behavior of that person, and the environment within which the behavior is performed is called *reciprocal determinism.* Behavior is not simply the result of the environment and the person, just as the environment is not simply the result of the person and behavior. Instead, these three components are constantly interacting. A change in one component has implications for the others (Bandura, 1978, 1986). Reciprocal determinism is accepted within SCT as a principle or a postulate and is not submitted to empirical test.

Environments and Situations

The term *environment* refers to an objective notion of all the factors that can affect a person's behavior but that are physically external to that person. Examples of the social environment include family members, friends, and peers at work or in the classroom. The physical environment might include the size of a room, the ambient temperature, or the availability of certain foods. The term *situation* refers to the cognitive or mental representation of the environment (including real, distorted, or imagined factors) that may affect a person's behavior. The situation is a person's perception of the environment and may include place, time, physical features, activity, participants, and his or her own role in the situation. This concept of situation corresponds to Lewin's notion of the life space ([1942] 1951) or Bronfenbrenner's idea of microsystem (1977). Environment and situation provide an ecological framework for understanding behavior (Parraga, 1990).

On the one hand, the environment can affect behavior without a person's awareness (Moos, 1976). For example, if preferred fresh fruits and vegetables are made available in a child's environment, the child will probably learn to include those foods in his or her diet. However, when a person is not aware of important opportunities in the environment, the influence of the environment on behavior will be correspondingly limited. The situation, on the other hand, guides and limits thinking and behavior. For example, the social situation and physical situation provide cues about acceptable types of behavior (Rotter, 1955). If nonfat milk is not merely available but is also perceived by the child as something that classmates drink and value for its healthfulness, the child may begin to drink it, too. A situation may also pose certain problems that require immediate attention, or it may preclude and limit types of behavior.

Characteristics of the environment are usually the result of personal and behavioral interactions between people. Thus, the self-injection equipment available in the home of a person with diabetes usually reflects the financial resources available and the actions of one or more family members in acquiring them. A model of family reciprocal determinism (Taylor, Baranowski, and Sallis, 1994; Baranowski, 1996) has been proposed to capture this complexity. The habitual patterns of interaction between family members constitute an aspect of the environment: *emergent family characteristics* (Baranowski, 1996). For example, when habitual family interactions are characterized as conflicts, whether and how family members seek information or assistance from one another will consistently vary from interactions characterized as supportive. Within this model, behavior is a function of a shared environment with other family members and their behaviors and personal characteristics, all of which function within a larger environment. Thus, a child's eating certain foods is in part a result of the child's preferences for those foods (Domel and others, 1993b), what foods are available in the home, certain prompts by parents to eat those foods (Iannotti, O'Brien, and Spillman, 1994), and what foods are available in the local region or particular season (Sallis, 1986).

The environment has become increasingly important in health behavior change. State and worksite policies restricting smoking have enhanced smoking prevention and cessation (Biener, Abrams, Follick, and Dean, 1989). The unavailability of targeted foods in the home precludes their increased consumption (Kirby and others, 1995). Modifying the food in the school cafeteria increases student consumption of low-fat meals (Simons-Morton and others, 1991). Table 8.3 identifies common categories of environments, their likely physical and social characteristics, and a preliminary delineation of categories of influence on health behavior. Each possible category of influence must influence behavior through one of the theoretical processes specified here. The organizational and family climate characteristics are contextual variables that moderate how other influences affect behavior.

Observational Learning

The environment is important in Social Cognitive Theory in part because it provides *models* for behavior. A person can learn from other people not only by receiving reinforcements from them but also through observing them. *Observational learning* occurs when a person watches the actions of another person and the reinforcements that the person receives. This process has also been called vicarious reward or vicarious experience (Bandura, 1972, 1986).

Observational learning is a more efficient approach than operant learning for learning complex behaviors. In the operant approach, a person must perform a behavior that is subsequently reinforced. Through a trial-and-error process, the person continues to perform behaviors that come progressively closer to the desired performance. Trial and error is an inefficient process. In observational learning,

TABLE 8.3. ASPECTS OF THE ENVIRONMENT IN RECIPROCAL DETERMINISM.

Environment	Physical Location	Actors	Categories of Influence
Institutional	Government offices	Lawmakers Bureaucrats Clients	Laws, rules, regulations, policies Organizational climate Peer interpersonal influences Agency-client interpersonal influences Agency cafeteria (see below) Agency programs (see below)
Neighborhood	Area around home	Neighbors, peers	Neighborhood climate Peer interpersonal influences
Occupational	Worksite, school	Managers Staff, employees Teachers Clients, customers, students	Rules, regulations, policies Organizational climate Wellness programs (see below) Teacher-student interpersonal influences Peer interpersonal influences Company-client interpersonal influences
Consumer	Grocery store Convenience store Fast-food eatery Restaurant Employee cafeteria	Managers Employees Customers, patrons	Rules, regulations, policies Organizational climate Peer interpersonal influences Store-customer interpersonal influences
Wellness programs	Wellness center or worksite	Managers Staff, employees Clients	Rules, regulations, policies Organizational climate Change program techniques
Family	Home	Parents Spouses, partners Children, siblings	Rules, regulations, policies Emergent family characteristics Spousal interpersonal relationship Socialization practices

the observer does not need to go through this time-consuming process in uncertain circumstances. Instead, the learner discovers rules that account for the behavior of others by observing the behavior and the reinforcements the others receive for their behavior. The person learns what is appropriate by observing the behaviors, successes, and mistakes of others.

Many types of behavior can be learned through observational learning (Bandura and Walters, 1963; Bandura, 1972, 1986). This process accounts for family members' often having common behavioral patterns. Children observe their parents when they eat, smoke, drink, and use seat belts, and they see the various rewards or penalties the parents receive for these activities. Some children observe other children smoking at school and notice the rewards and punishments that the smokers receive. If the smokers get responses that the observers consider rewarding (acceptance from peers or a desirable image), the observers become more likely to smoke.

Behavioral Capability

Behavior is complex and can be viewed at many levels (Frederiksen, Martin, and Webster, 1979), from having a meal, to eating a specific food, to taking a certain number of bites to chew a mouthful of food, for example. Health educators must clearly specify the targeted behavior. The concept of *behavioral capability* maintains that if a person is to perform a particular behavior, he or she must know what the behavior is (knowledge of the behavior) and how to perform it (skill). The concept of behavioral capability enables a distinction between learning and performance because a task can be learned yet not performed whereas performance presumes learning.

Behavioral capability is the result of the individual's training, intellectual capacity, and learning style. The skills training technique called mastery learning provides cognitive knowledge of what is to be performed, practice in performing the activities, and feedback to refine successful performance until the person performs the behavior at a predefined level of acceptability (Block, 1971).

Reinforcement

Reinforcement is the primary construct in the operant form of learning theory. *Positive reinforcement,* or reward, is a response to a person's behavior that increases the likelihood that the behavior will be repeated. In traditional operant theory, the reinforcement works in an unknown mechanistic way to affect behavior. For example, providing a positive comment ("Nice job!") will increase the likelihood that someone will repeat the praised behavior, especially if the person doing the behavior values the commentator's opinion. Negative reinforcement also increases the likelihood of a behavior but by withdrawal of a negative stimulus when the desired behavior is performed. For example, smoking is negatively reinforcing because the inhaled nicotine removes negative affect (depression, anxiety, and anger, for example), withdrawal, and craving. Punishment may simply reduce the likelihood that a particular behavior will be performed in those situations in which a person expects to receive punishment but not in other situations. Exercise among obese children was increased both by reinforcing active behaviors and reinforcing decreased time in sedentary behaviors (Epstein, Saelens, and O'Brien, 1995).

SCT incorporates three types of reinforcement: direct reinforcement (as in operant conditioning), vicarious reinforcement (as in observational learning), and self-reinforcement (as in self-control). SCT further categorizes these types of reinforcement into external (or extrinsic) and internal (or intrinsic) reinforcement (Lepper and Green, 1978). External reinforcement is the occurrence of an event or act known to have predictable reinforcement value. Internal reinforcement is a person's own experience or perception that an event has some value. Internal reinforcement accounts for behavior that is not reinforced externally or may even be negatively reinforced externally. For example, a person may choose to return $10 that was given in error as change, because it is the "right" thing to do, even though the $10 would have fulfilled some personal desire, an external reinforcement. Educational programs that are intrinsically reinforcing result in more learning, retention, and interest in the subject matter (Lepper and Cordova, 1992). Participants who reported higher intrinsic than extrinsic motivation were more likely to achieve abstinence from smoking (Curry, Wagner, and Grothaus, 1990).

The difference in reward mechanisms is particularly important in the area known as the *overjustification effect*. If a person is given an external reward for a task that is intrinsically interesting, he or she may find that task less intrinsically interesting in the future (Lepper and Green, 1978). Thus, if a person who usually enjoys jogging were to be paid to jog for a week, he or she might find that jogging was no longer as enjoyable (valuable) as it was before the payment was provided. Researchers have shown that any external constraint imposed on behavior may reduce the level of internal motivation (Lepper and Green, 1978). Health educators and behavioral scientists may do well not to provide external rewards for all health promotion activities, in order to ensure that the internal appeal of these activities will be maintained. Practitioners can, however, use external rewards for behaviors that are part of a behavioral change program—for example, maintaining daily diet records, which can be discontinued at the end of a program—while they emphasize the intrinsic rewards of the behavioral change itself (Perry and others, 1988).

Outcome Expectations

Outcome expectations are the anticipatory aspects of behavior that Bandura (1977b, 1986) called *antecedent determinants* of behavior. A person learns that certain events are likely to occur in response to his or her behavior in a particular situation and then expects them to occur when the situation arises again. For behavior that is not habitual, people anticipate many aspects of the situation in which the behavior might be performed, develop and test strategies for dealing with the situation, and anticipate what will happen as a result of their behavior in this situation. In this way, people develop expectations about a situation and expectations for outcomes of their behavior before they actually encounter the situation. In most cases, this anticipatory behavior reduces their anxiety and increases their ability to handle the situation. Expectations are learned in four ways: (1) from previous experience in similar situations (performance attainment), (2) from observing others in similar situations (vicarious experience), (3) from hearing about similar situations from other people or social persuasion, and (4) from emotional or physical responses to behaviors (physiological arousal).

Adolescent smoking prevention offers an example of how expectations may develop and be changed. Generally, an adolescent learns to expect, from advertising, older peers, or adult role models, that smoking can be a fun or exciting experience or that he or she can attain a grown-up or even sexy appearance by smoking. In a health education program, adolescent peers can be taught to direct discussions on the negative social consequences of smoking and on how to handle pressure to smoke from other adolescents. This approach has been successful in deterring smoking onset (Flay, 1985). It succeeds, in essence, because negative social consequences (negative outcome expectations) for these young adolescents have changed.

Outcome Expectancies

Outcome expectancies (called *incentives* by Bandura, 1977b, 1986) are different from expectations in that expectancies are the *values* that a person places on a particular outcome. Expectancies have magnitude, a quantitative value that can be positive or negative and is usually represented on a continuum from −1 to +1. Expectancies influence behavior according to the hedonic principle; that is, if all other things are equal, a person will choose to perform an activity that maximizes a positive outcome or minimizes a negative outcome. Mischel (1973) proposed that expectancies explained classical conditioning. For example, when teaching weight reduction skills to overweight adults, one may need to help those adults replace the positive outcomes of food consumption with negative outcomes. This can be done by stressing the attractiveness or healthfulness of weight reduction or, even more overtly, by paying money for weight loss. In a recent study, positive outcome expectancies for smoking predicted the severity of withdrawal symptoms, and both positive and negative outcome expectancies predicted success of attempts at smoking cessation (Wetter and others, 1994). Food preferences and tastes can be considered immediate outcome expectancies of eating. Preference was the only predictor of consumption of fruits and vegetables among children (Domel and others, forthcoming), and taste was a primary predictor of consumption of beverages among adults (Lewis, Sims, and Shannon, 1989).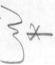

A person's positive expectancies should be assessed early in any project designed to promote changes in health behavior, in order to identify motivators for that behavior. Many researchers have observed, for example, that people are more likely to engage in physical activity to achieve short-term benefits (to become physically attractive, to feel better, or to compete with friends in tennis) than to achieve long-term gains (for example, to avoid a heart attack thirty years from now). McAlister and others (1980) showed that smoking prevention programs for adolescents are more successful if they emphasize the immediate negative effects of smoking such as bad breath or unattractiveness rather than the long-term effects such as morbidity and mortality from cancer and heart disease. Thus, an emphasis on immediate positive expectancies may more likely influence the initiation of some desired behaviors than may an emphasis on long-range expectancies.

Self-Efficacy

Self-efficacy is the confidence a person feels about performing a particular activity, including confidence in overcoming the barriers to performing that behavior. Bandura and colleagues (Bandura, 1977a, 1978, 1982, 1986) proposed that self-efficacy is the most important prerequisite for behavioral change, because it affects how much effort is invested in a given task and what level of performance is attained (Ewart, Taylor, Reese, and Debusk, 1983). Self-efficacy was a primary predictor of intention to engage in eight healthy dietary practices among office staff (Sheeshka, Woolcott, and MacKinnon, 1993) and of healthy food choices among third- and fourth-grade students (Parcel and others, 1995).

Both observational and interactive (participatory) learning techniques can be used in introducing and promoting each sequence of a targeted behavior (Bandura, 1986). Repetition of the performance of a single task builds a person's self-efficacy through changing the person's performance expectations. Through repeated successful enactment of incremental tasks, the person acquires enhanced expectations of success in the task, which in turn affects task persistence, initiation, and endurance and thus promotes behavioral change. Therefore, health professionals who are training people with diabetes to self-inject insulin, for example, may divide the self-injection process into a number of small steps, each of which individuals can learn through repetition (for example, filling the syringe with the correct amount of insulin, ensuring that all items remain sterilized, seeing that no bubbles get into the syringe, and making sure that the fluid is at the precise marker on the syringe). Simplifying each step and allowing individuals to practice each step in isolation, with many repetitions, enables them to build self-efficacy about performing each step. When persons are self-confident about each step, they can progressively put the steps together and build self-efficacy about the entire task. Measurement of self-efficacy must be specific to the target behavior and to the barriers faced by the target audience and audience members' understanding and capabilities (Maibach and Murphy, 1995).

Self-Control of Performance

The term *performance* refers to human behavior focused on achievement of a goal. One of the goals of health education is to bring the performance of health behavior under the control of the individual. Bandura (1991) proposed that the self-control system has several component subfunctions. These subfunctions include monitoring of one's own behavior and its determinants and effects; comparison of behavior and its outcomes to personal standards, especially self-set goals; and self-reward, especially affective self-reaction. Self-efficacy has an important role in self-control, affecting a person's selection of the extent of behavioral change and his or her practice in building confidence in self-regulation. The setting of a criterion of performance, or a goal, may be the most important factor. Promotion of self-control requires a focus on a specific type of behavior. In a weight control program, for example, a target of "cutting down on sweets" would be too vague to produce observable results because a person in the program might become confused about actual goals or might make only small changes that conformed to the target but did not lead to weight loss. A person might cut down on sweets, for example, by aiming to eat eight instead of eleven cookies a day.

Management of Emotional Arousal

Bandura (1977b) recognized that excessive emotional arousal inhibits learning and performance, and he proposed that certain stimuli give rise to fearful thoughts (*stimulus-outcome expectancies*). These fearful thoughts produce emotional arousal and trigger defensive behaviors. As the defensive behaviors deal effectively with stimuli, the fear, anxiety, hostility, or emotional arousal is reduced.

Categories of behavioral management for emotional and physiological arousal were identified by Moos (1976). One category includes psychological defenses (denial, repression, and sublimation). Another category includes more cognitive techniques, such as problem restructuring. A third category includes stress management techniques (progressive relaxation or exercise) that treat the symptoms of the emotional distress. A fourth category includes methods for solving problems effectively (clarifying a problem and identifying, selecting, and implementing solutions for the causes of the emotional arousal). SCT constructs and methods are usually employed to learn these behavioral management skills.

Although many programs employ behavioral management strategies, these strategies vary across individuals and cultures (Diaz-Guerrero, 1979). For example, severely overweight people may find it difficult to deny or repress their condition. People often react negatively to overweight people, and these reactions can increase anxiety about being overweight (Hudson and Williams, 1981). For some obese people, this anxiety causes further overeating (Slochower and Kaplan, 1980).

Heightened anxiety also makes it difficult for people to attend to the health messages coming from health professionals (Ley and Spelman, 1965). Therefore, health educators and behavioral scientists may do well to help people learn methods that aid in minimizing emotional arousal before they help them change their behavior, or to postpone interventions until anxiety has subsided.

Reciprocal Determinism Revisited

It is instructive to return to the concept of reciprocal determinism and examine it in the light of the component Social Cognitive Theory constructs just discussed. If a characteristic of a person, environment, or behavior changes, the situation changes, and the behavior, situation, and person are reevaluated. For example, a man may be so opposed to exercise that his friends come to expect him to maintain a sedentary lifestyle. The man has strengthened this expectation about exercise by avoiding any physical or social environments in which he might be expected to exercise (for example, gyms or playing fields). At some point, however, a dramatic event (for example, the death of a close family member from a heart attack and exposure to information that heart attacks may be caused in part by a sedentary lifestyle) may occur in this man's life and make him decide to start exercising. However, the man will now encounter the expectations of his sedentary friends, who may pressure him not to exercise. To avoid these negative pressures, he may seek new friends (a new social environment) who value exercise and support his new behavior (reciprocal effect). This change, in turn, may motivate a sedentary friend to begin to exercise as well (a reciprocal effect to that friend), and that friend will then either change the exercise habits of other sedentary friends or acquire new friends who are interested in exercise.

This kind of behavioral change underscores how important it is for professionals to avoid the simplicity of *single direction of change* thinking. Reciprocal determinism may be used to advantage in developing programs that do not focus on behavior in isolation but focus on changes in the environment and in the individual instead. A recent health promotion program based on social cognitive theory that included environmental and individual changes is the Child and Adolescent Trial for Cardiovascular Health (CATCH), which was designed to improve nutrition and physical activity behavior. In this multicenter trial, interventions for third- through fifth-grade students were tested for their influence in changing cognitive factors through classroom instruction and environmental changes. The interventions modified the food service program and the physical education program and were predicated on reciprocal determinism, addressing behavioral capability, self-efficacy, and perceived norms in the classroom. They provided an opportunity for children to practice the new behaviors in the school cafeteria and in physical education and provided reinforcement from important others in the child's environment (teachers and parents). The evaluations indicated significant changes in cognitive variables, environmental conditions, and nutrition and physical activity behavior (Luepker and others, 1996; Edmundson and others, forthcoming).

To provide more examples of the use of these SCT concepts, the following section describes how SCT was used in the design of two health education programs.

Case Study: Project Northland's Amazing Alternatives!

Social Cognitive Theory provided the conceptual foundation for the development of a communitywide program, Project Northland, to prevent alcohol use among young adolescents in grades 6 through 9 (ages eleven through fifteen). The research design and intervention programs in the sixth grade have been described in detail elsewhere (Perry and others, 1993; Williams and others, 1995). The design and results of the intervention program in the seventh grade (Amazing Alternatives!) are summarized here. A major challenge of Project Northland was to translate SCT concepts into creative and developmentally appropriate educational and environmental programs (see Table 8.4) that would effectively deter young adolescents from beginning to drink alcohol.

Project Northland involved twenty-four school districts and twenty-eight adjoining communities in northeastern Minnesota, an area with high levels of alcohol-related problems (Perry and others, 1993). The school districts were blocked by size and randomized to either an intervention or a delayed program condition. The project focused on the Class of 1998, that is, those who were sixth-grade students in the 1991–92 school year ($n = 2,351$). In the intervention communities, Class of 1998 students participated in four years of school-based behavioral health curricula, parental involvement programs, peer leadership activities, and community-wide task force activities (Wagenaar and Perry, 1994).

During the seventh grade, 1992–93, the Amazing Alternatives! Program was implemented. This program consisted of (1) a kick-off evening for students and their parents at each of the intervention schools (the Awesome Autumn Party) as a model for a fun alcohol-free event; (2) an eight-week eight-session peer-led social influences curriculum, based on that used in a World Health Organization study (Perry and others, 1989) and the Saving Lives Program (Hingson, Howland, and Schiavone, 1991); (3) a peer participation program, T.E.E.N.S. (The Exciting and Entertaining Northland Students), in which Class of 1998 student volunteers planned alternative alcohol-free activities for their peers outside of class (Komro,

TABLE 8.4. EXAMPLES OF SOCIAL COGNITIVE CONSTRUCTS IN PROJECT NORTHLAND'S AMAZING ALTERNATIVES!

SCT Constructs	Examples of Construct Use
Environment	Alcohol-free alternative activities offered for teens at school and in the community (Awesome Autumn Party). Parents are involved in the Amazing Alternatives! Home Program.
Situation	Audiocassettes are played of four teen role models, part of the curriculum to create negative perceptions of alcohol use.
Behavioral capabilities	Students develop skills during the curriculum to resist influences to use alcohol. Students develop skills in T.E.E.N.S. to create alcohol-free social events.
Expectations	Peer leaders direct discussion on negative consequences of drinking.
Expectancies	Curriculum activities portray alcohol use as not cool, attractive, or functional.
Self-control	Students write time capsules at the end of Amazing Alternatives! about remaining alcohol free.
Observational learning	Elected and trained peer leaders conduct the curriculum. Four audiotaped teens tell their alcohol-related stories. T.E.E.N.S. groups create parties for their peers.
Reinforcement	T.E.E.N.S. T-shirts are designed and distributed to students.
Self-efficacy	Curriculum activities include role-plays and group activities on resisting influences to use alcohol.
Reciprocal determinism	Students learn skills to deal with social influences to drink. The social environment changes so there are fewer opportunities to drink. Fewer students drink, so there are fewer influences to drink.

Perry, Veblen-Mortenson, and Williams, 1994); and (4) four booklets sent to parents of the Class of 1998 that included activities and discussion topics for parents and their seventh-graders (the Amazing Alternatives! Home Program).

SCT guided the development of Amazing Alternatives! as summarized in Table 8.4. The name Amazing Alternatives! derived from the motif that linked the four levels of the program together. Multiple age-appropriate role models (peer leaders, peers telling their stories on audiotape, and T.E.E.N.S. participants) and experiential activities (at home, through alternative parties, and in the classroom) and the extension of what was taught in the classroom to both the home and community environments were unique SCT-based components in this health promotion program to deter adolescent alcohol use.

Project Northland was evaluated by annual Class of 1998 surveys from the beginning of sixth grade (fall 1991) through the end of ninth grade (spring 1995).

Data from the spring of 1994 were available from 81 percent of the baseline Class of 1998 students ($n = 1,901$). Students in the intervention districts had statistically significant lower past-month and past-week alcohol use than those in the reference school districts and communities (Perry and others, forthcoming). Among intervention students, 23.6 percent reported drinking in the past month compared with 29.2 percent of the reference students; 10.5 percent of the intervention students reported drinking in the past week compared with 14.8 percent of the reference students. It is important that Project Northland significantly changed many of the factors identified by SCT among the intervention students, including alcohol use expectancies, peer role models and peer influence, self-efficacy to resist offers to drink, and outcome expectations of drinking. Thus, the application of SCT at the community level appears to have yielded results in deterring young adolescents from beginning to drink.

Case Study: Gimme 5!
Fruits and Vegetables for Fun and Health

Fourth- and fifth-grade children are not eating sufficient numbers of servings of fruits and vegetables (Baranowski and others, 1993; Kirby and others, 1995). Social Cognitive Theory was used first to define the nature of this problem (McLeroy and others, 1994) and then to design a creative intervention to remedy the identified factors (Domel and others, 1993a).

Several dietary guidelines for the United States recommend that everyone should be eating five to nine servings of fruits and vegetables every day (Domel and others, 1993c); however, recent data revealed that children are eating somewhere between 1.8 and 2.5 servings per day (Domel and others, 1994). Focus group discussions predicated on SCT were conducted in four geographic areas around the country (Baranowski and others, 1993; Kirby and others, 1995). The discussions revealed that children were not eating fruits and vegetables due to environmental, personal, and behavioral factors. Environmental issues were that fruits and vegetables were not available in the homes of lower-income families and not accessible in all the homes—for example, cut up in a glass of water on the front of a shelf in the refrigerator within easy reach for a child. Personal factors included children's not having positive outcome expectancies, especially preference or taste, for eating vegetables. Behavioral factors were that children were responsible for making their own snacks and some of their own meals but did not have a repertoire of recipes for making their favorite fruit and vegetable dishes. An analysis of a baseline survey of the students revealed that the primary predictor of fruit and vegetable consumption was preference for fruits and vegetables (Domel and others, forthcoming).

A school curriculum called Gimme 5! was designed to help remedy these influencing factors and thereby increase fruit and vegetable consumption (Domel and others, 1993a). The intervention attempted to increase availability and accessibility of fruits and vegetables through "asking skills." That is, skills training activities including role-playing were designed to encourage children to go home and ask to purchase their favorite fruits and vegetables at the grocery store, to have their favorite fruits and vegetables available at meals and snacks, and to select fast-food eateries that offer a variety of fruits and vegetables. Gimme 5! attempted to increase preference for fruits and vegetables by developing and pretasting FaSST (fast, simple, safe, and tasty) recipes that children were likely to enjoy; increasing exposure to fruits and vegetables through taste testings in the classroom (Birch, 1987); and by associating fun participative activities (for example, a rap song or role-playing) with fruits and vegetables. The children's ability to prepare fruit and vegetable dishes was addressed by preparing FaSST recipes in the classroom and sending the recipes home in newsletters to the family, with homework assignments to prepare them at home. Self-regulation skills were promoted by having students monitor their fruit and vegetable consumption, set goals for eating more fruits and vegetables at specific meals or snacks, problem solve when goals were not achieved, and receive rewards when goals were achieved. Rewards came in the form of congratulations and applause from the teacher and students and small toys given to those children who achieved all their goals. The pilot test of the curriculum revealed that children experienced a 50 percent increase in their fruit consumption and changed their most frequently consumed vegetable from french fries (undesired because they are high in fat) to green salad (Domel and others, 1993a). Further analyses revealed that all these changes occurred at school, that is, children took more advantage of the fruits and vegetables offered in school lunches but did not change eating habits at home. Examples of the use of SCT constructs in Gimme 5! are found in Table 8.5.

The ensuing implementation of the Gimme 5! curriculum has attempted to target the home environmental variables of availability, accessibility, and consumption of fruits and vegetables more effectively (Havas and others, 1995). The same conceptual analysis has been employed, but the attempts to reach parents have been expanded to include, first, a more detailed weekly newsletter with many tips for helping children eat more fruit and vegetable recipes and, second, three fifteen-minute videotapes per year with an MTV format, a local professional basketball player as the VJ, and children and parents from the local schools as actors modeling many of the desired behaviors. Point-of-purchase education at the local grocery stores has also been added, addressing parental concerns about how to select low-cost and unlikely to perish fruits and vegetables and offering taste testings and free samples through coupons and prizes as incentives to attend the evening sessions in the stores.

TABLE 8.5. EXAMPLES OF SOCIAL COGNITIVE CONSTRUCTS IN GIMME 5!

SCT Constructs	Examples of Construct Use
Environment	Increase availability and accessibility of fruits and vegetables at home.
Behavioral capability	Students develop skills to make FaSST recipes.
	Students develop skills to ask for more fruits and vegetables at home and at fast-food eateries.
Outcome expectancies	Students learn that eating more fruits and vegetable will enhance their at-school performance but will not impair their acceptance by peers.
Self-control	Students set goals to eat more fruits and vegetables at targeted meals and snacks.
Observational learning	Students observe the teacher set goals for his or her own dietary change.
Reinforcement	Students receive congratulations for attaining all dietary change goals.
	Students receive small prizes (for example, neon shoelaces, fruit and vegetable refrigerator magnets) for completing all homework assignments.
Self-efficacy	Students role-play situations to enhance their confidence to ask for fruits and vegetables.
Reciprocal determinism	Students ask for more of their favorite fruits and vegetables to be available and accessible at home; as the fruits and vegetables become more available and accessible, children eat more of them because their preferences for fruits and vegetables have increased; the increased exposure to fruits and vegetables further increases preferences for fruits and vegetables.

Teachers constitute part of the environment for students. The curriculum can work only if delivered as designed. A process evaluation involving in-classroom observations of teacher implementation of the curriculum revealed that in spite of substantial teacher training, teacher fidelity to the curriculum was less than 50 percent, with teachers least likely to employ the goal-setting activities (18 percent). Greatest fidelity was attained among teachers who preferred vegetables the most. Thus, a personal teacher variable affected the environment of the students.

Limitations of Social Cognitive Theory

Some health educators and behavioral scientists have complained that Social Cognitive Theory has been too comprehensive in its formulation. There are so many constructs that some authors have found a way to explain almost any phenomenon using one or another of the constructs. When a theory explains everything, it explains nothing. That is, a good theory must be falsifiable. There must be ways of testing ideas to clearly identify the range of phenomena to which they apply and the range to which they do not apply. If negative findings can always be explained by other ideas in the theory, then the theory is no longer falsifiable and does not explain. Proponents of SCT must, therefore, clearly specify the range of phenomena to which tests apply, clearly recognize where the theory applies, and not make claims about the utility of SCT that are not supported by empirical evidence.

All current behavioral theories are limited in their ability to predict behavior. The percentage of variance accounted for in a measure of behavior is one way to think about the ability of a theory to predict behavior. Stafleu, deGraaf, vanStaveren, and Schroots (1991–1992) recently reviewed twenty-one survey research studies, each of which attempted to predict some aspect of consumption of fat in the diet. None of these studies, including two based on SCT, were able to predict more than 30 percent of the variance in dietary behavior. Part of this low predictiveness is due to limitations of measurement of both the independent and dependent variables, but there is also a severe limit in the extent to which any of the commonly used health behavior theories predict behavior. SCT constructs have not appeared frequently in survey research (Stafleu, deGraaf, vanStaveren, and Schroots, 1991–1992). More frequent use in survey research may help refine measurement of the constructs and our understanding of their relationships to behaviors.

Existing health behavior theories do not appear to capture the nonlinearities in life. Sometimes things get better for us, and sometimes, for no apparent reason, they get worse. There are nonlinear occurrences of events and relationships over time. All the single constructs in SCT, however, propose linear relationships: in theory, the more of one construct (for example, positive outcome expectancies about eating fruits and vegetables), the more likely a behavior is to occur (for example, fruit and vegetable consumption). The principle of reciprocal determinism suggests the nonlinear relationships among environmental, personal, and behavioral factors. For example, a woman who wants to lower her fat consumption changes the home environment and no longer keeps high-fat desserts there. However, she still really enjoys such desserts and has to eat out often during working hours. As a result, she may eat more high-fat desserts when eating away from home, thereby vitiating the home restrictions. At this time, there is no clear guidance from SCT for anticipating such reciprocal nonlinear relationships. Furthermore, Bandura's writing suggests that multiplicative interaction terms should account for behavior. For example, self-efficacy should predict behavior primarily when positive outcome expectations are high. Along these lines, self-efficacy predicted smoking cessation in an interaction term with internal locus of control (Strecher, DeVellis, Becker, and Rosenstock, 1986). However, such interaction terms have not usually been found (Domel and others, forthcoming; Resnicow and others, forthcoming). More attention needs to be paid to these non-linear aspects of SCT.

Several large funded intervention studies have been designed using SCT constructs but have not resulted in changed behavior (Carleton and others, 1995; Fortmann and others, 1993; Luepker and others, 1994). Although the lack of positive outcomes in these trials could be due to inadequacies in the theory, it could also be due to inadequate or noncreative uses of the theory by the program designers, lack of fidelity to the intervention by the people implementing it, contamination between experimental and control groups, problems in measurement of the constructs or in other issues of evaluation, among many other factors. The lack of positive outcomes emphasizes the need to (1) clearly state where and when SCT constructs apply; (2) creatively design interventions based on the constructs tailored to the characteristics of the target population; (3) do extensive process evaluations to learn where the program may be breaking down; and (4) carefully select, design, and pretest measures for use in evaluations (Maibach and Murphy, 1995). If we consider SCT constructs as mediators of the effects of an intervention, their usefulness can be assessed in future intervention research by (1) clearly specifying the extent to which interventions change the SCT-specified mediating variables and, in turn, (2) specifying the extent to which changes in these mediating variables predict behavioral change outcomes. We may find that our interventions are not successfully changing the SCT mediating variables or that changes in the SCT constructs are not closely related to changes in behavior.

Work with SCT needs to pursue new avenues to better understand health behavior. People are often faced with choices between alternative behaviors. Thus, a young adult is not only faced with the choice of using contraception or not but of choosing the best type of contraception in the circumstances. SCT constructs have most often been applied to doing a single behavior or not. For example, a person may have high outcome expectancies and self-efficacy for use of a condom, suggesting a high probability that the person will use a condom in the future. However, the person may possess even higher outcome expectations and self-efficacy for the early withdrawal method, an ineffective contraceptive technique. Research and programs based on SCT should be expanded to predict selections from among the multiple behavioral choices facing people.

Environmental factors are increasingly seen as important influences on behavior. Although the environment is an important component within reciprocal determinism, the nature of the predicted relationships has not been well specified. In particular, research must address whether self-efficacy, outcome expectancies, and behavioral capability account for all the ways in which the environment affects personal and behavioral characteristics.

A final lead for future development of SCT involves more micro-analyses of behavior. For example, availability and accessibility of various foods provide important constraints on what foods children can eat. There is a long series of steps that influence what foods become available, from availability at stores in the neighborhood (Sallis and others, 1986), to parental selection of foods at those stores, to parental food preparation practices at home (Baranowski, 1996). At each of these steps, there is the potential for interplay between environmental, personal, and behavioral characteristics. Better understanding of these influences should lead to more effective dietary intervention programs.

Continuing research will enable us to revise SCT to better understand targeted behaviors and to find the areas or the conditions under which SCT does not apply.

Conclusion

This chapter has focused on Social Cognitive Theory and its relevance in the design of health education programs. By incorporating a concern for environment, people, and behavior, SCT provides a framework for designing and implementing comprehensive behavioral change programs.

SCT is attractive for health education and health promotion programs because it not only illuminates the dynamics of individual behavior but also gives direction to the design of intervention strategies to influence behavioral change. Great emphasis is placed currently on the importance of multicomponent interventions in the development of health promotion programs. Recent interventions address not only behavioral change at the individual level but also change within the environment to support behavioral change (Simons-Morton and others, 1991). SCT applies to a multilevel change strategy because it includes environmental, personal, and behavioral constructs.

SCT is a robust theory that can be applied to health education and health promotion activities. However, it is sometimes inappropriately applied because intervention methods are oversimplified or derive from single concepts, not the total theory. To guard against such oversimplification, intervention designers should clearly specify the desired behavioral outcomes and then identify the SCT variables most likely to influence each behavior. SCT intervention methods can be matched with the targeted SCT variables. Evaluations of programs based on SCT should use measures of relevant SCT constructs to ensure that the interventions are having the desired effects and to alert program planners to program components they can improve.

References

Abrams, D. B., and Follick, M. J. "Behavioral Weight-Loss Intervention at the Worksite: Feasibility and Maintenance." *Journal of Consulting and Clinical Psychology*, 1983, *51*, 226–233.

Abrams, D. B., and others. "Social Learning Principles for Organizational Health Promotion: An Integrated Approach." In M. F. Cataldo and T. J. Coates, *Health and Industry: A Behavioral Medicine Perspective*. New York: Wiley, 1986.

Bandura, A. "Social Learning Through Imitation." In M. R. Jones (ed.), *Nebraska Symposium on Motivation*. Vol. 10. Lincoln: University of Nebraska Press, 1962.

Bandura, A. *Principles of Behavior Modification*. Austin, Tex.: Holt, Rinehart and Winston, 1969.

Bandura, A. *Psychological Modeling: Connecting Theories*. Chicago: Aldine/Atherton, 1972.

Bandura, A. "Self-Efficacy: Toward a Unifying Theory of Behavior Change." *Psychological Review*, 1977a, *84*, 191–215.

Bandura, A. *Social Learning Theory*. Englewood Cliffs, N.J.: Prentice Hall, 1977b.

Bandura, A. "The Self System in Reciprocal Determinism." *American Psychologist*, 1978, *33*, 344–358.

Bandura, A. "Self-Efficacy Mechanism in Human Agency." *American Psychologist*, 1982, *37*, 122–147.

Bandura, A. *Social Foundations of Thought and Action: A Social Cognitive Theory*. Englewood Cliffs, N.J.: Prentice Hall, 1986.

Bandura, A. "Social Cognitive Theory of Self Regulation." *Organizational Behavior and Human Decision Processes*, 1991, *50*, 248–285.

Bandura, A. *Self-Efficacy in Changing Societies*. New York: Cambridge University Press, 1995.

Bandura, A., and Walters, R. H. *Social Learning and Personality Development*. Austin, Tex.: Holt, Rinehart and Winston, 1963.

Baranowski, T. "Families and Health Action." In D. S. Gochman (ed.), *Handbook of Health Behavior Research*. Vol. 1. New York: Plenum, 1996.

Baranowski, T., and others. "Increasing Fruit and Vegetable Consumption Among 4th and 5th Grade Students: Results from Focus Groups Using Reciprocal Determinism." *Journal of Nutrition Education*, 1993, *25*, 114–120.

Biener, L., Abrams, D. B., Follick, M. J., and Dean, L. "A Comparative Evaluation of a Restrictive Smoking Policy in a General Hospital." *American Journal of Public Health*, 1989, *79*, 192–195.

Birch, L. L. "Children's Food Preferences: Developmental Patterns and Environmental Influences." *Annals of Child Development*, 1987, *4*, 171–208.

Block, J. H. (ed.). *Mastery Learning: Theory and Practice*. Austin, Tex.: Holt, Rinehart and Winston, 1971.

Bronfenbrenner, U. "Toward an Experimental Ecology of Human Development." *American Psychologist*, 1977, *32*, 513–553.

Carleton, R. A., and others. "The Pawtucket Heart Health Program: Community Changes in Cardiovascular Risk Factors and Projected Disease Risk." *American Journal of Public Health*, 1995, *85*(6), 777–785.

Curry, S. J., Wagner, E. H., and Grothaus, L. C. "Intrinsic and Extrinsic Motivation for Smoking Cessation." *Journal of Consulting and Clinical Psychology*, 1990, *58*, 310–316.

Diaz-Guerrero, R. "The Development of Coping Style." *Human Development*, 1979, *32*, 320–331.

Domel, S. B., and others. "Development and Evaluation of a School Intervention to Increase Fruit and Vegetable Consumption Among 4th and 5th Grade Students." *Journal of Nutrition Education,* 1993a, *25,* 345–349.

Domel, S. B., and others. "Measuring Fruit and Vegetable Preferences Among Fourth and Fifth Grade Students." *Preventive Medicine,* 1993b, *22,* 866–879.

Domel, S. B., and others. "To Be or Not to Be . . . Fruits and Vegetables." *Journal of Nutrition Education,* 1993c, *25*(6), 352–358.

Domel, S. B., and others. "Fruit and Vegetable Food Frequencies by Fourth and Fifth Grade Students: Validity and Reliability." *Journal of the American College of Nutrition,* 1994, *13*(1), 1–7.

Domel, S. B., and others. "Psychosocial Predictors of Fruit and Vegetable Consumption Among Elementary School Children." *Health Education Research: Theory and Practice,* forthcoming.

Edmundson, E., and others. "The Effects of Child and Adolescent Trial for Cardiovascular Health upon Psychosocial Determinants of Diet and Physical Activity Behavior." *Preventive Medicine,* forthcoming.

Epstein, L. H., Saelens, B. E., and O'Brien, J. G. "Effects of Reinforcing Increases in Active Behavior Versus Decreases in Sedentary Behavior for Obese Children." *International Journal of Behavioral Medicine,* 1995, *2,* 41–50.

Ewart, C. K., Taylor, C. B., Reese, L. B., and Debusk, R. F. "Effects of Early Postmyocardial Infarction Exercise Testing on Self-Perception and Subsequent Physical Activity." *American Journal of Cardiology,* 1983, *51,* 1076–1080.

Farquhar, J. W., and others. "Community Education for Cardiovascular Health." *Lancet,* 1977, *1,* 1192–1195.

Flay, B. R. "What We Know About the Social Influences Approach to Smoking Prevention: Review and Recommendations." In C. S. Bell and R. J. Battjes (eds.), *Prevention Research: Deterring Drug Abuse Among Children and Adolescents.* National Institute for Drug Abuse Research Monograph, no. 63. Washington, D.C.: National Institute for Drug Abuse, 1985.

Fortmann, S. P., and others. "Effect of Community Health Education on Plasma Cholesterol Levels and Diet: The Stanford Five-City Project." *American Journal of Epidemiology,* 1993, *137,* 1039–1055.

Frederiksen, L. W., Martin, J. E., and Webster, J. S. "Assessment of Smoking Behavior." *Journal of Applied Behavior Analysis,* 1979, *12,* 653–664.

Havas, S., and others. "5-A-Day for Better Health." *Public Health Reports,* 1995, *110*(1), 68–79.

Hingson, R. H., Howland, J., and Schiavone, T. "The Massachusetts Saving Lives Program: Six Cities Widening the Focus from Drunk Driving to Speeding, Reckless Driving, and Failure to Wear Safety Belts." *Journal of Traffic Medicine,* 1991, *18,* 123–132.

Hudson, A., and Williams, S. G. "Eating Behavior, Emotions, and Overweight." *Psychological Reports,* 1981, *48,* 669–760.

Hull, C. L. *Principles of Behavior.* Englewood Cliffs, N.J.: Appleton-Century-Crofts, 1943.

Iannotti, R. J., O'Brien, R. W., and Spillman, D. M. "Parental and Peer Influences on Food Consumption of Preschool African-American Children." *Perceptual and Motor Skills,* 1994, *79,* 747–752.

Kirby, S., and others. "Children's Fruit and Vegetable Intake: Socioeconomic, Adult Child, Regional, and Urban-Rural Influences." *Journal of Nutrition Education,* 1995, *27,* 261–271.

Komro, K. A., Perry, C. L., Veblen-Mortenson, S., and Williams, C. L. "Peer Participation in Project Northland: A Community-Wide Alcohol Use Prevention Project." *Journal of School Health,* 1994, *64,* 318–322.

Lepper, M. R., and Cordova, D. I. "A Desire to Be Taught: Instructional Consequences of Intrinsic Motivation." *Motivation and Emotion,* 1992, *16,* 187–208.

Lepper, M. R., and Green, D. (eds.). *The Hidden Costs of Reward: New Perspectives on the Psychology of Human Motivation.* Hillsdale, N.J.: Erlbaum, 1978.

Lewin, K. "Field Theory and Learning." In K. Lewin, *Field Theory in Social Science: Select Theoretical Papers* (D. Cartwright, ed.). New York: HarperCollins, 1951. (Originally published 1942.)

Lewis, C. J., Sims, L. S., and Shannon, B. "Examination of Specific Nutrition/Health Behaviors Using a Social Cognitive Model." *Journal of the American Dietetic Association,* 1989, *89,* 194–202.

Ley, P., and Spelman, M. S. "Communications in an Out-Patient Setting." *British Journal of Social and Clinical Psychology,* 1965, *4,* 114–116.

Luepker, R. V., and others. "Community Education for Cardiovascular Disease Prevention: Risk Factor Changes in the Minnesota Heart Health Program." *American Journal of Public Health,* 1994, *84,* 1383–1393.

Luepker, R. V., and others. "Outcomes of a Trial to Improve Children's Dietary Patterns and Physical Activity: The Child and Adolescent Trial for Cardiovascular Health (CATCH)." *Journal of the American Medical Association,* 1996, *275,* 768–776.

Maibach, E., and Murphy, D. A. "Self-Efficacy in Health Promotion Research and Practice: Conceptualization and Measurement." *Health Education Research,* 1995, *10,* 37–50.

McAlister, A., and others. "Pilot Study of Smoking, Alcohol, and Drug Abuse Prevention." *American Journal of Public Health,* 1980, *70,* 719–721.

McLeroy, K. R., and others. "Social Science Theory in Health Education: Time for a New Model?" *Health Education Research,* 1994, *9,* 305–312.

Miller, N. E., and Dollard, J. *Social Learning and Imitation.* New Haven, Conn.: Yale University Press, 1941.

Mischel, W. "Toward a Cognitive Social Learning Reconceptualization of Personality." *Psychological Review,* 1973, *80,* 252–283.

Moos, R. H. *The Human Context: Environmental Determinants of Behavior.* New York: Wiley, 1976.

Parcel, G., and Baranowski, T. "Social Cognitive Theory and Health Education." *Health Education,* 1981, *12,* 14–18.

Parcel, G. S., and others. "Measurement of Self-Efficacy for Diet-Related Behaviors Among Elementary School Children." *Journal of School Health,* 1995, *65,* 23–27.

Parraga, I. M. "Determinants of Food Consumption." *Journal of the American Dietetic Association,* 1990, *90,* 661–663.

Perry, C. L., and others. "Parent Involvement with Children's Health Promotion: The Minnesota Home Team." *American Journal of Public Health,* 1988, *78,* 1156–1160.

Perry, C., and others. "WHO Collaborative Study on Alcohol Education and Young People: Outcomes of a Four-Country Pilot Study." *International Journal of the Addictions,* 1989, *4,* 1145–1171.

Perry, C. L. and others. "Background, Conceptualization, and Design of a Community-Wide Research Program on Adolescent Alcohol Use: Project Northland." *Health Education Research,* 1993, *8*(1), 125–136.

Perry, C. L., and others. "Outcomes of a Community-Wide Alcohol Use Prevention Program During Early Adolescence: Project Northland." *American Journal of Public Health,* forthcoming.

Resnicow, K., and others. "Psychosocial Correlates of Fruit and Vegetable Consumption." *Health Psychology,* forthcoming.

Rotter, J. B. *Social Learning and Clinical Psychology.* Englewood Cliffs, N.J.: Prentice Hall, 1954.

Rotter, J. B. "The Role of the Psychological Situation in Determining the Direction of Human Behavior." In M. R. Jones (ed.), *Nebraska Symposium on Motivation.* Lincoln: University of Nebraska Press, 1955.

Rotter, J. B. "Generalized Expectancies for Internal Versus External Control of Reinforcement." *Psychological Monographs,* 1966, *80*(1), 1–28.

Sallis, J. F., and others. "San Diego Surveyed for Heart-Healthy Foods and Exercise Facilities." *Public Health Reports,* 1986, *101,* 216–219.

Sheeshka, J. D., Woolcott, J. D., and MacKinnon, N. J. "Social Cognitive Theory as a Framework to Explain Intentions to Practice Healthy Eating Behaviors." *Journal of Applied Social Psychology,* 1993, *23,* 1547–1573.

Simons-Morton, B. G., and others. "Promoting Diet and Physical Activity Among Children: Results of a School Based Intervention Study." *American Journal of Public Health,* 1991, *81,* 986–991.

Slochower, J., and Kaplan, S. P. "Anxiety, Perceived Control, and Eating in Obese and Normal Weight Persons." *Appetite,* 1980, *1,* 75–83.

Stafleu, A., deGraaf, C., vanStaveren, W. A., and Schroots, J.J.F. "A Review of Selected Studies Assessing Social-Psychological Determinants of Fat and Cholesterol Intake." *Food Quality and Preference,* 1991–1992, *3,* 183–200.

Stokols, D. "The Reduction of Cardiovascular Risk: An Application of Social Learning Perspectives." In A. J. Enelow and J. B. Henderson (eds.), *Applying Behavioral Science to Cardiovascular Risk.* Dallas, Tex.: American Heart Association, 1975.

Strecher, V. J., DeVellis, B. M., Becker, M. H., and Rosenstock, I. M. "The Role of Self-Efficacy in Achieving Health Behavior Change." *Health Education Quarterly,* 1986, *13*(1), 73–91.

Strecher, V. J., and others. "Goal Setting as a Strategy for Health Behavior Change." *Health Education Quarterly,* 1995, *22,* 190–200.

Taylor, W., Baranowski, T., and Sallis, J. "Family Determinants of Childhood Physical Activity: A Social Cognitive Model." In R. K. Dishman (ed.), *Exercise Adherence: Its Impact on Public Health.* Champaign, Ill.: Human Kinetics, 1994.

Wagenaar, A. C., and Perry, C. L. "Community Strategies for the Reduction of Youth Drinking: Theory and Application." *Journal of Research on Adolescence,* 1994, *4,* 319–345.

Wallston, K. A., and Wallston, B. S. "Locus of Control and Health: A Review of the Literature." *Health Education Monographs,* 1978, *6*(2), 107–117.

Wetter, D. W., and others. "Smoking Outcome Expectancies: Factor Structure, Predictive Validity, and Discriminant Validity." *Journal of Abnormal Psychology,* 1994, *103,* 801–811.

Williams, C., and others. "A Home-Based Prevention Program for Sixth Grade Alcohol Use: Results from Project Northland." *Journal of Primary Prevention,* 1995, *16,* 125–147.

Zifferblatt, S. M. "Increasing Patient Compliance Through the Applied Analysis of Behavior." *Preventive Medicine,* 1975, *4,* 173–182.

CHAPTER NINE

SOCIAL NETWORKS AND SOCIAL SUPPORT

Catherine A. Heaney
Barbara A. Israel

Ecological approaches to health education emphasize the importance of the social context within which individuals live and work (McLeroy, Bibeau, Steckler, and Glanz, 1988; Stokols, 1992). Indeed, numerous studies have shown that the extent and nature of one's social relationships affect one's health (House, Umberson, and Landis, 1988). An understanding of the impact of social relationships on health status, health behaviors, and health decision making contributes to the design of effective interventions for preventing the onset or reducing the negative consequences of a wide array of diseases. Although there is no one theory that adequately explicates the link between social relationships and health, various conceptual models and theories have guided research in this area. This chapter provides a conceptual overview of the link between social relationships and health and briefly reviews the empirical support for that link, discusses intervention implications, and presents two cases illustrating how the health-enhancing potential of social relationships has been incorporated into health education practice.

Definitions and Terminology

Various conceptualizations and operationalizations of the health-enhancing components of social relationships exist. The term *social integration* has been used to refer to the existence or quantity of social ties (House, Umberson, and Landis, 1988). The term *social network* refers to a person-centered web of social relationships (Israel, 1982; Israel and Rounds, 1987). The provision of *social support* is one of the important functions of social relationships. Thus, social networks are linkages between people that may (or may not) provide social support and that may serve other functions in addition to that support.

The structure of social networks can be described in terms of dyadic characteristics (that is, the characteristics of each relationship between the focal individual and another person in the network) and in terms of the characteristics of the network as a whole (Israel, 1982; House, Umberson, and Landis, 1988). Examples of dyadic characteristics include the extent to which resources and support are both given and received in a relationship (reciprocity), the extent to which a relationship is characterized by emotional closeness (intensity), and the extent to which a relationship serves a variety of functions (complexity). Examples of characteristics that describe a whole network include the extent to which network members are similar in terms of demographic characteristics such as age, race, and socioeconomic status (homogeneity); the extent to which network members live in close proximity to the focal person (geographical dispersion); and the extent to which network members know and interact with each other (density).

Social support has been defined and measured in numerous ways. According to House (1981), social support is the functional content of relationships (that is, social networks), which can be categorized along four broad types of supportive behaviors or acts. *Emotional support* involves the provision of empathy, love, trust, and caring. *Instrumental support* involves the provision of tangible aid and services that directly assist a person in need. *Informational support* is the provision of advice, suggestions, and information that a person can use in addressing problems. *Appraisal support* involves the provision of information that is useful for self-evaluation purposes, that is, constructive feedback, affirmation, and social comparison. Although these four types of support can be differentiated conceptually, relationships that provide one type often also provide other types, thus making it difficult to study them empirically as separate constructs (House and Kahn, 1985; Israel and Rounds, 1987). For a comprehensive review of measurement and methodological issues, see Heitzmann and Kaplan, 1988; House and Kahn, 1985; O'Reilly, 1988. Table 9.1 summarizes the key concepts and their definitions.

Social support can be distinguished from other functions of social relationships. Social support is always intended (by the sender of it) to be helpful, thus distinguishing it from intentional negative interactions. Whether or not the intended support is perceived or experienced as helpful by the receiver is an empirical question, and indeed, negative perceptions and consequences of well-intended interpersonal exchanges have been identified (for example, Wortman and Lehman,

TABLE 9.1. TYPES AND CHARACTERISTICS OF SOCIAL NETWORKS AND SOCIAL SUPPORT.

Concepts	Definitions
Social network	A person-centered web of social relationships
Selected social network characteristics:	
Reciprocity	Extent to which resources and support are both given and received in a relationship
Intensity	Extent to which social relationships offer emotional closeness
Complexity	Extent to which social relationships serve many functions
Density	Extent to which network members know and interact with each other
Social support	Aid and assistance exchanged through social relationships and interpersonal transactions
Types of social support:	
Emotional support	Expressions of empathy, love, trust and caring
Instrumental support	Tangible aid and service
Informational support	Advice, suggestions, and information
Appraisal support	Information that is useful for self-evaluation

Source: Based on Israel, 1982; House, 1981.

1985). In addition, social support is consciously provided by the sender, which sets it apart from the social influence exerted through simple observation of the behavior of others (Bandura, 1986) and from receiver-initiated social comparison processes (Taylor, Buunk, and Aspinwall, 1990). Lastly, although the provision of social support, particularly informational support, can attempt to influence the thoughts and behaviors of the receiver, such informational support is provided in an interpersonal context of caring, trust, and respect for each person's right to self-determination. This quality distinguishes social support from some other types of social influence that derive from the ability to provide or withhold desired resources or approval.

Although many investigations of the effects of social relationships on health have narrowly focused on the provision of social support, a broader social network approach has several advantages. First, a social network approach can incorporate functions or characteristics of social relationships other than social support. For example, there is increasing evidence that negative interpersonal interactions, such as those characterized by mistrust, hassles, criticism, and domination, are more strongly related to psychiatric morbidity than is a lack of social support (Rook, 1984). Furthermore, these negative interactions occur independently of levels of social support (Israel and others, 1989). Second, whereas a social support approach usually focuses on one relationship at a time, a social network approach allows for the study of how changes in one social relationship affect other relationships. Third, a social network approach facilitates the investigation of how the structural and interactional characteristics of networks (reciprocity or density, for example) influence the quantity and quality of social support that is exchanged (Israel, 1982; Gottlieb and McLeroy, 1994). This information may be important for the development of effective support-enhancing interventions.

Background of the Concepts

Barnes's (1954) pioneering work in a Norwegian village first presented the concept of the social network to describe patterns of social relationships that were not easily explained by more traditional social units such as extended families or work groups. Much of the early work on social networks was exploratory and descriptive. The findings from these studies provided a knowledge base that facilitated the identification of the network characteristics mentioned earlier. In general, it was found that close-knit networks exchange more affective and instrumental support and also exert more social influence upon members to conform to network norms. Homogenous networks, networks with more reciprocal linkages, and networks with closer geographic proximity were also more effective in providing affective and instrumental support (see Israel, 1982, for a review).

The study of social support owes much to the work of social epidemiologist John Cassel (1976). Drawing from numerous animal and human studies, Cassel posited that social support serves as a key psychosocial "protective" factor that reduces individuals' vulnerability to the deleterious effects of stress on health. He further specified that psychosocial factors such as social support are likely to play a nonspecific role in the etiology of disease. Thus, social support may influence the incidence and prevalence of a wide array of health outcomes.

From the definitions and background provided, it is clear that the terms social network and social support do not connote theories per se. Rather, they are concepts that describe the structure, processes, and functions of social relationships. Various sociological and social psychological theories (such as exchange theory, attachment theory, and symbolic interactionism) have been used to explain the basic interpersonal processes that underlie the association between social relationships and health. Israel and Rounds (1987) provide a concise review of these theoretical considerations.

Conceptual Model of the Relationship of Social Networks and Social Support to Health

The various mechanisms through which social networks and social support may have positive effects on physical, mental, and social health are presented in Figure 9.1. Although we concentrate in this chapter on social networks and social support as the starting point or initiator of a causal flow toward health outcomes, several of the relationships hypothesized in Figure 9.1 entail reciprocal influence. For example, health status will influence the extent to which one is able to maintain and mobilize a social network.

Pathway 1 in Figure 9.1 represents a hypothesized direct effect of social networks and social support on health. By meeting basic human needs for companionship, intimacy, a sense of belonging, and reassurance of one's worth as a person, supportive ties enhance well-being and health regardless of stress levels (Berkman, 1984). Pathways 2 and 4 represent a hypothesized effect of social networks and social support on individual coping resources and community resources, respectively. For example, social networks and social support can enhance an individual's ability to access new contacts and information and to identify and solve problems. If the support provided helps to reduce uncertainty and unpredictability or helps to produce desired outcomes, then a sense of personal control over specific situations and life domains will be enhanced (Wallston, Alagna, DeVellis, and DeVellis, 1983). In addition, the theory of symbolic interactionism suggests that human behavior is based on the meaning that people assign to events. This meaning is derived, in large part, from their social interactions (Israel, 1982). Thus, people's social network linkages may help them to reinterpret events or problems in a more positive, constructive light (Thoits, 1986).

The potential effects of social networks and social support on organizational and community competence are less well studied. However, strengthening social networks and enhancing the exchange of social support may increase a community's ability to garner its resources and solve problems. Several community-level interventions have shown how intentional network building and the strengthening of social support within communities are associated with enhanced community capacity and control (Minkler, 1985; Eng and Parker, 1994).

Resources at both the individual and community levels may have direct health-enhancing effects and may also diminish the negative effects on health due to exposure to stressors. When people experience stressors, the availability of enhanced individual or community resources increases the likelihood that stressors will be handled or coped with in a way that reduces both short-term and long-term adverse health consequences. This *buffering effect* is reflected in pathways 2a

FIGURE 9.1. CONCEPTUAL MODEL OF THE RELATIONSHIP OF SOCIAL NETWORKS AND SOCIAL SUPPORT TO HEALTH.

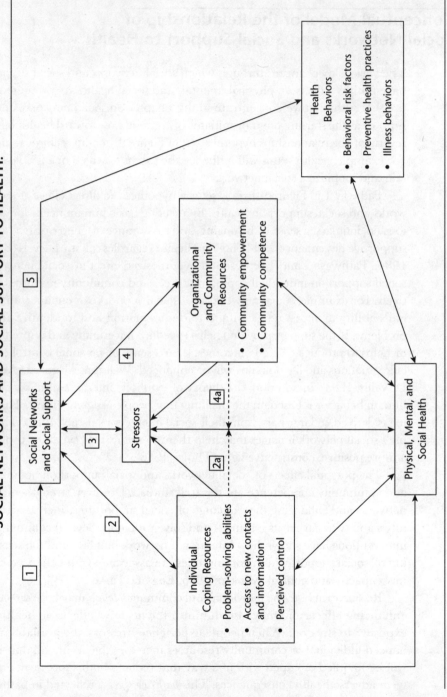

and 4a. Research involving people going through major life transitions (such as loss of a spouse or birth of a child) has illustrated how social networks and social support influence the coping process and buffer the effects of the stressor on health (Rhodes, Contreras, and Mangelsdorf, 1994; Hirsch and DuBois, 1992; Walker, MacBride, and Vachon, 1977).

Pathway 3 suggests that social networks and social support may influence the frequency and duration of exposure to stressors. For example, a supportive supervisor may ensure that an employee is not given more work to do than time allows to be completed (House, 1981). Similarly, having a social network that is able to provide information about new jobs may reduce the likelihood that a person will suffer from long-term unemployment. Reduced exposure to stressors is then, in turn, associated with enhanced mental and physical health.

Pathway 5 reflects the potential effects of social networks and social support on health behaviors. Through the interpersonal exchanges within a social network, individuals are influenced and supported in their health behavior choices. Through influences on behavioral risk factors, preventive health behavior, and illness behavior, pathway 5 makes explicit that social networks and social support may have an impact on the incidence of, diagnosis of, and recovery from disease.

Empirical Evidence on the Influence of Social Relationships

Several reviews of the empirical studies that address the influence of social relationships on health have been published (Antonucci, 1990; Berkman, 1984; House, Umberson, and Landis, 1988; Israel, 1982; Israel and Rounds, 1987; Turner and Marino, 1994). There are some inconsistencies in this body of research and some differences among the conclusions of the reviews. However, few would disagree with the following summary: "Although the results of individual studies are usually open to alternative interpretations, the pattern of results across the full range of studies strongly suggests that what are variously termed social relationships, social networks, and social support have important causal effects on health, exposure to stress, and the relationship between stress and health" (House, 1987).

Prospective epidemiological studies, most often using measures of social integration, have consistently found a relationship between a lack of social relationships and all-cause mortality (see Berkman, 1984; House, Umberson, and Landis, 1988; Israel and Rounds, 1987, for reviews). The evidence for buffering effects is less conclusive, but studies do suggest that social support mobilized to help a person cope with a stressor does reduce the negative effects of the stressor on health (Cohen and Wills, 1985). Although the direct effects and the buffering effects of social networks and social support were initially investigated as either/or relationships, evidence suggests that social support and social networks have both types of effects, and that the predominance of one effect over the other depends on the target population, the situation being studied, and the ways in which the social relationship concepts are measured (Cohen and Syme, 1985; Cohen and Wills, 1985; House, Umberson, and Landis, 1988; Israel and Rounds, 1987).

The effect of social relationships on all-cause mortality supports the hypothesis, first put forth by Cassel (1976), that the effect of social relationships on health is not specific to any one disease process. This nonspecific role may explain why studies of the effect of social relationships on specific morbidities have not been conclusive (House, Umberson, and Landis, 1988). Although evidence for a link between social networks and social support and the incidence of particular diseases is not strong, a positive role for affective support in the processes of coping with and recovering from serious illness has been consistently found (Spiegel, Bloom, Kraemer, and Gottheil, 1989; Spiegel, 1992; Wallston, Alagna, DeVellis, and DeVellis, 1983).

The association between social relationships and health does not follow a linear dose-response curve. Rather, very low levels of social integration are most deleterious, with higher levels being less advantageous once a threshold level has been reached (House, 1981). Having at least one strong intimate relationship is an important predictor of good health. Of the several types of support that can be exchanged among network members, affective support is most strongly and consistently associated with good health and well-being (Israel and Rounds, 1987). Research also suggests that social relationships influence health behavior in the areas of compliance with medical regimens (Levy, 1983), help-seeking behavior (McKinlay, 1980; Starrett and others, 1990), infant feeding practices, smoking (Cohen and others, 1988), and weight loss (Epstein and Wing, 1987), to name but a few.

The social network characteristics of reciprocity and intensity have been somewhat consistently linked to positive mental health (Israel, 1982). Networks characterized by few ties, high-intensity relationships, high density, and close geographical proximity are most suited to the maintenance of social identity and the exchange of affective support; thus, these networks prove to be most health enhancing when these social network functions are needed. However, during times of transition and change, networks that are larger, more diffuse, and composed of less intense ties may be more adaptive, because they are better at facilitating social outreach and the exchange of informational support (Israel, 1982; House, Umberson, and Landis, 1988).

Demographically defined subgroups maintain qualitatively different social networks and experience varying health benefits from those networks. Shumaker and Hill (1991) reviewed gender differences in the link between social support and physical health. They suggested that the prospective epidemiological studies investigating the effect of social relationships on mortality found a weaker health protective effect for women than for men. In addition, women of a particular age group (usually over fifty years of age) experienced a positive association between high levels of social support and high levels of mortality. Noting that women tend to cast a "wider net of concern" (that is, maintain more strong ties), are more likely to be both the providers and recipients of social support, and are more responsive to the life events of others than are men, the authors suggest that further study is needed to explore the impact of these differences on the health protective potential of women's social networks.

Both Berkman (1984) and House, Umberson, and Landis (1988) noted that social integration is more prevalent, but less predictive of mortality, in smaller rural communities than in urban centers. Berkman hypothesized that some communities may be so cohesive and well integrated that few of their citizens are placed at risk for ill health due to social isolation or a lack of social support. House, Umberson, and Landis called for further research on urban-rural differences in network structures and characteristics such as density, homogeneity, and reciprocity.

People in different age groups tend to maintain different social networks, with older people having smaller, denser networks (Depner and Ingersoll-Dayton, 1988). Interestingly, these social network differences have not translated into clear differences in the levels or types of social support available across age groups (Turner and Marino, 1994).

Translating Theory and Research into Practice

The conceptual and empirical literature summarized here has important implications for health education practice. The consistent links between social network characteristics and health status, as well as the evidence showing that certain types of networks are best suited to the provision of certain types of support, confirm that a social network approach to investigating the association between social relationships and health has important strengths. Results also suggest that any support-enhancing intervention needs to begin with an assessment of the social networks that are maintained by the target population (Israel, 1982). Such assessments can diagnose aspects of existing social networks that are not meeting the needs of the focal individuals as well as point out the strengths of the networks. Several network mapping and assessment tools are available (House and Kahn, 1985; Kahn and Antonucci, 1980; McCallister and Fischer, 1978; Tardy, 1985; O'Reilly, 1988). The evidence for the health-enhancing effects of affective support suggests that, whenever possible, interactions with potential helpers should facilitate expressions of trust, closeness, and caring. In addition, the importance of reciprocity for well-being suggests that helping relationships should be founded on a basis of mutual interdependence and exchange.

Although the literature does provide some clear implications for practice, health educators who wish to incorporate social network enhancement into their practices face several difficult decision points. House (1981) summarized these decision points in a single question: In order to effectively enhance the health-protective functions of social networks, *who* should provide *what* to *whom* (and *when*)? The issues of who, what, and when will be discussed briefly below.

Who

Social support can be provided by many types of people in both a natural or informal network (for example, family, friends, coworkers, and supervisors) and in a more formal helping network (for example, health care professionals and human service workers). Different network members are likely to provide differing amounts and types of support (Gottlieb and McLeroy, 1994; House, 1981; Lanza and Revenson, 1993; Wenger, 1994). In addition, the effectiveness of the support provided may depend, in part, on the source of the support (House, 1981).

Some researchers have focused on the differences between kin and nonkin sources of support (for example, Wenger, 1994). For example, long-term assistance is most often provided by family members, with neighbors and friends more likely to provide short-term aid (Gottlieb and McLeroy, 1994). In occupational settings, differences in the types and effectiveness of social support provided by coworkers and supervisors have been investigated, with supervisor support often proving to be the most important in terms of health (House, 1981; Israel and others, 1989).

A more comprehensive approach to defining an effective source of support has been offered by Thoits (1986). The effective provision of support is likely to stem from people who are socially similar to the support recipient and who have experienced similar stressors or situations (Thoits, 1986). These characteristics enhance the *empathic understanding* of the support provider, making it more likely that the support proffered is in concert with the needs and values of the recipient. In addition, the person who desires the support is more likely to overcome any stigma attached to needing help and to seek or mobilize support when the social network member is perceived to be empathic and understanding. Empathic understanding is particularly relevant to the exchange of emotional support but also matters in instrumental and informational support.

Long-standing intimate social network ties have unique capabilities to provide social support (House, 1981; Gottlieb and Wagner, 1991). However, there can be a downside to depending on these types of relationships for support, particularly informational support. For example, Gottlieb and Wagner (1991) describe the process of exchanging support in close relationships. They note that often people in close relationships are distressed by the same stressor and that the nature and quality of the support provided are affected by the distress levels of the helper. Also, because the support providers are very interested in the well-being of the support recipients, when support attempts are not well received or do not result in positive changes in the receiver, the helpers can experience negative reactions. Interestingly, this was most true when information and advice were provided. When the support provided entailed supportive listening and expressions of empathy and caring, helpers did not often exhibit negative consequences due to their support attempts. Perhaps close intimate ties are best used for emotional support, but other relationships are better suited to the exchange of informational support (Lanza and Revenson, 1993).

Considerable debate surrounds the question of whether professional helpers are effective sources of social support. Health education interventions may attempt to enhance the social support available to participants by linking them with professional helpers. Professional helpers often have access to information and resources that are not otherwise available in the social network (Lanza and Revenson, 1993; Walker, 1987). However, when mapping their social networks, few people include professional helpers as members of their networks (Veroff, Douvan, and Kulka, 1981), and professional helpers are rarely available to provide social support over long periods of time. Additionally, professional-lay relationships are not often characterized by reciprocity and often entail large power differentials and a lack of the empathic understanding just described. (For further discussion of this relationship, see Chapter Ten.) Walker (1987) suggests that people may be best served when there is a partnership between formal and informal helpers. In such a partnership, each type of helper brings different skills and strengths to the helping process.

What

The extent to which social interactions provide support has usually been addressed from the point of view of the support recipient. Indeed, it is the perception of the support recipient, rather than the objective behaviors involved in the interaction, that are most strongly linked to the recipient's health and well-being (Wethington and Kessler, 1986). However, in order to design interventions aimed at enhancing social support, it is necessary to identify the factors that may influence whether behaviors are likely to be perceived as supportive. These factors include previous experiences that the support recipient has had with the helper, the social context of the relationship (for example: are the two people in competition for resources? does one have the power to reward or punish the other?), role expectations, and individual preferences for types and amounts of social support. Thus, even though knowledge about supportive interactions has been amassed through the observation and study of professional helping relationships (Gottlieb, 1983), the extent to which these behaviors (for example, active listening and providing constructive feedback) generalize across sources of support and situations is not likely to be great.

Given the multitude of factors that affect how social interactions will be perceived by participants, a priori assumptions about what specific behaviors will increase perceived social support may be ill advised. As a corollary, efforts to train social network members in professional helping skills may have little likelihood of success (Weisenfeld and Weis, 1979). Instead, the ways in which social network members can be more supportive may be best identified through target population participation in program development. Discussion among the interested parties about previous successful support efforts and support efforts that have gone awry may generate a set of desired social behaviors and skills specific to the population and problem being addressed. For example, a program designed to enhance coworker and supervisor support among human service workers employed a group format through which, with the guidance of trained facilitators, the employees gleaned suggestions for modifying their behavior from the stories of other employees' effective, supportive social interactions (Heaney, 1991).

When

Research has suggested that the types of social networks and social support that effectively enhance well-being and health differ according to the age or developmental stage of the support recipient (Kahn and Antonucci, 1980). In addition, people who are experiencing a major life transition or stressor benefit from different types of support during the different stages of coping with the stressor (Thoits, 1986). For example, people whose spouses have just died may benefit from a closely knit, dense social network able to provide strong affective support to the bereaved. However, as the widowed individuals modify their lives in order to adapt to their losses, more diffuse networks that offer access to new social ties and diverse informational support may be most helpful. As another example, patients for whom surgery has been recommended may need different types of support as they anticipate surgery, undergo hospitalization and the surgical procedure, and then experience recovery and rehabilitation.

Social Network and Social Support Interventions

Several typologies of social network and social support interventions have been suggested (Israel, 1982; Gottlieb, 1988; Vaux, 1988; Gottlieb and McLeroy, 1994).

Table 9.2 presents a typology that has four categories of interventions: enhancing existing social network linkages, developing new social network linkages, enhancing networks through the use of indigenous natural helpers, and enhancing networks at the community level through participatory problem-solving processes. A fifth category could be composed by combining types of the interventions described in Table 9.2.

One strategy important to all social network interventions is to enhance awareness among the members of the target population of the health-enhancing qualities of social relationships. Just as someone who understands the benefits of antibiotics is more likely to adhere to a prescribed antibiotic regimen, someone who fully appreciates the importance of social relationships to good health is more likely to be motivated to engage in the processes of providing and receiving support. This has been the rationale for mass media campaigns such as the Friends Can Be Good Medicine campaign in California, which attempted to increase awareness among the general population of the importance of friendship to a person's quality of life and to increase people's confidence in their abilities to initiate and maintain friendships (Hersey, Klibanoff, Lam, and Taylor, 1984). Such educational messages and activities are included in many social relationship interventions. In addition to this common component, each category of intervention outlined in Table 9.2 has some unique features, as described briefly in the following paragraphs.

Enhancing existing social network linkages. Existing network linkages often offer much untapped potential. Interventions aimed at enhancing these ties either try to change the attitudes and behaviors of the support recipient, the support provider, or both. The transactional nature of social exchanges suggests that the latter will be most effective, and some research supports this notion (Heaney, 1991). In addition to enhancing participants' awareness of social network and social support concepts, interventions often include skill-building activities in behaviors associated with effective support mobilization, provision, and receipt.

Interventions may focus on enhancing the quality of specific social ties to provide support across many different situations. For example, a worksite intervention might address the potential of coworker and supervisory relationships to be supportive on a day-to-day basis at work. Some interventions have attempted to mobilize social support from an existing network in response to specific health behavior needs. For example, family members can provide instrumental aid (monitoring blood pressure) and affective support to those with hypertension (Earp and Ory, 1979; Morisky and others, 1985). Partners or significant others have been incorporated into smoking cessation programs (Cohen and others, 1988), weight loss programs (Epstein and Wing, 1987), and treatment programs for alcohol abuse (Marlatt and Gordon, 1985).

TABLE 9.2. TYPOLOGY OF SOCIAL NETWORK INTERVENTIONS.

Intervention Type	Examples of Intervention Activities	Selected References
Enhancing existing social network linkages	• Training of network members in skills for support provision	Heaney, 1991 Morisky and others, 1985 Sandler and others, 1992
	• Training of focal individual in mobilizing and maintaining social networks	
	• Systems approach (for example, marital counseling or family therapy)	
Developing new social network linkages	• Creating linkages to mentors	Katz, 1993 Sosa and others, 1980
	• Developing buddy systems	
	• Coordinating self-help groups	
Enhancing networks through the use of indigenous natural helpers	• Identification of natural helpers in the community	Eng and Hatch, 1991 Eng and Young, 1992 Meister, Warrick, DeZapien, and Wood, 1992
	• Analysis of natural helpers' existing social networks	
	• Training of natural helpers in health topics and community problem-solving strategies	
Enhancing networks at the community level through participatory problem-solving processes	• Identification of overlapping networks within the community	Minkler, 1985
	• Examination of social network characteristics of members of the selected need or target area	
	• Facilitation of ongoing community problem identification and problem solving	

Some of the challenges encountered in this type of intervention include identifying existing network members who are committed to providing support and have the resources to sustain the commitment; identifying the changes in attitudes and behaviors that will result in increased perceived support on the part of the support recipient; and intervening in ways that are consistent with established norms and styles of interaction.

Developing new social network linkages. Interventions designed to develop new social network linkages are most useful when the existing network is small, overburdened, or unable to mobilize for the provision of effective support. Sometimes new ties are introduced to alleviate chronic social isolation such as that experienced by the rural elderly (Hooyman, 1980). Most often new ties are introduced in response to a major life transition or specific stressor, and they access important resources to be passed on to others in need. Some interventions introduce *mentors* or *advisers,* people who have already coped with or traversed the situation being experienced by the focal individual. In the Widow-to-Widow program, women who have successfully coped with the loss of a spouse are trained to provide emotional and informational support to new widows (Silverman, 1986). In Alcoholics Anonymous, one member of the group is designated as a fellow alcoholic's "sponsor" and commits to helping that fellow alcoholic deal with the challenges of recovery (Kurtz, 1990). Other interventions introduce *buddies* who are experiencing the stressor or life transition at the same time as the focal individual. For example, in some smoking cessation programs and weight control programs, each participant is encouraged to "buddy up" with one other participant so the two of them can support and encourage each other (Cohen and others, 1988). Rather than introducing a single new social tie, self-help or mutual aid groups provide a new *set* of network ties. Usually, people come together in self-help groups because they are facing a common stressor or because they want to bring about similar changes, either at the individual level (for example, individual weight loss) or at a community level (for example, increased access to health care in one's community). In self-help or mutual aid groups, the roles of support provider and support recipient are mutually shared among the members. Thus, the ties often entail high levels of reciprocity. Although a full description of self-help groups is beyond the scope of this chapter, several good reviews and descriptions exist (Lee, 1988; Katz, 1993; Katz and others, 1992).

The use of indigenous natural helpers. Natural helpers are members of social networks to whom other network members naturally turn for advice, support, and other types of aid (Israel, 1982). They are usually respected and trusted network members who are responsive to the needs of others. In addition to providing support directly to network members, natural helpers can serve an important linking capacity, linking social network members to each other and to resources outside the network. One of the first tasks in natural helper interventions is to identify the people who currently fill these helping roles. Although various strategies have been employed to do this (Eng and Young, 1992; Meister, Warrick, DeZapien, and Wood, 1992), they commonly entail asking people in the target population for the names of people who demonstrate the characteristics of natural helpers. Those people whose names are repeatedly mentioned can be contacted and recruited. The participation of the target population in the identification process is critical. Once the natural helpers are recruited, the health professional can provide information on specific health topics, health and human service resources available in the community, and community problem-solving strategies and can engage in a consultative relationship with the natural helpers. The goal of this consultation is to enhance the skills and support provided by the helpers to their network members, without altering the nature of their helping relationships. Involving natural helpers in both the analysis of the social networks existing in the target community and the development of their own training activities is likely to increase the effectiveness of natural helper programs.

Natural helper interventions have been conducted in a number of different communities, including inner-city neighborhoods, rural counties, residential institutions for the elderly, and church congregations (Salber, 1979; Israel, 1985; Eng and Hatch, 1991; Meister, Warrick, DeZapien, and Wood, 1992; Wilkinson, 1992). For example, the Black Churches Project (Eng and Hatch, 1991; Eng, Hatch, and Callan, 1985) identified natural helpers within congregations of black churches in North Carolina and provided training in health promotion concepts and skills to the identified helpers. The goals of the project were to enhance the health behaviors of members of the congregations by having the natural helpers provide information, advice, emotional support, and access to resources.

Enhancing networks through community problem-solving. Interventions that involve community members in identifying and resolving community problems may have the indirect consequence of strengthening the social networks that exist in the community (Israel, 1982). Such interventions use community organizing techniques with the goals of (1) enhancing the ability of a community to resolve its own problems; (2) increasing the community's role in making decisions that have important implications for community life; and (3) resolving specific problems. Through participating in collective problem-solving processes, community members forge new network ties and strengthen existing ones. For example, in the Tenderloin Senior Outreach Project, elderly residents in the Tenderloin district of San Francisco formed groups and coalitions to address safety and health concerns. Through participation in these groups, the residents became less socially isolated and began to turn to each other for information, advice, and support (Minkler, 1985).

Although community problem-solving interventions often affect social networks only indirectly, social network strategies could be more explicitly incorporated into both the assessment and implementation stages of these interventions (Israel, 1985). The community assessment could determine how people gain information, resources, and support as well as identify potential problem areas. Examining the extent to which people's networks overlap may aid in the diffusion of new information throughout the community.

Combined strategies. Some programs have incorporated a combination of the intervention strategies described earlier in order to improve program impact. For example, a program that enhances existing ties and also forges new ties can benefit both from the power of well-established social relationships and the infusion of new social resources. In the Family Bereavement Program (Sandler and others, 1992), members of families that have experienced a loss attend workshops during which they explore ways in which family members can provide support to each other. During the workshops, the participants also engage in supportive interactions with other bereaved families. After participating in the workshops, each family is matched with a family adviser. This adviser then provides ongoing emotional and informational support, shoring up over-burdened family sources of support.

Combining natural helper interventions with community problem solving is another potentially effective strategy (Eng and Hatch, 1991). The natural helpers can address the needs of the individual network members, and the community-level strategy can address some of the broader social, legal, and economic problems facing the community. This results in a more comprehensive ecological approach to enhancing the health of the community. Lay health advisers can also enhance the effectiveness of community-level cooperative problem solving by working to integrate community residents more fully into the life of the community, and more specifically, into cooperative problem-solving efforts.

Health Education Applications

The two cases described below illustrate in more detail how social network and social support concepts have been applied in health education interventions. Both cases explicitly incorporate stress buffering and health behavior change mechanisms. The first case exemplifies a support intervention involving a professional helper and the second case describes the use of natural helpers.

Case Study: Latin American Trial of Psychosocial Support During Pregnancy

Under the auspices of the Latin American Network for Perinatal and Reproductive Research, a randomized trial was conducted to evaluate the impact of an intervention to enhance the social support available to pregnant women at high risk for delivering a low birth weight or preterm infant (Villar and others, 1992). Epidemiological studies have shown that high stress levels and low levels of social support during pregnancy are associated with adverse effects on maternal and child health (Oakley, 1988). In addition, the provision of a supportive companion during labor and delivery has resulted in enhanced perinatal outcomes (Kennell and others, 1991; Sosa and others, 1980). The major components of this intervention included (1) providing emotional support through a professional home visitor; (2) strengthening existing social ties by including a significant other or support person in the home visits; (3) providing oral and printed health information during home visits; and (4) facilitating appropriate use of health services by providing guided hospital tours and a telephone information hotline. The program developers hypothesized that these activities would enhance health-related behavior, reduce psychological distress, and reduce adverse maternal and infant health outcomes (Langer and others, 1993).

The target population for this intervention was high-risk pregnant women who sought prenatal care by the twenty-second week of their pregnancies at one of the four participating medical centers in Argentina, Brazil, Cuba, and Mexico. The intervention consisted of four to six home visits conducted by specially trained social workers or nurses. Each participant was asked to select a support person from her social network and to invite this person to be present during the home visits. During the visits, the home visitor provided both emotional support (through expressions of empathy and caring) and informational support (through discussions of health behaviors and descriptions of medical care system characteristics and regulations). In order to strengthen the naturally occurring social networks of the pregnant women, the home visitor encouraged the pregnant women and their support persons to reflect on the stressors involved in pregnancy and the ways in which social network members could be supportive (for example, helping with heavy housework and providing child care during labor and delivery). Support persons were asked to "remain involved with the woman throughout the pregnancy, to participate in the decision-making process, to help the woman resolve personal problems, to promote healthful behavior, and to encourage attendance at visits for prenatal care" (Villar and others, 1992). Although the home visitors used a standardized decision-making flowchart to guide their visits, each home visit could be tailored to the problems and resources of the participant. For example, if there were limited support available to a participant, the home visitor could suggest the establishment of new linkages.

Ninety percent of the 1,115 women assigned to the intervention group received at least one visit, with 83 percent of the women receiving the planned four to six home visits. Support persons were present at 66 percent of the visits. Process data suggests that, although discussion of the planned topics occurred in a high proportion of the visits, conversation about health-related topics (for example, diet and weight, physical activity, biological changes during pregnancy) was more frequent than conversation about the availability, mobilization, and maintenance of the participants' social networks (Langer and others, 1993).

The intervention had no discernable effect on perinatal health outcomes. The risks of having low birth weight babies, preterm delivery, and intrauterine growth retardation among women in the intervention group were similar to the risks experienced by the women who received routine care. In addition, the intervention had no effect on the type of delivery, length of hospital stay, perinatal mortality, or infant morbidity during the first forty days of life. Even among the participants with the highest baseline stress levels or the least naturally occurring social support available to them at the beginning of the study, the intervention did not affect these maternal and child health outcomes.

The impact of the intervention on the participants' social networks and social support is not reported in the published accounts of the intervention. Given the positive results of some other social support interventions for enhancing maternal and infant health (Oakley, 1988), the extent to which the Latin American program was effective in terms of enhancing social support should be investigated. To what extent did the participants perceive the home visitors as supportive? Did the persons selected by the participants to be helpers or supporters perform the supportive behaviors suggested during the visits? Were the women any better able to mobilize support as a consequence of the home visits? The fact that a number of pregnant women did not (or could not) elicit the participation of a helper may indicate that their social networks were not suitable for this type of intervention. In addition, the emphasis of the home visitors on health behavior and health care use topics during home visit discussions may indicate a "professional bias" (Langer and others, 1993). The home visitors may not have been able fully to incorporate the participants' and the support persons' expertise about their social networks and social norms into the home visit discussions. Rather than taking the time "to first gauge the ways that ordinary people help one another and then try to strengthen the helping processes that work for them" (Gottlieb, 1985), the home visitors may have inadvertently been overly prescriptive and directive. A more extensive assessment of the women's social networks, building on the strengths of those networks, and less emphasis on professionally defined problems (for example, inadequate use of health services) might have enhanced the effectiveness of the program.

Case Study: Save Our Sisters Project

Although the incidence of breast cancer is no higher among African American women than among white women in the United States, the five-year survival rates for African American women are lower than for white women. Differences in survival may be due, in part, to African American women's being diagnosed at a later stage of the disease. Indeed, a racial gap in the use of mammography screening does exist and appears to be widening (Vernon and others, 1992). In an effort to reduce this racial disparity among older African American women in a rural county of North Carolina, the Save Our Sisters (SOS) Project employed a natural helper intervention for increasing mammography screening (Eng, 1993; Eng and Smith, 1995).

Fourteen focus group interviews were conducted as an initial qualitative investigation of the mammography use behavior of African American women in the targeted county. Two major themes relevant to the social networks of this population emerged from the focus group data: the women tended to seek support from other women in the community when dealing with matters of women's health, and many of the women belonged to social groups that were an important aspect of the community's vitality (Tessaro, Eng, and Smith, 1994). These themes suggested that building on the strengths of the social networks of these women through the use of natural helpers who would serve as "lay health advisors" (LHAs) might be an effective strategy for exchanging informational, emotional, and instrumental support relevant to mammography screening (Eng and Young, 1992). Specifically, those best positioned in African American communities to assist older women to overcome prevailing fears and reticence about breast cancer were likely to be other women who were slightly younger active members of community organizations that put them in contact with women from all income groups, and known for their good judgment, discretion, and willingness to help others.

The SOS Project attempted to create a structure and context within which LHAs could effectively support women in the community in their efforts to learn about and gain access to mammography screening. The project included the following components: identification of LHAs; recruitment of LHAs; provision of training to the LHAs to increase their knowledge of breast cancer and mammography and to enhance their interpersonal and group process skills; ongoing consultation with the LHAs for the purpose of exchanging informational and emotional support through community projects; and evaluation. All these components were implemented in a manner that facilitated community participation and ownership of the project.

A woman from the African American community in the county was hired as project coordinator. She identified African American members of social networks to which she herself did not belong (thereby expanding the reach of the project) and invited them to serve on a twelve-member Community Advisory Group (CAG). The coordinator and the CAG organized the requisite focus group interviews.

Based on the results of these interviews, they developed a recruitment strategy and a plan for training potential LHAs. The recruitment strategy built on the existing networks of the coordinator and CAG members. Each member of the CAG group invited two women from the community to a house party during which the background and goals of the SOS Project were described. Invitees were chosen based on the extent to which they demonstrated the qualities of natural helpers in this community, as described in the focus groups (Eng, 1993). Each of the attendees was then encouraged to invite two more women to another similar event.

After attending the house party, those interested in project participation completed a five-session training course (called Peace of Mind). This training provided information about breast cancer, mammography, and the health care system; addressed the potential roles of lay health advisors; and provided opportunities to build skills in interpersonal counseling and small-group facilitation. Over the course of three years, ninety-five women have completed this LHA training.

Process evaluation data, collected through telephone interviews with LHAs every four months, showed that a level of sixty active volunteer LHAs could be maintained. Inactivity was typically temporary and due to personal illness or a family member's needing special care. Active LHAs were engaged in at least one of the following roles: providing informational and emotional support to social network members, creating a bridge between the lay community and the medical care system, and mobilizing the resources of the community to sustain a commitment to breast cancer prevention (Eng and Smith, 1995). For example, in addition to providing advice and counseling about mammography to social network members, the LHAs have organized mobile mammography screening campaigns, raised funds from community agencies for women who need financial assistance in order to obtain a mammogram, and developed a video for community education purposes. The activities of the LHAs indicate that the SOS Project has been successful in breaking the silence surrounding breast cancer in this community. No data are yet available on the effectiveness of the SOS Project on reducing racial disparities in mammography use.

As in the Latin American intervention described above, little information is available through the published literature on how interactions with the SOS helpers (in this case, the LHAs) were experienced by the support recipients. Although it is important to gain an understanding of the interpersonal transactions through the eyes of the support providers, the perceptions of the support recipients are most strongly associated with health behavior and health status (Wethington and Kessler, 1986; Wortman and Lehman, 1985). Unfortunately, it is difficult to gather such information while maintaining the trust of the LHAs and protecting the LHAs' reputations for confidentiality in their social networks.

Conclusion and Future Directions for Research and Practice

Although descriptive studies have supported many of the hypothesized relationships suggested in Figure 9.1, the health protective effects of social networks and social support have not been consistently translated into effective interventions. For example, descriptive research clearly indicates that receiving social support enhances the likelihood that a smoker will successfully quit. However, smoking cessation interventions that incorporate social network or social support enhancement have not been able to positively affect quit rates (Cohen and others, 1988). How can we improve our ability to incorporate social networks and social support into health education practice?

There is unlikely to be a generic effective social network intervention. Instead, as with other types of health education interventions, effective social network programs need to be tailored to the needs and resources of the participants. Thus, establishing participatory assessment processes during which participants describe and identify the strengths and weaknesses of their social networks will help structure programs so as to be truly supportive. A fair amount of research, including the Latin American intervention trial described in this chapter, suggests that we cannot assume that we have identified the most appropriate helpers nor that behaviors that are intended to be supportive are experienced as supportive by the receiver (see for example, Wortman and Lehman, 1985; Peters-Golden, 1982). Only through dialogue with participants about these issues can we gain the insights necessary for effective health education interventions.

Evaluation of carefully designed and meticulously implemented theory-informed social network interventions will advance our ability to answer the question posed earlier: In order to effectively enhance the health-protective functions of social networks, *who* should provide *what* to *whom* (and *when*)? Recognizing the need for and value of ecological approaches to health education, social network interventions that combine strategies across multiple units of practice (for example, the individual, family, and community) deserve the greatest attention in future research and practice. In keeping with recommendations for the evaluation of health education interventions (Israel and others, 1995), it is important to evaluate both intervention processes and outcomes. As the two cases presented illustrate, understanding of key issues in the development of effective social network interventions will be advanced through (1) careful description of the intervention activities intended to enhance social relationships; (2) monitoring of the effects of these activities on the amount and quality of social support that is both delivered to and experienced by the target population; and (3) assessment of changes in factors such as knowledge, health behaviors, community competence, and health status of the target population.

The complexity of the structure and function of social networks makes the development of effective social network interventions challenging. The conceptual framework and research reviewed in this chapter suggest that the health-enhancing potential of such interventions is substantial.

References

Antonucci, T. C. "Social Supports and Social Relationships." In R. H. Binstock and L. K. George (eds.), *Handbook of Aging and the Social Sciences.* Orlando, Fla.: Academic Press, 1990.

Bandura, A. *Social Foundations of Thought and Action: A Social Cognitive Theory.* Englewood Cliffs, N.J.: Prentice Hall, 1986.

Barnes, J. A. "Class and Committees in a Norwegian Island Parish." *Human Relations,* 1954, *7,* 39–58.

Berkman, L. "Assessing the Physical Health Effects of Social Networks and Social Support." *Annual Review of Public Health,* 1984, *5,* 413–432.

Cassel, J. "The Contribution of the Social Environment to Host Resistance." *American Journal of Epidemiology,* 1976, *104,* 107–123.

Cohen, S., and Syme, S. L. (eds.). *Social Support and Health.* Orlando, Fla.: Academic Press, 1985.

Cohen, S., and Wills, T. A. "Stress, Social Support, and the Buffering Hypothesis." *Psychological Bulletin,* 1985, *98*(2), 310–357.

Cohen, S., and others. "Social Support Interventions for Smoking Cessation." In B. H. Gottlieb (ed.), *Marshaling Social Support: Formats, Processes, and Effects.* Thousand Oaks, Calif.: Sage, 1988.

Depner, C. E., and Ingersoll-Dayton, B. "Supportive Relationships in Later Life." *Psychology and Aging,* 1988, *3,* 348–357.

Earp, J. A., and Ory, M. G. "The Effects of Social Support and Health Professionals' Home Visits on Patient Adherence to Hypertension Regimens." *Preventive Medicine,* 1979, *8,* 155–165.

Eng, E. "The Save Our Sisters Project: A Social Network Strategy for Reaching Rural Black Women." *Cancer,* 1993, *72,* 1071–1077.

Eng, E., and Hatch, J. W. "Networking Between Agencies and Black Churches: The Lay Health Advisor Model." *Prevention in Human Services,* 1991, *10,* 123–146.

Eng, E., Hatch, J. W., and Callan, A. "Institutionalizing Social Support Through the Church and into the Community." *Health Education Quarterly,* 1985, *12,* 81–92.

Eng, E., and Parker, E. "Measuring Community Competence in the Mississippi Delta: The Interface Between Program Evaluation and Empowerment." *Health Education Quarterly,* 1994, *21,* 199–220.

Eng, E., and Smith, J. "Natural Helping Functions of Lay Health Advisors in Breast Cancer Education." *Breast Cancer Research and Treatment,* 1995, *35,* 23–29.

Eng, E., and Young, R. "Lay Health Advisors as Community Change Agents." *Family and Community Health,* 1992, *15,* 24–40.

Epstein, L. H., and Wing, R. R. "Behavioral Treatment of Childhood Obesity." *Psychological Bulletin,* 1987, *101,* 331–342.

Gottlieb, B. H. *Social Support Strategies: Guidelines for Mental Health Practice.* Thousand Oaks, Calif.: Sage, 1983.

Gottlieb, B. H. "Social Networks and Social Support: An Overview of Research, Practice, and Policy Implications." *Health Education Quarterly,* 1985, *12,* 5–22.

Gottlieb, B. H. "Marshaling Social Support: The State of the Art in Research and Practice." In B. H. Gottlieb (ed.), *Marshaling Social Support: Formats, Processes, and Effects.* Thousand Oaks, Calif.: Sage, 1988.

Gottlieb, B. H., and McLeroy, K. R. "Social Health." In M. P. O'Donnell and J. S. Harris (eds.), *Health Promotion in the Workplace.* (2nd. ed.) Albany, N.Y.: Delmar, 1994.

Gottlieb, B. H., and Wagner, F. "Stress and Support Processes in Close Relationships." In J. Eckenrode (ed.), *The Social Context of Coping.* New York: Plenum, 1991.

Heaney, C. A. "Enhancing Social Support at the Workplace: Assessing the Effects of the Caregiver Support Program." *Health Education Quarterly,* 1991, *18,* 477–494.

Heitzmann, C. A., and Kaplan, R. M. "Assessment of Methods for Measuring Social Support." *Health Psychology,* 1988, *7*(1), 75–109.

Hersey, J. C., Klibanoff, L. S., Lam, D. J., and Taylor, R. L. "Promoting Social Support: The Impact of California's 'Friends Can Be Good Medicine' Campaign." *Health Education Quarterly,* 1984, *11,* 293–311.

Hirsch, B. J., and DuBois, D. L. "The Relation of Peer Social Support and Psychological Symptomatology During the Transition to Junior High School: A Two-Year Longitudinal Analysis." *American Journal of Community Psychology,* 1992, *20,* 333–347.

Hooyman, N. R. "Mutual Help Organizations for Rural Older Women." *Educational Gerontology: An International Quarterly,* 1980, *5,* 429–447.

House, J. S. *Work Stress and Social Support.* Reading, Mass.: Addison-Wesley, 1981.

House, J. S. "Social Support and Social Structure." *Sociological Forum,* 1987, *2,* 135–46.

House, J. S., and Kahn, R. L. "Measures and Concepts of Social Support." In S. Cohen and L. Syme (eds.), *Social Support and Health.* Orlando, Fla.: Academic Press, 1985.

House, J. S., Umberson, D., and Landis, K. R. "Structures and Processes of Social Support." *Annual Review of Sociology,* 1988, *14,* 293–318.

Israel, B. A. "Social Networks and Health Status: Linking Theory, Research, and Practice." *Patient Counselling and Health Education,* 1982, *4,* 65–79.

Israel, B. A. "Social Networks and Social Support: Implications for Natural Helper and Community Level Interventions." *Health Education Quarterly,* 1985, *12*(1), 65–80.

Israel, B. A., and Rounds, K. A. "Social Networks and Social Support: A Synthesis for Health Educators." *Advances in Health Education and Promotion,* 1987, *2,* 311–351.

Israel, B. A., and others. "The Relation of Personal Resources, Participation, Influence, Interpersonal Relationships and Coping Strategies to Occupational Stress, Job Strains and Health: A Multivariate Analysis." *Work and Stress,* 1989, *3,* 163–194.

Israel, B. A., and others. "Evaluation of Health Education Programs: Current Assessment and Future Directions." *Health Education Quarterly,* 1995, *22,* 364–389.

Kahn, R. L., and Antonucci, T. C. "Convoys over the Life Course: Attachments, Roles and Social Support." In P. B. Baltes and O. Brim (eds.), *Life Span Development and Behavior.* Vol. 3. Orlando, Fla.: Academic Press, 1980.

Katz, A. H. *Self-Help in America: A Social Movement Perspective.* New York: Twayne, 1993.

Katz, A. H., and others. *Self-Help: Concepts and Applications.* Philadelphia: Charles Press, 1992.

Kennell, J., and others. "Continuous Emotional Support During Labor in a US Hospital: A Randomized Controlled Trial." *Journal of the American Medical Association,* 1991, *265,* 2197–2201.

Kurtz, L. F. "Twelve-Step Programs." In T. J. Powell (ed.), *Working with Self-Help.* Silver Spring, Md..: National Association of Social Workers Press, 1990.

Langer, A., and others. "The Latin American Trial of Psychosocial Support During Pregnancy: A Social Intervention Evaluated Through an Experimental Design." *Social Science and Medicine,* 1993, *36,* 495–507.

Lanza, A. F., and Revenson, T. A. "Social Support Interventions for Rheumatoid Arthritis Patients: The Cart Before the Horse?" *Health Education Quarterly,* 1993, *20,* 97–117.

Lee, D. L. "The Support Group Training Project." In B. H. Gottlieb (ed.), *Marshaling Social Support: Formats, Processes, and Effects.* Thousand Oaks, Calif.: Sage, 1988.

Levy, R. "Social Support and Compliance: A Selective Review and Critique of Treatment Integrity and Outcome Measurement." *Social Science and Medicine,* 1983, *17,* 1329–1338.

Marlatt, G. A., and Gordon, J. R. (eds.). *Relapse Prevention.* New York: Guilford Press, 1985.

McCallister, L., and Fischer, C. S. "A Procedure for Surveying Personal Networks." *Sociological Methods and Research,* 1978, *7,* 131–149.

McKinlay, J. B. "Social Network Influences on Morbid Episodes and the Career of Help Seeking." In L. Eisenberg and A. Kleinman (eds.), *The Relevance of Social Science for Medicine.* Boston: Reidel, 1980.

McLeroy, K. R., Bibeau, D., Steckler, A., and Glanz, K. "An Ecological Perspective on Health Promotion Programs." *Health Education Quarterly,* 1988, *15,* 351–377.

Meister, J. S., Warrick, L. H., DeZapien, J. G., and Wood, A. H. "Using Lay Health Workers: Case Study of a Community-Based Prenatal Intervention." *Journal of Community Health,* 1992, *17,* 37–51.

Minkler, M. "Building Supportive Ties and Sense of Community Among the Inner-City Elderly: The Tenderloin Senior Outreach Project." *Health Education Quarterly,* 1985, *12*(4), 303–314.

Morisky, D. E., and others. "Evaluation of Family Health Education to Build Social Support for Long-Term Control of High Blood Pressure." *Health Education Quarterly,* 1985, *12,* 35–50.

Oakley, A. "Is Social Support Good for the Health of Mothers and Babies?" *Journal of Reproductive and Infant Psychology,* 1988, *6,* 3–21.

O'Reilly, P. "Methodological Issues in Social Support and Social Network Research." *Social Science and Medicine,* 1988, *26,* 863–873.

Peters-Golden, H. "Breast Cancer: Varied Perceptions of Social Support in the Illness Experience." *Social Science and Medicine,* 1982, *16,* 483–491.

Rhodes, J. E., Contreras, J. M., and Mangelsdorf, S. C. "Natural Mentor Relationships Among Latina Adolescent Mothers: Psychological Adjustment, Moderating Processes, and the Role of Early Parental Acceptance." *American Journal of Community Psychology,* 1994, *22,* 211–227.

Rook, K. S. "The Negative Side of Social Interaction: Impact on Psychological Well-Being." *Journal of Personality and Social Psychology,* 1984, *46,* 1097–1108.

Salber, E. J. "The Lay Advisor as a Community Health Resource." *Journal of Primary Prevention,* 1979, *3,* 116–132.

Sandler, I. N., and others. "Linking Empirically Based Theory and Evaluation: The Family Bereavement Program." *American Journal of Community Psychology,* 1992, *20,* 491–521.

Shumaker, S. A., and Hill, D. R. "Gender Differences in Social Support and Physical Health." *Health Psychology,* 1991, *10,* 102–111.

Silverman, P. *Widow to Widow.* New York: Springer, 1986.

Sosa, R., and others. "The Effect of a Supportive Companion on Perinatal Problems, Length of Labor, and Mother-Infant Interactions." *New England Journal of Medicine,* 1980, *303,* 597–600.

Spiegel, D. "Effects of Psychosocial Support on Patients with Metastatic Breast Cancer." *Journal of Psychosocial Oncology,* 1992, *10,* 113–120.

Spiegel, D., Bloom, J., Kraemer, H. C., and Gottheil, E. "Effects of Psychosocial Treatment on Survival of Patients with Metastatic Breast Cancer." *Lancet,* 1989, *2,* 888–891.

Starrett, R. A., and others. "The Role of Environmental Awareness and Support Networks in Hispanic Elderly Persons' Use of Formal Social Services." *Journal of Community Psychology,* 1990, *18,* 218–227.

Stewart, M. J. "Social Support: Diverse Theoretical Perspectives." *Social Science and Medicine,* 1989, *28,* 1275–1282.

Stokols, D. "Establishing and Maintaining Healthy Environments: Toward a Social Ecology of Health Promotion." *American Psychologist,* 1992, *47*(1), 6–22.

Tardy, C. H. "Social Support Measurement." *American Journal of Community Psychology,* 1985, *13,* 187–202.

Taylor, S. E., Buunk, B. P., and Aspinwall, L. G. "Social Comparison, Stress, and Coping." *Personality and Social Psychology Bulletin,* 1990, *16,* 74–89.

Tessaro, I., Eng, E., and Smith, J. "Breast Cancer Screening in Older African-American Women: Qualitative Research Findings." *American Journal of Health Promotion,* 1994, *8,* 286–293.

Thoits, P. A. "Social Support as Coping Assistance." *Journal of Consulting and Clinical Psychology,* 1986, *54,* 416–423.

Turner, R. J., and Marino, F. "Social Support and Social Structure: A Descriptive Epidemiology." *Journal of Health and Social Behavior,* 1994, *35,* 193–212.

Vaux, A. *Social Support: Theory, Research, and Intervention.* New York: Praeger, 1988.

Vernon, S. W., and others. "Breast Cancer Screening Behaviors and Attitudes in Three Racial/Ethnic Groups." *Cancer,* 1992, *69,* 165–174.

Veroff, J., Douvan, E., and Kulka, R. A. *The Inner American: A Self-Portrait from 1957 to 1976.* New York: Basic Books, 1981.

Villar, J., and others. "A Randomized Trial of Psychosocial Support During High-Risk Pregnancies. The Latin American Network for Perinatal and Reproductive Research." *New England Journal of Medicine,* 1992, *327,* 1266–1271.

Walker, A. "Enlarging the Caring Capacity of the Community: Informal Support Networks and the Welfare State." *International Journal of Health Services,* 1987, *17,* 369–386.

Walker, K. N., MacBride, A., and Vachon, M.L.S. "Social Support Networks and the Crisis of Bereavement." *Social Science and Medicine,* 1977, *11,* 35–41.

Wallston, B. S., Alagna, S. W., DeVellis, B. M., and DeVellis, R. F. "Social Support and Physical Health." *Health Psychology,* 1983, *2,* 367–391.

Weisenfeld, A. R., and Weis, H. M. "A Mental Health Consultation Program for Beauticians." *Professional Psychology,* 1979, *10,* 786–792.

Wenger, G. C. *Support Networks of Older People: A Guide for Practitioners.* Bangor, Wales: University of Wales Print Unit, 1994.

Wethington, E., and Kessler, R. C., "Perceived Support, Received Support, and Adjustment to Stressful Life Events." *Journal of Health and Social Behavior,* 1986, *27,* 78–89.

Wilkinson, D. Y., "Indigenous Community Health Workers in the 1960s and Beyond." In R. L. Braithwaite and S. E. Taylor (eds.), *Health Issues in the Black Community.* San Francisco: Jossey-Bass, 1992.

Wortman, C. B., and Lehman, D. R. "Reactions to Victims of Life Crises: Support Attempts That Fail." In I. G. Sarason and B. R. Sarason (eds.), *Social Support: Theory, Research, and Applications.* Dordrecht, Netherlands: Martinus Nijhoff, 1985.

CHAPTER TEN

PATIENT-PROVIDER COMMUNICATION

Debra L. Roter
Judith A. Hall

Communication is both the most basic and the most powerful vehicle of health care. It is the fundamental instrument by which the patient-provider relationship is crafted and by which therapeutic goals are achieved. Without the talk that organizes a patient's history and symptoms and puts them in a meaningful context, complicated technology and sophisticated treatment are of limited value. The talk of the medical visit, the words that are used, the facts exchanged, the advice given, and the social amenities that tie the conversation together are what we most often think of when communication between patient and health care provider is considered. But communication also goes beyond words to the whole repertoire of nonverbal expressions and cues that pass between doctor and patient. Smiles and head nods of recognition, the grimaces of pain, frowns of dis-

A portion of this chapter appeared in D. L. Roter and J. A. Hall, "Studies of Doctor-Patient Interaction" and is reproduced, with permission, from the *Annual Review of Public Health*, Volume 10, ©1989, by Annual Reviews Inc. A portion of this chapter also appeared in D. L. Roter and J. A. Hall, "Health Education Theory: An Application to the Process of Patient-Provider Communication," *Health Education Research Theory and Practice*, 1991, *6*, 185–193, and is reproduced here by permission of Oxford University Press. A further portion of this chapter appeared in D. L. Roter and J. A. Hall, *Doctors Talking to Patients/Patients Talking to Doctors: Improving Communication in Medical Visits* (1992), and is reproduced here by permission of Auburn House, an imprint of Greenwood Publishing Group, Inc., Westport, Connecticut.

approval, and the high-pitched voice of anxiety all give context and enhanced meaning to the words spoken.

Taken together the verbal and nonverbal exchanges of the medical dialogue reflect the dynamics of the relationship between the health care provider and his or her patient. The relationship is complicated by the diversity of functions it serves and the dynamic of patients' needs and circumstances over time, as well as shifts in societal values and cultural norms. This chapter reviews the historical roots of concepts of communication within the patient-provider relationship, with particular emphasis on the physician-patient relationship. An emphasis on communication within the physician-patient relationship reflects the bulk of research to date and serves as a point of departure for research on communication between patients and other health care providers as well.

Historical Perspective

"A physician to slaves never gives his patient any account of his illness. . . . [T]he physician offers some orders gleaned from experience with an air of infallible knowledge, in the brusque fashion of a dictator. . . . The free physician, who usually cares for free men, treats their diseases first by thoroughly discussing with the patient and his friends his ailment. This way he learns something from the sufferer and simultaneously instructs him" (Plato, cited in Hamilton and Cairns, 1961).

In contrasting medical paternalism and patient autonomy, Plato's characterization of the physician's relationship to free men and to slaves anticipated the core of the modern debate on the nature of the patient-physician relationship (Emanuel and Emanuel, 1992).

There are two views regarding the character of the potential clash between patient autonomy and physician paternalism in the doctor-patient relationship. The first is that it can take the form of consensual accommodation and the second is that it is outright conflict. The consensual view has been articulated by Parsons (1951), who argued that conflict is managed and diffused by well-defined societal expectations for both patient and physician conduct, as specified by the patient's sick role and the physician's professional obligations. In contrast, Freidson (1970) sees conflict as ongoing and fundamental to the doctor-patient relationship. The most fully discussed area of this autonomy-paternalism clash concerns medical knowledge.

In some respects, the argument over medical knowledge may be reduced to a question of ownership. Parsons argues that inherent in the definition of *physician* is the dedication of a lifetime to the mastery of knowledge and the gaining of experience in the application of that knowledge. The fund of medical knowledge is so vast and complex, the schooling so intense and grueling, and the daily experience so unique, that an unbridgeable competence gap exists between physicians and the lay world. Medical knowledge is thus earned and owned by doctors. Moreover, this knowledge is impossible to share fully. However, there are protections afforded patients because they must accept most medical practice on faith. Central to these protections is a higher order of moral conduct that physicians are held to, including a code of ethics defining the special duty of physicians to protect the interests of their patients. Patients, for their part, rely on physician adherence to this moral code and therefore cooperate with the doctor's orders. A patient who resists doctor's orders risks potential loss of standing as a patient and being stigmatized as a malingerer or a fake; no patient can truly want to get well if he or she does not cooperate with the doctor (Parsons, 1951).

A different view about the conflict over medical knowledge is articulated by Freidson (1970). While agreeing with Parsons that the core definition of professionalism is the mastery of expert knowledge and experience, Freidson sees the disinclination of physicians to share information with patients less as a function of an irrevocable competence gap than as a safeguard for physicians' high status and professional standing. Moreover, a less knowledgeable patient is unlikely to second-guess the doctor or detect medical errors (Freidson, 1970). Medical knowledge per se is not all that is gained during training. Physicians also learn and internalize a worldview that includes a way of thinking based on the biomedical model of disease (Engel, 1977). The predominant view a physician brings to medical practice is one anchored in the world of biochemistry and technology. In contrast, a patient's world comprises a complex web of personality, culture, living situations, and relationships, which color and define the illness experience (Kleinman, 1980; Mishler, 1984). The conflict, then, is between incomplete perspectives: the biomedical view loses the context of the patient's life, while the patient's experience lacks insight into science and potential medical intervention. Thus, a contest of definitions ensues between doctor and patient. The physician wants a biomedical definition of the patient's illness, posed as a disease with known physical manifestations, which implies medical ownership of those manifestations, while the patient wants the definition to be his or her own in terms of his illness experience (Mishler, 1984; Cassell, 1976). The physician who dismisses a debilitating flu as "only the flu" may miss, from the patient's perspective, the full impact of the illness experience and its meaning. The patient may see the flu as an indication of a compromised immune system and an early sign of cancer. A physicians' failure to appreciate this kind of significance arises from a fundamental difference between doctors and patients in their worldviews.

It is through manipulation of information and definition of the problem that the nature and conduct of the medical visit are determined—what will be said and done, when, and how. Patients have some measure of power over how the medical visit will proceed, although expression of that power is usually more subtle than the physician's corresponding expression of power. Patients can, of course, request and insist on certain procedures or prescriptions, ask questions and probe the physician's clinical reasoning, or refuse to go along with a recommended test or treatment. Direct confrontation between doctor and patient, however, is the exception rather than the rule. Far more common are maneuvers and negotiations that span a broad spectrum of power relations.

It is along this negotiated spectrum that patient autonomy and physician and health care provider authority are defined in any given relationship. Because of the great variability in patients' ability to negotiate in this realm, ethicists have identified the potential for medical coercion as a central question in medical ethics. Indeed, since the 1960s, patient autonomy has become a tenet of medical ethics, with almost universal regard that it is a necessary and important element of medical care (President's Commission for the Study of Ethical Problems in Medicine and Biomedical and Behavioral Research, 1982).

Patient-Physician Control Prototypes

To further explore the varying perspectives on the doctor-patient relationship, we can examine alternative ideal types. Figure 10.1 illustrates the four archetypal forms of doctor-patient relationship: paternalism, consumerism, mutuality, and default and lists the authors most closely associated with them. A more detailed discussion of the prototypes can be found in Roter (1987), Roter and Hall (1992), and Emanuel and Emanuel (1992). Although the referent is to the physician-patient relationship, the archetypal forms potentially relate to other health care providers as well.

The prototype of paternalism is shown in the upper left quadrant, illustrating a relationship of high physician control and low patient control. Paternalism is widely regarded as the traditional form of the doctor-patient relationship and it is still seen as the most common one (Parsons, 1951; Szasz and Hollender, 1956; President's Commission, 1982). A passive patient and dominant physician as the idealized therapeutic relationship is most clearly articulated by Parsons in his classic writings on the sick role (Parsons, 1951). Parsons saw the doctor and patient as fulfilling necessary functions in a well-balanced and maintained social structure. Sickness in this model is considered a necessary, occasional respite providing a brief exemption for patients from societal responsibilities. However, for society to continue to function, this respite must be controlled. By defining the terms of the illness and its privileges, physicians provide this controlling force.

FIGURE 10.1. DOCTOR-PATIENT RELATIONSHIP PROTOTYPES.

High Physician Control

Paternalism
 	
Parsons, 1951
Szasz and Hollender, 1956
Ende and others, 1990
	Mutuality
	
	Engel, 1970
	   (biopsychosocial approach)
	McWhinney, 1992
	   (patient-centered relationship)
	Kleinman, 1980
	   (patients' explanatory
	   framework)

Default Roter and Hall, 1992	**Consumerism** Freidson, 1970 Reeder, 1972 Haug and Lavin, 1983

Low Patient Control   High Patient Control

Low Physician Control

When sick, a patient is allowed the privilege of convalescence—he or she is not held responsible for poor health and is excused from everyday responsibilities. However, in order to enjoy these privileges, the patient must seek technically competent help and comply with medical advice. The patient's role then is passive and dependent. In contrast, the doctor's role is defined as professionally dominant and autonomous. The doctor legitimates the patient's illness and determines the course of treatment. In doing so, the physician is compelled by professional ethics to act only in his or her sphere of expertise, to maintain an emotional detachment and distance from the patient, and to act in the patient's best interest.

In addition to the social control function that the paternalism model affords, there are significant nurturing and supportive aspects to this type of relationship. Patients may draw comfort and support from a doctor-father figure. Indeed, the supportive nature of paternalism appears to be all the more important when patients are very sick and at their most vulnerable (Ende, Kazis, Ash, and Moskowitz, 1989). Relief of the burden of worry is curative in itself, some argue, and the trust and confidence implied by this model allow the doctor to do "medical magic." Classic placebo studies have also demonstrated that the idealization of the physician can have an important therapeutic effect (Lasagna, Mosteller, von Feisinger, and Beecher, 1954).

Consumerism, in the lower right quadrant, is the opposite of paternalism, reversing the power relationship between doctor and patient. The advent of medical consumerism in the United States has been attributed to several significant societal changes since the 1960s (Reeder, 1972). The first of these changes is the shift from curative to preventive services. Reeder notes that in a system dominated by curative or emergency care, there is a "seller's market," and the relationship tends to be characterized by the patient as supplicant. However, when prevention of illness is emphasized, the patient is less a supplicant than a skeptic. Part of the doctor's job is to convince the patient of the necessity of noncurative services such as periodic checkups. Under these circumstances, there are elements of a "buyer's market" and a tendency for the "customer to be right."

Another feature of societal change, also described by Reeder, is the development of consumerism as a social movement and the redefinition of the person as consumer rather than as patient. A concurrent critical focus on the bureaucratization of the system of medical care delivery and its spiraling costs has resulted in increasing use of *health care provider* to replace the more traditional terminology of *doctor*. Redefinition of the doctor-patient relationship as a consumer-provider exchange is more than a matter of simple semantics because it refocuses the traditional perspective and changes the very nature of the social relationship between the medical profession and the lay world (Reeder, 1972). Several authors have defined consumerism as a patient challenge to unilateral decision making by physicians when reaching closure on diagnosis and treatment plans (Haug and Lavin, 1983). Inherent in this definition is a challenge to physician authority, because the definition reverses the basic nature of the power relationship, focusing "on the purchaser's (patient's) rights and seller's (physician's) obligations, rather than on physician's rights (to direct) and patient obligations (to follow directions). . . . In a consumer relationship, the seller has no particular authority; if anything, legitimated power rests in the buyer, who can make the decision to buy or not to buy, as he or she sees fit" (Haug and Lavin, 1983).

While still stressing patient control, the prototype of mutuality shown in the upper right quadrant proposes a more moderate alternative to the polar extremes of paternalism and consumerism. In mutuality, each participant brings recognized strengths and resources to the relationship. Inasmuch as power in the relationship is balanced, decisions are the result of what may be considered a meeting between equals. The patient's job, in this model, is to become part of a joint venture, and the physicians' job is to recognize the centrality of the patient in patient care. The writings of Engel (1977, 1988) in the United States and McWhinney in Canada (1988, 1989) refocused a largely biomedical-centric profession to a more patient-centered endeavor. Likewise, contributions by medical anthropologists such as Kleinman (1980), sociologist Mishler (1984), and social epidemiologist Cassell (1976), among others, have brought the patients' perspective to the forefront of patient care.

What happens when patient and physician expectations are at odds or when the need for change in the relationship cannot be negotiated? A possible consequence of poor fit, or failure to change the relationship as needs and circumstances change, is relationship default, represented in the lower left quadrant and characterized by a total lack of control. In this case, the patient may ritualistically continue visits to the doctor but fail to make a commitment to the therapeutic regimen or assume responsibility for seeking alternative care. Physicians may likewise abandon a patient by similarly continuing a ritualistic schedule of visits while ceasing to engage, educate, or influence the patient.

Significance of Physician-Patient Communication to Patient Outcomes

Systematic study of doctor-patient communication, documenting the association between what is said during the medical interview and patients' attitudes and behaviors has been relatively recent. Nonetheless, the positive benefits to be derived from good doctor-patient communication have been found to span a spectrum from immediate and obvious effects during the medical visit to long-term effects following the visit and involving symptom and pain experience, compliance with therapeutic regimens, physiological changes, speed of recovery, and functional status (Roter and Hall, 1992). The virtually unanimous finding from two and a half decades of research in the area is the strong relationship of communication to patient satisfaction (Hall, Roter, and Katz, 1988). Satisfaction with medical care has been studied more than any other patient outcome; it is studied in its own right as a legitimate reflection of met patient needs but also in its relationship to other consequences.

Studies of objective records of doctor-patient communication reveal that the social climate established in the medical visit appears to be a major determinant of satisfaction. Satisfaction is increased when physicians treat patients in a more partner-like manner, when more positively toned words are spoken (such as statements of agreement), when fewer negative words are spoken (such as criticisms), when more social conversation occurs (such as greetings and nonmedical chitchat), and when the physician treats the patient in a warmer and more immediate nonverbal manner (such as sitting closer or engaging in more eye contact) (Hall, Roter, and Katz, 1988). All of these behaviors suggest the way people act when they like someone. Indeed, research shows that when doctors like their patients more, their patients are more satisfied with them (Hall, Epstein, DeCiantis, and McNeil, 1993; Like and Zyzanski, 1987).

The emotional climate is not the only factor that predicts patient satisfaction. The strongest predictor is how much information is given to the patient about diagnosis, the causes and course of a disease, or possible treatments and what they entail. Patients who get more information are more satisfied than patients who get less information (Hall, Roter, and Katz, 1988). This speaks to the high value placed on information by patients. The correlation of information to satisfaction could reflect not only patients' desire for information per se but also patients' feelings about doctors who give more information. Patients may reason that a doctor who gives more information is nicer or more concerned about them as people than is a physician who gives less information. Thus, two values may operate simultaneously—the value placed by patients on medical information and the value placed on having a humane and involved physician.

Another doctor trait associated with patient satisfaction is nonverbally communicated affect toward the patient. Physicians who feel critical and rejecting toward particular patients convey these feelings through their tone of voice. The doctor who speaks about patients in a coldly autocratic way tends also to speak to them in the same manner; physicians who speak about patients in a warm and caring way tend to speak to them in a warm and honest tone of voice (Rosenthal, Vannicelli, and Blanck, 1984).

Compliance has also been positively associated with a variety of communication skills. We know that when the doctor offers more information, engages in more positive talk and less negative talk, and asks fewer questions overall (but more questions about compliance in particular), the more likely a patient is to be compliant (Hall, Roter, and Katz, 1988). The association of less question asking to more compliance is consistent with research finding that question asking is inversely related to information giving (Hall, Roter, and Katz, 1987).

Finally, there is evidence that physicians' communication behaviors are associated with patient recall. Recall is best predicted by information giving, less question asking, more positive talk, and more partnership building (Hall, Roter, and Katz, 1987).

It is one thing to argue that good doctor-patient communication leads to higher patient satisfaction and even compliance with recommendations, but quite another to link communication to specific health outcomes. However, this link has been established in both hospital and outpatient studies. Doctor-patient communication has been associated with improved recovery from surgery, decreased use of pain medication, and shortened hospital stays (Devine, 1992) as well as physiological changes in blood pressure and blood sugar (Kaplan, Greenfield, and Ware, 1989).

Dynamics of Patient-Provider Communication: A Theoretical Framework

Despite the overwhelming evidence associating aspects of the therapeutic relationship to patients' health behavior and outcomes, little theorizing on the mechanisms of effect have been discussed. Reviews of empirical studies of doctor-patient communication underscore the atheoretical nature of the literature (Roter and Hall, 1992; Inui and Carter, 1985). The fragmented and predominantly exploratory nature of this research produces an overwhelming number of results almost impossible to interpret. Inui and Carter (1985) characterize the literature as a "Rorschach test" for readers, in which overall interpretations are as apt to reveal something about the reader as about the results themselves.

Limitations of the literature are especially striking when viewed from a health education perspective. Lack of attention to theoretical issues relevant to the doctor-patient relationship may be attributed, at least in part, to the nature and application of the field's predominant models or frameworks (Mullen, Hersey, and Iverson, 1987). The emphasis on antecedents or consequences of health behavior inherent in these models has discouraged researchers from addressing processes of change within the medical encounter. This point is well illustrated by the results of a comprehensive review of the history of the oldest and most popular of health education models, the Health Belief Model (Janz and Becker, 1984). While the forty-six studies detailed in the review address the prediction of patient behavior in regard to use of health services and compliance with prescribed regimens, none addresses the possible influences of the actual medical encounter on patient behavior. Thus, the explanatory mechanisms for understanding the process of communication during medical encounters is most often allocated to the proverbial "black box."

We propose a theoretical model that suggests a perspective for viewing the dynamics and consequences of patients' and providers' behavior within the medical visit. Our theoretical model is derived loosely from social exchange (Emerson, 1976) and reciprocity theory (Gouldner, 1960) focusing on the trade of valued resources through the social interaction processes of the medical visit. First described by Gouldner (1960) and elaborated in the medical context by Davis (1969), the reciprocity hypothesis places the exchange of information during the medical encounter within the context of an exchange of rights and obligations. Patients' obligation to cooperate with the physician, for instance by complying with medical recommendations may be contingent on satisfaction of patients' rights to feedback and information regarding their condition. Failure of the physician to satisfy patient's rights to information may lead to patient failure in regard to the obligation of compliance.

We have elaborated this notion of reciprocity beyond information giving to suggest that all physicians' behaviors can be seen broadly to reciprocate parallel patient behaviors. We see physician behaviors as falling within two complementary behavioral domains: a task-focused technical realm and a socioemotional realm. Furthermore, these domains of provider behavior inspire parallel patient behaviors, similarly reflecting task and socioemotional domains.

Task Domain

Physicians' task behaviors are defined as technically based skills used in problem solving that constitute the base of the "expertness" for which a physician is consulted. Task behaviors are essentially those behaviors that define the role of the physician and are close to the role conceptualizations proposed by Parsons (1951) and others (Bloom, 1963; Ben-Sira, 1980). Included are such tasks as data gathering, medical information giving, and patient counseling as well as other markers of clinical proficiency such as accurate diagnosis and appropriate treatment.

These technical functions are important not only in furthering the physicians' clinical agenda to diagnose and treat but also in furthering the patient's agenda to understand and make sense of the frightening vulnerability of illness as well as to feel that his or her experience and perspective are understood. Therefore, some task-focused behaviors may be considered vehicles for the patient agenda (that is, *patient centered*), and others may be more directly linked to the physicians' agenda (that is, *physician centered*). Information giving and patient counseling are examples of the former, and question asking, especially of the closed-ended questions that often dominate data-gathering efforts, is an example of the latter (Roter and Hall, 1992).

We suggest that patient behavior also has a task dimension that reflects problem-solving skills. For instance, patient task behaviors include accurate and full reporting of current and past symptoms and medically relevant experiences; attentiveness, comprehension, and recall; and active participation in the care process. Further, although not directly articulated within the medical encounter, behaviors such as compliance and use of care or services are influenced by the dynamics of the encounter and may also be numbered among patients' task functions.

Socioemotional Domain

The socioemotional dimension of communication behavior is more complex than the task dimension. Conceptualization of the appropriate expression of physicians' affect has varied tremendously, from Parsons' view of affective neutrality (1951), in which affect is controlled or ignored, to models in which expression of affect and task are distinguished as different types of communication that are both present during an interaction but are largely independent of one another (Bloom, 1963).

Our conceptualization differs from these models. It is premised on the belief that all face-to-face behavior, even that which is ostensibly neutral, carries affective content. This is true of both physicians' and patients' behavior. The affective character of the interaction may be seen on three levels: (1) intrinsic, (2) conveyed, and (3) interpreted. The *intrinsic* level consists of verbal exchanges with explicit socioemotional content such as social conversation, agreements, criticisms, statements of concern, reassurance, legitimation, partnership, and empathy. The basis of identification for these exchanges is face validity, that is, the obvious and literal content of a communication.

The *conveyed* level of affect consists of qualities of voice tone that carry emotional content. Our assessment process for conveyed affect is to filter out the verbal content from audiotapes by passing them through an electronic band filter. This process preserves voice qualities such as syncopation, rhythm, and speed but obscures the verbal content. It is like listening to a conversation through a closed door—one can hear only sounds, not individual words. Independent raters have been shown to substantially agree on ratings of voice quality measured in this manner (Hall, Roter, and Rand, 1981). This conveyance of affect occurs during verbal exchanges that are intrinsically affective as well as those that involve task behaviors such as giving information, counseling, and question asking.

Finally, the *interpreted*, or attributed, level of affect reflects the total impression created in the receiver of a communication. Particular communications may gain affective significance even when that attribution or interpretation is not warranted by their intrinsic content or the way they are conveyed. For example, physicians who give information may be perceived as interested irrespective of whether they have expressed or conveyed interest through any other messages they may communicate to patients, or a patient may be perceived as bored or disinterested because of silence or a downward gaze of the eyes.

In addition to socioemotional expression, interpersonal attitudes and satisfaction with the therapeutic relationship are also reflections of the socioemotional domain.

Application: A Patient-Analogue Study

The framework just described may be viewed as a comprehensive matrix for hypothesis generation. With this framework in mind, we have conducted a patient-analogue study, predicting relationships between patient and provider socioemotional domains and patient and provider task domains and relationships crossing patient and provider socioemotional and task domains based on our previous studies (Hall, Roter, and Katz, 1987; Roter, Hall, and Katz, 1987).

The data sources for these studies were audiotapes and transcripts of two different standardized patient cases presented by trained patient simulators to forty-three primary care physicians. The simulated patients were four men in their late fifties with medical histories consistent with the scripted cases. The two cases were designed to reflect a patient with chronic bronchitis in the first instance and emphysema in the second. Both cases were exacerbated by smoking and prior noncompliance. The simulators were trained to fully represent the particulars of the scripted case and to otherwise react as they would in a medical encounter. They were instructed to answer questions in an open manner but not to initiate discussion regarding their medical history. Training was conducted by a team including a pulmonary specialist and behavioral scientists.

Transcripts of the resulting audiotapes were scored based on criteria generated by pulmonary experts to determine physician proficiency in history taking, physical examination, patient education, accuracy of diagnosis, and appropriate drug prescription. Transcripts were also subjected to analysis to assess the process and explicit content of the communication using the Roter Interaction Analysis System (RIAS) (Roter, 1995). The RIAS codes task-related categories such as information giving and patient counseling, as well as socioemotional categories such as agreements, compliments, jokes, concern, reassurance, and social remarks.

The expert-based physician proficiency scores and the RIAS scores reflecting information giving and patient counseling were used as indicators of physicians' task behaviors. Because no actual patients participated in this study, an attempt was made to create a proxy for likely patient reactions to the physicians' behavior in the recorded visits. We recruited three different subjects to listen to each of the eighty-six audiotapes (total $N = 258$). The subjects were instructed to imagine that they were the patient while listening to the audiotape. Afterward, they were asked to complete an extensive recall measure of the medical information communicated to them during the visit. This recall measure was used as an indicator of the patients' task behaviors.

The subjects were also asked to rate their satisfaction in three ways: (1) a one-item global satisfaction assessment, (2) a five-item satisfaction assessment of each physician's technical performance, and (3) a six-item satisfaction assessment of each physician's interpersonal skills. These satisfaction ratings constituted the patients' socioemotional measure.

The physicians' socioemotional measure was based on two different kinds of ratings. The positive socioemotional composite of the RIAS coding (agreements, compliments, jokes, concern, reassurance, and social remarks) represented the first measure of physicians' socioemotional behavior and reflected the expression of explicit or intrinsic affect. Physicians' affect may also be conveyed through voice tone. We used electronically filtered excerpts, as described earlier, of the physicians' remarks to assess voice tone. These filtered speech clips were played to a group of thirty-seven independent judges, who assessed physician emotion through voice quality. The voice ratings reflect conveyed affect by the physicians and represent the second of the physicians' socioemotional measures. The resulting relationships between patient and physician task and socioemotional domains are shown in Table 10.1.

In the task domain, we hypothesized that physician task behaviors would predict parallel patient task behaviors. Our findings were quite convincing from the perspective of the role-playing patients and the performance of the simulated patients. Correlations between role-playing patient recall of medical information communicated to them and physician technical proficiency, information giving, and counseling ranged from .27 to .71, all significant at the .01 level or lower. Only question asking was unrelated to recall. These findings suggest that patient and physician task domains are substantially related.

Within the socioemotional domain, we similarly hypothesized that physicians' socioemotional behaviors (explicitly positive talk and emotion conveyed through filtered voice tone) would be associated with patients' satisfaction. As mentioned earlier, satisfaction was measured by a single global item and two independent scales, one reflecting satisfaction with interpersonal skills and the other satisfaction with technical performance.

Explicit socioemotional talk was significantly correlated with both satisfaction dimensions but in opposite directions. Socioemotional talk was positively associated (although missing significance) with satisfaction with interpersonal skill $(.21, p < .1)$ but negatively associated with satisfaction with technical performance $(-.21, p < .1)$. There was no relationship between socioemotional talk and global satisfaction.

We also found that the role-playing patient ratings of satisfaction were related to the aspects of affect measured through the filtered tapes of physician conversation. Excerpts rated high on anger and boredom were negatively correlated with satisfaction (with anger being significantly related). When satisfaction was defined in terms of the two subscales, anger was negatively correlated with interpersonal skill $(-.27, p < .05)$ but not significantly so with technical performance $(-.08, p > .25)$. However, boredom was negatively correlated with technical performance $(-.30, p < .05)$ but not significantly with interpersonal skill $(-.02, p > .25)$.

This implies that a physician who sounds angry will jeopardize patient satisfaction with interpersonal skills, while a physician who sounds bored may jeopardize patient satisfaction with technical performance. Since the measures of voice quality and of explicit talk were made by different judges and uncorrelated, these effects are independent and not two expressions of the same relationship. The

TABLE 10.1. CORRELATIONS BETWEEN PROVIDER AND PATIENT BEHAVIORAL DOMAINS.

Provider Domain	Patient Domain	Correlation
Task	*Task*	
Proficiency	Recall	.46
Information giving	Recall	.27
Counseling	Recall	.39
Medical information	Recall	.71
Question asking	Recall	−.15
Task	*Socioemotional*	
Proficiency	Satisfaction (global)	.57
	Interpersonal skills	.29
	Technical performance	.59
Information giving	Satisfaction (global)	.53
	Interpersonal skills	.27
	Technical performance	.62
Counseling	Satisfaction (global)	.52
	Interpersonal skills	.28
	Technical performance	.57
Question asking	Satisfaction (global)	.24
	Interpersonal skills	.21
	Technical performance	.22
Socioemotional	*Task*	
Socioemotional talk	Recall	−.36
Filtered speech		
Anger	Recall	−.12
Boredom	Recall	−.13
Calm	Recall	−.14
Socioemotional talk	Satisfaction (global)	−.04
	Interpersonal skills	.21
	Technical performance	−.22
Filtered speech		
Anger	Satisfaction (global)	−.27
	Interpersonal skills	−.31
	Technical performance	.08
Boredom	Satisfaction (global)	−.16
	Interpersonal skills	−.02
	Technical performance	−.30
Calm	Satisfaction (global)	−.01
	Interpersonal skills	−.16
	Technical performance	.13

Note: Correlations of .25 are significant at $p = .10$; .30 at $p = .05$; .37 at $p < .01$; and .47 at $p < .001$.

results mean that physicians who engage in socioemotional conversation and *sound* bored are most likely to inspire patient dissatisfaction. This is reflected particularly in dissatisfaction with technical performance of care, implying that patients interpret this combination as a lack of technical proficiency rather than a lack of interpersonal skill.

Most notable in this study are the cross-domain findings. As illustrated in the third quadrant of Table 10.1, there was a significant negative relationship $(-.36, p < .05)$ between physicians' socioemotional talk and role-playing patients' recall. The relationship to voice tone was not significant. The second quadrant of Table 10.1 illustrates the many significant relationships between the physicians' proficiency, information giving, and counseling and the role-playing patients' satisfaction. Global satisfaction was strongly related to these variables (range .52 to .57), as well as satisfaction with technical performance (range .57 to .62). Interpersonal skill satisfaction was also related but at more modest levels (range .27 to .29). Only question asking was not statistically significant in its relation to patient satisfaction.

It is also interesting that physicians' task behaviors created a strong affective impression on raters (not illustrated in the table). The clinically proficient physician created an impression of interest $(.54, p < .001)$, calm $(.48, p < .001)$, and friendliness $(.28, p < .1)$. Physicians who communicated relatively more medical information and devoted more communication to counseling were also perceived as interested and less bored than the others $(.39, .46, p < .01$, and $.28, p < .1$, respectively).

We conclude from these findings that the manner in which task behaviors were performed was anything but neutral in its effect on patients. Substantial variation in physician voice quality *conveys* affective messages to patients during the performance of such routine task behaviors as information giving and counseling. Moreover, patients *interpret* or attribute affective meaning to these behaviors; they see information giving and counseling as behaviors that reflect physician interest in them.

In sum, these cross-domain findings are perhaps counterintuitive. Patient satisfaction with and affective impressions of the physician were more strongly predicted by the ostensibly neutral task-oriented communications than by the explicitly socioemotional communications or by nonverbal voice quality. We maintain that words reflecting socioemotional communication are not nearly as effective in conveying a consistent message of interest and concern as are words reflecting task-oriented communication. Moreover, not all task behaviors are equivalent in their effect on patients. The patient-centered behaviors, information giving and counseling, are more positive in their effect than physician-centered behaviors such as question asking.

These positive effects of patient-centered behaviors are consistent with a growing literature demonstrating the efficacy of information giving for a variety of therapeutic effects including shortened hospital stays, decreased use of analgesics, and reduced patient and anxiety, among others (Devine, 1992). We suggest that the mechanism by which information achieves its therapeutic effects involves *both* the explicit content and the interpreted message of interest and caring.

Our findings support the results of another study designed to measure physician behavior along the technical and affective dimension. Willson and McNamara (1982) designed an analogue study in which providers' technical competence and courtesy were manipulated in taped vignettes. The investigators report that the viewers of the videotape were able to discriminate fairly subtle behavioral variations in both the technical and interpersonal domains with respectable accuracy. Furthermore, it appeared that the affective manipulation influenced the perception of courtesy and general medical satisfaction while the competence manipulation influenced perceived competence and anticipated compliance as well as perceived courtesy and general medical satisfaction. Ratings in the two domains were moderately correlated, but subjects did not appear to confuse the domains, as evidenced by their accurate ratings of the videotapes.

Application: Meta-Analysis Study of Communication Dynamics

Using the same framework we described earlier, we examined relationships within the results of a meta-analysis of provider communication during medical visits (Hall, Roter, and Katz, 1988). The meta-analysis was performed following standard procedures, using studies retrieved through Medline searches of 1966 to 1985 bibliographies and hand searches of key journals and our reprint files. Forty-one independent studies, described in fifty-five articles, containing correlates of objectively measured provider behaviors were included in the final analysis. Using quantitative methods to summarize the research findings, we extracted effect sizes, expressed as correlations, from each study. A special challenge in this review was to group the many conceptual variables used to describe communication, 247 in all, in a meaningful and interpretable way. Many of these communication variables were conceptual equivalents of one another. For instance, information giving was variously articulated as "gives opinion," "gives suggestion," "gives medical information," "informative nonevaluativeness," "volunteers explanation," "statement of information or opinion," "edifies," and "gives direction," among many others. The conceptual grouping was accomplished through a process of consensus sorting by the two lead authors of the review. Five broad conceptual groupings of communication variables emerged from this process and accounted for virtually all the 247 variables: (1) information giving (in general; in relation to treatment, procedures, and physical exam; and illness or symptom specific); (2) question asking (in general, with closed and open questions, and for compliance monitoring); (3a) competence (technical proficiency); (3b) competence (interpersonal proficiency); (4) partnership building (encouragement of patient participation in the dialogue, use of "we" as a sentence stem, not dominating the visit verbally, producing global affect judgments of low dominance or high submissiveness); (5) socioemotional behavior (including positive talk such as social conversation, agreements, approvals, and laughter and humor and negative talk).

Three of these groupings were further seen to reflect physicians' task-focused behaviors: information giving, technical competence, and question asking. The first two of these are patient centered, while the third is physician centered. The remaining three groupings—interpersonal competence, partnership building, and socioemotional behaviors—all reflect physicians' socioemotional domain. Table 10.2 reflects these measures and their division into provider and patient task and socioemotional domains.

The dependent variables in the reviewed studies were less variable than the communication measures and most often reflected patient satisfaction, recall of medications or understanding of the medical problem, and compliance. Also, as reflected in Table 10.2, satisfaction measures can be considered a socioemotional outcome, while recall and compliance can be considered task-related outcomes.

The correlations displayed in Table 10.2 reflect the mean relationships found between communication variables within conceptual groupings and each given dependent variable, as reported in the meta-analysis (Hall, Roter, and Katz, 1988). More detail regarding the methodology is provided in Hall, Roter, and Katz, 1988.

Using the same framework as described for the analogue study, we found the strongest relationships in our meta-analysis between parallel domains. Inspection of the task-task domain (the first quadrant of Table 10.2) reflects significant correlations between the physician task of information giving and the patient task behaviors of compliance and recall. Question asking showed a negative relationship to patient outcomes. This relationship, as well as the negative relationship between question asking and recall found in the analogue study (see Table 10.1), may reflect the special nature of questions as a physician-centered task behavior.

The correlations between physician socioemotional behaviors (positive, social, and negative talk, interpersonal competence and partnership building) and patient satisfaction, shown in the fourth quadrant of Table 10.2, were stronger than the relationships in any other quadrant. All individual correlations, except the one between negative talk and satisfaction, are significant.

Relationships across domains present a somewhat different pattern of association. Physicians' task behaviors and patient satisfaction showed a positive re-

TABLE 10.2. CORRELATIONS BETWEEN PROVIDER INTERACTION AND PATIENT BEHAVIOR: META-ANALYSIS STUDY.

Provider Domain	Patient Domain	Mean Correlation	Combined Z
Task	*Task*		
Information giving	Compliance	.12(8)	3.63
Information giving	Recall	.31(8)	5.71
Questions	Compliance	−.12(4)	3.68
Questions	Recall	−.09(4)	2.14
Task	*Socioemotional*		
Information giving	Satisfaction	.25(12)	6.31
Questions	Satisfaction	−.06(7)	.91
Technical competence	Satisfaction	.17(4)	3.73
Socioemotional	*Task*		
Partnership building	Compliance	−.03(7)	1.19
Partnership building	Recall	.20(3)	3.50
Positive talk	Compliance	.05(6)	1.26
Positive talk	Recall	.04(4)	1.84
Negative talk	Compliance	−.03(5)	2.88
Socioemotional	*Socioemotional*		
Partnership building	Satisfaction	.17(8)	4.19
Positive talk	Satisfaction	.19(10)	3.65
Negative talk	Satisfaction	.008(6)	1.40
Social talk	Satisfaction	.17(3)	2.84
Interpersonal competence	Satisfaction	.33(5)	6.80

Note: Combined Z of 1.96, $p < .05$; 2.55, $p < .01$; 2.85, $p < .001$; 4.0 and greater, $p < .0001$ (two-tailed).

lationship. Information giving and technical competence were significantly related to patient satisfaction, and question asking was not and, indeed, again showed a relationship in a negative direction.

Finally, the relationship between physicians' socioemotional and patients' task behaviors showed a weaker pattern than variables in the other quadrants. Here, partnership showed a positive relationship to recall, and negative talk showed a very small (but significant) negative relationship to compliance.

We believe that the explanatory mechanism for these result patterns is the same as that described in our earlier example. The weaker relation found in the meta-analysis between physicians' socioemotional behaviors and patients' task behaviors can be seen as a indication of weaker reciprocity between these domains.

In our view, physicians' socioemotional behaviors do not have sufficient task or technical significance to lead strongly or frequently to reciprocal task-relevant responses in patients. The physician who is socioemotionally expressive may inspire patient friendliness or liking, but this is not sufficient for a patient task response. Friendliness is not enough to motivate patients to attend to information, modify a lifestyle, or adhere to a therapeutic regimen.

Conclusion

The basic characteristics of the patient-provider relationship may be undergoing substantial evolutionary change (Inui and Carter, 1985). Patients are becoming more like consumers in their orientation, and physicians may be accommodating their patients with more egalitarian relationships and greater tolerance for patient participation in decision making (Roter and Hall, 1992). Changes in the direction of increased patient participation in medical affairs and increased consumerism have been generally regarded as positive, with anticipated consequences for an expansion of the medical dialogue to include patients as full partners in negotiating and evaluating medical services (Brody, 1980; Quill, 1983; Speedling and Rose, 1985).

Assessment of the dynamics of these changes and their implications should be of key interest to health educators. However, health education as a field has not yet developed a well-articulated perspective or a theoretical base to guide research and practice in this arena. Such a perspective, Pratt (1976) has argued, would include two elements: first, that health care be approached as a problem-solving endeavor that requires active coping rather than passivity and submission and, second, that the patient-physician relationship be viewed as an organized system of social behavior that can be entered into to negotiate for services. We believe that the concept of reciprocity in medical exchange is very much in keeping with the consumer perspective and will be useful in furthering this line of research. It assumes active and conscious patient judgment of the value of provider behavior and a rational and predictable patient response along attitudinal and behavioral lines.

References

Ben-Sira, Z. "Affective and Instrumental Components in the Physician-Patient Relationship: An Additional Dimension of Interaction Theory." *Journal of Health and Social Behavior,* 1980, *21,* 170–180.

Bloom, S. *The Doctor and His Patient: A Sociological Interpretation.* New York: Russell Sage Foundation, 1963.

Brody, D. S. "The Patient's Role in Clinical Decision-Making." *Annals of Internal Medicine,* 1980, *93,* 718–722.

Cassell, E. J. *The Healer's Art.* Cambridge, Mass.: MIT Press, 1976.

Davis, M. "Variations in Patients' Compliance with Doctors' Advice: An Empirical Analysis of Patterns of Communication." *American Journal of Public Health,* 1969, *58,* 274–288.

Devine, E. "Effects of Psychoeducational Care for Adult Surgical Patients: A Meta Analysis of 191 Studies." *Patient Education and Counseling,* 1992, *19,* 129–142.

Emanuel, E. J., and Emanuel, L. L. "Four Models of the Physician-Patient Relationship." *Journal of the American Medical Association,* 1992, *267,* 2221–2226.

Emerson, R. M. "Social Exchange Theory." *Annual Review of Public Health,* 1976, *2,* 335–362.

Ende, J., Kazis, L., Ash, A., and Moskowitz, M. A. "Measuring Patients' Desire For Autonomy: Decision Making and Information-Seeking Preferences Among Medical Patients." *Journal of General Internal Medicine,* 1989, *4,* 23–30.

Engel, G. L. "The Need For a New Medical Model: A Challenge For Biomedicine." *Science,* 1977, *196,* 129–136.

Engel, G. "How Much Longer Must Medicine's Science Be Bound by a Seventeenth Century World View?" In K. L. White (ed.), *The Task of Medicine: Dialogue at Wickenburg.* Menlo Park, Calif.: Henry J. Kaiser Family Foundation, 1988.

Freidson, E. *Professional Dominance.* Chicago: Aldine Press, 1970.

Gouldner, A. W. "The Norm of Reciprocity: A Preliminary Statement." *American Sociological Review,* 1960, *26,* 161–179.

Hall, J. A., Epstein, A. M., DeCiantis, M. L., and McNeil, B. J. "Physicians' Liking for Their Patients: More Evidence for the Role of Affect in Medical Care." *Health Psychology,* 1993, *12,* 140–146.

Hall, J. A., Roter, D. L., and Katz, N. R. "Task Versus Socioemotional Behaviors in Physicians." *Medical Care,* 1987, *25,* 399–412.

Hall, J. A., Roter, D. L., and Katz, N. R. "Meta-Analysis of Correlates of Provider Behavior in Medical Encounters." *Medical Care,* 1988, *26,* 657–675.

Hall, J. A., Roter, D. L., and Rand, C. S. "Communication of Affect Between Patient and Physician." *Journal of Health and Social Behavior,* 1981, *22,* 18–30.

Hamilton, E., and Cairns, H. (eds.). *Plato: The Collected Dialogues* (E. J. Emanuel, trans.). Princeton, N.J.: Princeton University Press, 1961.

Haug, M., and Lavin, B. *Consumerism in Medicine: Challenging Physician Authority.* Thousand Oaks, Calif.: Sage, 1983.

Inui, T. S., and Carter, W. B. "Problems and Prospects for Health Services Research on Provider-Patient Communication." *Medical Care,* 1985, *23,* 521–538.

Janz, N. K., and Becker, M. H. "The Health Belief Model: A Decade Later." *Health Education Quarterly,* 1984, *11,* 1–47.

Kaplan, S. H., Greenfield, S., and Ware, J. E., Jr. "Assessing the Effects of Physician-Patient Interactions on the Outcomes of Chronic Disease." *Medical Care,* 1989, *27,* S110–S127.

Kleinman, A. *Patients and Healers in the Context of Culture.* Berkeley: University of California Press, 1980.

Lasagna, L., Mosteller, F., von Feisinger, J. M., and Beecher, H. K. "A Study of the Placebo Response." *American Journal of Medicine,* 1954, *37,* 770–779.

Like, R., and Zyzanski, S. J. "Patient Satisfaction and the Clinical Encounter: Social Psychological Determinants." *Social Science and Medicine,* 1987, *24,* 351–357.

McWhinney, I. "Through Clinical Method to a More Humanistic Medicine." In K. L. White (ed.), *The Task of Medicine: Dialogue at Wickenburg.* Menlo Park, Calif.: Henry J. Kaiser Family Foundation, 1988.

McWhinney, I. "The Need for a Transformed Clinical Method." In M. Stewart and D. L. Roter (eds.), *Communicating with Medical Patients.* Thousand Oaks, Calif.: Sage, 1989.

Mishler, E. G. *The Discourse of Medicine: Dialectics of Medical Interviews.* Norwood, N.J.: Ablex, 1984.

Mullen, P. D., Hersey, J. C., and Iverson, D. C. "Health Behavior Models Compared." *Social Science and Medicine,* 1987, *24*(11), 973–981.

Parsons, T. *The Social System.* New York: Free Press, 1951.

Pratt, L. *Family Structure and Effective Health Behavior: The Energized Family.* Boston: Houghton Mifflin, 1976.

President's Commission for the Study of Ethical Problems in Medicine and Biomedical and Behavioral Research. *Making Health Care Decisions: The Ethical and Legal Implications of Informed Consent in the Patient-Practitioner Relationship.* Vol 1. Washington, D.C.: U.S. Government Printing Office, 1982.

Quill, T. E. "Partnerships in Patient Care: A Contractual Approach." *Annals of Internal Medicine,* 1983, *98,* 228–234.

Reeder, L. G. "The Patient-Client as a Consumer: Some Observations on the Changing Professional-Client Relationship." *Journal of Health and Social Behavior,* 1972, *13,* 406–412.

Rosenthal, R., Vannicelli, M., and Blanck, P. "Speaking to and About Patients: Predicting Therapists' Tone of Voice." *Journal of Consulting and Clinical Psychology,* 1984, *52,* 679–686.

Roter, D. L. "Patient Participation in Clinical Decision Making." *Patient Education and Counseling,* 1987, *9,* 25–31.

Roter, D. L. *The Roter Interaction Analysis System (RIAS) Coding Manual.* Baltimore, Md.: Johns Hopkins School of Hygiene and Public Health, 1995. (Available upon request from the author.)

Roter, D. L., and Hall, J. A. "Studies of Doctor-Patient Interaction." *Annual Review of Public Health,* 1989, *10,* 163–180.

Roter, D. L., and Hall, J. A. "Health Education Theory: An Application to the Process of Patient-Provider Communication." *Health Education Research Theory and Practice,* 1991, *6,* 185–193.

Roter, D. L., and Hall, J. A. *Doctors Talking to Patients/Patients Talking to Doctors: Improving Communication in Medical Visits.* Westport, Conn.: Auburn House, 1992.

Roter, D. L., Hall, J. A., and Katz, N. R. "Relations Between Physicians' Behaviors and Analogue Patients' Satisfaction, Recall, and Impressions." *Medical Care,* 1987, *25,* 437–451.

Speedling, E. J., and Rose, D. N. "Building an Effective Doctor-Patient Relationship: From Patient Satisfaction to Patient Participation." *Social Science and Medicine,* 1985, *2,* 115–120.

Szasz, P. S., and Hollender, M. H. "A Contribution to the Philosophy of Medicine: The Basic Model of the Doctor-Patient Relationship." *Archives of Internal Medicine,* 1956, *97,* 585–592.

Willson, P., and McNamara, J. R. "How Perceptions of a Simulated Physician-Patient Interaction Influence Intended Satisfaction and Compliance." *Social Science and Medicine,* 1982, *16,* 1699–1704.

CHAPTER ELEVEN

PERSPECTIVES ON MODELS OF INTERPERSONAL HEALTH BEHAVIOR

Frances Marcus Lewis

Models of interpersonal health behavior are the focus of the chapters in Part Three. The basic assumption of the chapters is that individuals are socially embedded and are partly defined in terms of their interpersonal relationships. Concurrently, individuals are regarded as active, not passive, agents: they are not merely responding to their interpersonal environments; they are also affecting them. Interpersonal relationships create the context in which persons derive their sense of self-value and personal confidence over health matters and from which they obtain information, affirmation, or services that affect their health behavior and health status.

This chapter sums up key ideas that have been presented in Part Three and suggests some directions for future research into the influence of interpersonal relationships on health behavior.

The chapters in Part Three comprise one theory and two frameworks. Social Cognitive Theory is analyzed in Chapter Eight, social support and social networks are reviewed in Chapter Nine, and patient-provider communication is examined in Chapter Ten.

Social Cognitive Theory

Social Cognitive Theory, as chapter authors Baranowski, Perry, and Parcel describe, integrates both the operant conditioning and the cognitive branches of social learning theory. Seminal work in the operant conditioning branch was completed by Rotter (1954, 1966, 1975) and was extended into health behavior areas by Wallston (Wallston, Smith, Rye, and Burish, 1991). From the operant conditioning branch, we learned about the construct of locus of control, including health locus of control. Literally hundreds of professional papers have been published on the concept of locus of control or health locus of control as a predictor of health behavior (Lewis, 1987). Although these papers were helpful in describing and predicting who might be at risk for such problems as noncompliance (Lewis, Morisky, and Flynn, 1978) or alcoholic recidivism, studies using the construct of health locus of control did not yield consistent results, even as the measures for assessing the locus of control concept were increasingly refined (Wallston, Stein, and Smith, 1994). This may be because two key concepts were missing from Rotter's and Wallston's models—concepts that depicted the *cognitive frame of reference of the individual* and the *processes by which the individual's cognitive frame could be changed.* The cognitive branch of social learning theory responded to these theoretical limitations: it delineated concepts that added to our understanding of the individual's frame of reference and it described methods for changing both the cognitive frame and the behavior of the individual.

Social Cognitive Theory is a dynamic, multicomponent theory that posits that individuals derive an enhanced sense of self-efficacy or confidence over their health behavior through specific mechanisms: through modeling, through performance accomplishment, through persuasion, and through minimizing physiological arousal (O'Leary, 1985). Due to the delineation of these mechanisms for affecting self-efficacy, Social Cognitive Theory can guide development of finely targeted interventions in health education (Strecher, DeVellis, Becker, and Rosenstock, 1986). As seen in the applications in Chapter Eight, the theory has relevance to interventions focused on individuals as well as to community-focused interventions. Many others are also using Social Cognitive Theory as the basis for media-based interventions at the community or population level (Amezcua, McAlister, Ramirez, and Espinoza, 1990; Parcel and others, 1994; Maibach, Flora, and Nass, 1991).

Social Networks and Social Support

In Chapter Nine, Heaney and Israel analyze social support and social networks as applied to health behavior. Their chapter adds to our understanding of the importance of both social support and social networks in creating health-enhancing interpersonal environments. The authors draw on a substantial body of literature from a variety of disciplines to develop their framework, including sociology, psychology, epidemiology, and health education. Their model helps us understand both the processes as well as the outcomes of social support and social network characteristics, thereby helping us to open up the "black box" of causation. In delineating these explanatory processes, they help us to begin to answer the question: What is it about social support that *causes* enhanced health behavior and outcomes?

Social support and social networks are not a theory but a set of concepts that have been studied over a number of years. During that time, the dimensions of social support and social networks have been linked to both intermediate health behavior and long-range outcomes like health status, morbidity, and mortality. The literature on networks and support is almost limitless, and Figure 9.1 in Chapter Nine serves as a helpful heuristic in organizing this large array of prior studies.

Not content with a conceptual and empirical analysis of prior research in Chapter Nine, the authors also identify categories of interventions that hold promise for enhancing the effectiveness of both social support and social networks. These categories of intervention include developing or enhancing existing network linkages, augmenting networks by using indigenous natural helpers, and adding to participatory problem-solving processes at the network level in the community.

Patient-Provider Communication

Chapter Ten offers a new direction to research on patient-provider communication. The conceptualization of authors Roter and Hall veers from the traditional power-based models of interactions between provider and patient and instead casts communication within a mutual influence model. Joos and Hickam's review of the traditional literature on physician-patient communication (1990), published in the first edition of this book, is an important summary of the extant research and literature at that time; Roter and Hall's chapter suggests a complementary direction for research and intervention.

Like Chapter Nine, Chapter Ten is not about a fully developed theory but an evolving theoretical framework, with hypothesized relationships between a set of predetermined concepts. It is also highly linked to Roter and Hall's empirical model of physician-patient interaction, which builds on thousands of hours of observing and coding such interactions. Their two cases offer the reader examples of results that feed back to the theoretical framework, including results that raise questions about the conditions under which certain types of provider interactions have deleterious consequences.

Future Research

The two theoretical frameworks and one formal theory presented in Part Three suggest that multiple research agendas are needed to advance our understanding of interpersonal theories and their effects on health-related behavior and outcomes. All the chapters go well beyond broadly stated predictions to include an analysis of the explanatory mechanisms that need further elaboration and testing. The central sets of concepts in these chapters vary, however, in their level of development. Social Cognitive Theory is the only set of concepts that would meet the most stringent criteria for a hypothetical-deductive theory. It has also enjoyed over thirty years of research, including development in both experimental and clinical psychology as well as current applications in health education.

Three areas of needed future research are suggested by the authors of Part Three: further testing of the explanatory mechanisms of effect; further refinement of methods to change, not merely describe, health-related behavior; and further refinement of the conditions under which the theories or frameworks either do or do not apply, or need to be modified in order to apply better.

Further Testing of the Explanatory Mechanisms

Additional research is needed to further examine the mechanisms of effect in social networks and social support and in patient-provider communication. The mechanisms of effect in Social Cognitive Theory are well specified, not so yet in the two frameworks. It is through understanding the mechanisms of effect, not merely isolated variables, that scientists and practitioners alike have the greatest potential to tell us where to intervene and on what variables programs and services need to be developed in order to advance the health of individuals and of communities.

We need to better understand answers to the following questions about the mechanisms of effect in patient-provider communication: What interpersonal processes explain why certain provider behaviors result in optimal responses in the patient? What characteristics of the exchange foster health-enhancing behavior by both the provider and the patient, including mutual decision making (Kaplan and others, 1995)? What are the tolerances for error (inattentiveness, nonempathic response) in the provider that do not have deleterious consequences on the patient's behavior? Increasingly, we look to future work by Roter and Hall and others to help us answer these questions.

We also need to better understand the mechanisms of effect of social support: What are the essential properties of the exchange that help the person *perceive* the exchange as supportive or nonsupportive? (An answer to this question might help us understand why, for example, in the case application described by Heaney and Israel, the pregnant women who received support as defined by the support providers did not perceive support.) What are the tolerances for variability in the interpersonal exchange that still allow it to be perceived as supportive? What is it about a person's perception of connectedness with others that makes the difference between a healthy or unhealthy state for the person? Notice that these questions do not ask for more correlational research with social support; instead, they focus precisely on better understanding the *explanatory mechanisms* through which social support affects a person's health.

Refinement of Methods to Change Behavior

Theories of health behavior and health education can be descriptive and predictive. They can be behavioral change theories, or they can be a combination of descriptive, prescriptive, *and* behavioral change theories. In Part Three, Social Cognitive Theory is both a descriptive-predictive theory *and* a behavioral change theory; the social support and social networks framework includes both a descriptive-predictive component and suggestions for methods to enhance health behavior. Future research on social networks and support as well as on patient-provider communication will be increasingly challenged to build additional variables into these frameworks that will include or suggest behavioral change methods. Heaney and Israel offer the first step toward that goal when they identify broad areas in which networks can be used in interventions and programs. The editors of this book find this expansion into the realm of intervention, not just description, encouraging. It will be exciting over the next years to watch as these areas for intervention evolve into formal components of the model, thereby transforming the framework of description into a theory of change. We also hold hopes for Roter and Hall's model to expand increasingly into domains of intervention. Our hope is that other investigators will also attempt to answer these questions; there is room for the contributions of many scientists and practitioners.

Refinement and Extension of Theory into New Areas

The conditions under which the provision of certain types of social support are beneficial or potentially harmful are still to be understood. See, for example, Belle's analysis (1982) of the negative consequences of social support under the expectation of reciprocity. A cautious view of social support protects researchers and practitioners from an ideology of practice in health education in which social support is *inherently* valued and, worse yet, reified, in its importance. There is an emerging literature in feminist theory, for example, that raises serious questions about the conditions under which persons "silence" the self in interpersonal exchanges (Jack, 1991); such silencing may maintain membership in the network, may elicit supportive statements from an intimate partner, but may do so at excessive emotional and health cost to the individual. There is also beginning evidence from longitudinal descriptive research on the family's long-term adjustment to chronic illness that social support fails to significantly predict how the family adjusts to the illness, even when social support is available (Lewis, Woods, Hough, and Bensley, 1989; Lewis, Hammond, and Woods, 1993; Lewis and others, 1996). Early suggestive evidence indicates that some families do not want to use available support when they think it will negatively reflect on their own competencies, be interpreted by others as a failure to successfully manage, or otherwise label them as vulnerable or weak.

Both program planners and scientists need to know the conditions under which support, even when available, is not perceived, is not used, or fails to affect health outcomes. Still to be studied, too, are the methods needed to best fit the type, form, and frequency of support to the persons needing support (Nelles, McCaffrey, Blanchard, and Ruckdeschel, 1991). Also needed is identification of the most effective methods by which to positively affect the person's *perception of support.*

Refinements and extensions will enhance the theoretical framework offered by Roter and Hall. At present, their framework is focused on the micro-elements of interpersonal exchange between the physician and the patient. We look forward to the evolution of their model as a parsimonious and conceptual model in which the micro-elements of exchange are depicted as operational components of more abstract concepts. We hope, too, that their framework will evolve in ways that account for the counterintuitive findings obtained in the first application they describe. Ongoing research in patient-provider communication will also do well to include two additional directions: a systems approach and an interactional model of provider systems that are not limited to physician-dominated systems.

Patient-provider interactions should be studied in a context larger than face-to-face dyadic exchanges, one that includes the emotional and physical environment of the service delivery system. Continuing research that isolates patient-provider communications as simple dyadic phenomena may be appropriate for studying the micro-elements of exchange, but in the long run, this perspective will be enhanced by imbedding it within a model of the larger system. Providers and patients are not isolated in an office nor in a clinic encounter. A more inclusive model would imbed the patient-provider encounter within a larger framework of service delivery, including the receptivity of the health care system to the patient's expressed concerns; complementary methods, other than the face-to-face encounter, that the provider uses to augment, sustain, and foster self-management and self-care; the processes by which the patient is brought into the service delivery system; and the persons, other than the direct provider, with and from whom the patient interacts and receives service.

More research on various types of providers, not just physicians, needs to be conducted in the future. Currently there is an overdominance of research on physicians in studying the effects of patient-provider communication; future agendas need to include other providers as well. Recent research by Lowenberg (1993) on primary care services and nurse-run clinics offers promising new directions for alternative provider–based research. Expanding investigation to other types of patient-provider communication is also important because the physician's powerful status is a potential confounder in Roter and Hall's model. Studies of providers whom patients perceive to be more nearly equal in status to themselves could demonstrate the effect of status on patient-provider relationships.

Even though Social Cognitive Theory has enjoyed a rich and varied history of research, its increased application in health and illness situations begs for the theory's further extension and refinement. The following questions are currently unanswered: Under what conditions, if any, does self-efficacy generalize across behavioral areas? Research is needed to help us answer this question. Under what conditions can self-efficacy be enhanced in a person who is already taxed by the stress of an illness? An assumption of Social Cognitive Theory is that self-efficacy cannot be enhanced under conditions of arousal. When arousal cannot be diminished, does that mean self-efficacy cannot be enhanced, or are there critical levels of arousal that can be experienced without impeding the enhancement of self-efficacy? When arousal is related to illness and cannot be diminished, should health educators demure from intervening with self-efficacy? In the case of life-threatening or chronic life-threatening illness, is self-efficacy mutable? (See recent relevant work by Parcel and others, 1994). In asking these questions, we are asking for an examination of the conditions under which self-efficacy may or may not be mutable. Such questions also raise issues about the methods for inducing higher levels of self-efficacy in persons experiencing threats to their health.

Conclusion

The theory and frameworks in Part Three suggest targets and methods by which both health behavior and health outcomes can be enhanced. Moreover, they highlight the importance of the forms and methods of both communicating and interpersonally connecting with the persons whose health enhancement is the goal. All the chapters in this section support the use of these theoretical frameworks in the development and evaluation of health-related studies and programmatic interventions.

References

Amezcua, C., McAlister, A., Ramirez, A., and Espinoza, R. "A Su Salud: Health Promotion in a Mexican-American Border Community." In N. Bracht (ed.), *Health Promotion at the Community Level*. Thousand Oaks, Calif.: Sage, 1990.

Belle, D. *Lives in Stress: Women and Depression*. Thousand Oaks, Calif.: Sage, 1982.

Jack, D. C. *Silencing the Self*. Cambridge, Mass.: Harvard University Press, 1991.

Joos, S. K., and Hickam, D. H. "How Health Professionals Influence Health Behavior: Patient-Provider Interaction and Health Care Outcomes." In K. Glanz, F. M. Lewis, and B. K. Rimer (eds.), *Health Behavior and Health Education, Theory, Research, and Practice*. San Francisco: Jossey-Bass, 1990.

Kaplan, S., and others. "Patient and Visit Characteristics Related to Physicians' Participatory Decision-Making Style." *Medical Care*, 1995, *33*, 1176–1187.

Lewis, F. M. "The Concept of Control: A Typology and Health-Related Variables." *Advances in Health Education and Promotion*, 1987, *2*, 277–309.

Lewis, F. M., Hammond, M. A., and Woods, N. F. "The Family's Functioning with Newly Diagnosed Breast Cancer in the Mother: The Development of an Explanatory Model." *Journal of Behavioral Medicine*, 1993, *16*, 351–370.

Lewis, F. M., Morisky, D. E., and Flynn, B. S. "A Test of the Construct Validity of Health Locus of Control: Effects on Self-Reported Compliance for Hypertensive Patients." *Health Education Monographs*, 1978, *6*, 138–148.

Lewis, F. M., Woods, N. F., Hough, E. E., and Bensley, L. S. "The Family's Functioning with Chronic Illness in the Mother: The Spouse's Perspective." *Social Science and Medicine*, 1989, *29*, 1261–1269.

Lewis, F. M., and others. "The Functioning of Single Women with Breast Cancer and Their School-Aged Children." *Cancer Practice*, 1996, *4*, 1–10.

Lowenberg, J. "Interpretive Research Methodology: Broadening the Dialogue." *Advanced Nursing Science*, 1993, *16*, 57–69.

Maibach, E., Flora, J. A., and Nass, C. "Changes in Self-Efficacy and Health Behavior in Response to Minimal Contact Community Health Campaign." *Health Communication*, 1991, *3*, 1–15.

Nelles, W. B., McCaffrey, R. J., Blanchard, C. G., and Ruckdeschel, J. C. "Social Supports and Breast Cancer: A Review." *Journal of Psychosocial Oncology*, 1991, *9*, 21–34.

O'Leary, A. "Self-Efficacy and Health." *Behavioral Research Therapeutics*, 1985, *23*, 437–451.

Parcel, G. S., and others. "Self-Management of Cystic Fibrosis: A Structural Model for Educational and Behavioral Variables." *Social Science and Medicine*, 1994, *38*, 1307–1315.

Rotter, J. B. *Social Learning and Clinical Psychology*. Englewood Cliffs, N.J.: Prentice Hall, 1954.

Rotter, J. B. "Generalized Expectancies for Internal Versus External Control of Reinforcement." *Psychological Monographs*, 1966, *80*(1), 1–28.

Rotter, J. B. "Some Problems and Misconceptions Related to the Construct of Internal Versus External Control of Reinforcement." *Journal of Consulting and Clinical Psychology*, 1975, *43*, 56–67.

Strecher, V. J., DeVellis, B. M., Becker, M. H., and Rosenstock, I. M. "The Role of Self-Efficacy in Achieving Health Behavior Change." *Health Education Quarterly,* 1986, *13*(1), 73–91.

Wallston, K. A., Smith, M. S., Rye, P., and Burish, T. G. "Desire for Control and Choice of Anti-Emetic Treatment for Cancer Chemotherapy." *Western Journal of Nursing Research,* 1991, *13,* 12–23.

Wallston, K. A., Stein, M. J., and Smith, C. A. "Form C of the MHLC Scales: A Condition-Specific Measure of Locus of Control." *Journal of Personality Assessment,* 1994, *63,* 534–553.

PART FOUR

COMMUNITY AND GROUP INTERVENTION MODELS OF HEALTH BEHAVIOR CHANGE

Karen Glanz

An understanding of the functioning of groups, organizations, large social institutions, and communities is vital to health enhancement. Designing health promotion initiatives to serve communities and targeted populations, and not just single individuals, is at the heart of a public health orientation. The collective well-being of communities can be fostered by creating structures and policies that support healthy lifestyles and by reducing or eliminating health hazards and constraints in the social and physical environments. Both approaches require an understanding of how social systems operate, how change occurs within and among systems, and how community and organizational changes influence people's behavior and health.

Health promotion today exists in the context of rapid technological change and important policy debates. Health concerns such as substance abuse, AIDS prevention and education, smoking prevention and control, and new health care technologies raise issues that cannot be addressed adequately through individual or small-group interventions alone. Rather, health professionals need to view and understand health behavior and organizational changes in the context of social institutions and communities. The theories and frameworks in this part of *Health Behavior and Health Education* can help professionals understand the health behavior of large groups, communities, organizations, and coalitions, and can guide organization-wide and communitywide health promotion and education interventions. These social systems are both viable and essential units of practice when widespread and long-term maintenance of behavioral change and social change are important goals.

Community-level models are frameworks for understanding how social systems function and change, and how communities and organizations can be activated. They complement individually oriented behavioral change goals with broad aims that include advocacy and policy development. Community-level models suggest strategies and initiatives that are planned and led by organizations and institutions whose missions are to protect and improve health: schools, worksites, health care settings, community groups, and governmental agencies. Other institutions for whom health enhancement is not a central mission, such as the mass media, also play a critical role.

The chapters in this section represent state-of-the-art descriptions of four models for behavioral change in social systems or large populations. Some of the chapters address theoretical perspectives on changing the health behavior of populations, whereas other chapters are concerned primarily with conceptual frameworks for intervention methods that are *based on* theoretical foundations from the social sciences.

In Chapter Twelve, Minkler and Wallerstein provide a comprehensive overview of principles and methods of community organization and community building as they apply to health promotion and education. The authors discuss the main theoretical and conceptual bases of community organization, processes and models for community organization, and emerging concepts and methods of community building for health. They also discuss progress and tools for measuring and evaluating community organizing and community building. Minkler and Wallerstein then describe two case studies of community organization. The Tenderloin Senior Organizing Project for low-income elderly in San Francisco illustrates a community organization program that grew and developed over more than fifteen years. The Adolescent Social Action Program in New Mexico is a youth-centered experiential prevention program that involved a collaboration between university, schools, and numerous community and health organizations and that included empowerment education, leadership development, and community building.

In Chapter Thirteen, Oldenburg, Hardcastle, and Kok present diffusion of innovations theory, which addresses how new ideas, products, programs, and social practices spread within a society or from one society (or social system) to another. They then focus on how the diffusion of innovations framework was applied to increase primary care providers' adoption and implementation of cardiovascular risk reduction counseling and efforts to reduce excess alcohol consumption in Australia. An additional application examines Dutch secondary school teachers' adoption of AIDS prevention curricula.

In Chapter Fourteen, Goodman, Steckler, and Kegler analyze three theories of organizational change: stage theory, organizational development theory, and interorganizational relations theory. Each of these theories suggests specific intervention strategies directed at levels of a single organization or at coalitions of multiple organizations, thus improving adoption and implementation of health promotion programs and community strategies. Further, strategies based on each of the three theories can be used simultaneously to produce optimal effects. Goodman and colleagues then illustrate how these theories can be used as a basis for health promotion interventions in school settings and in public health action in the community.

Finnegan and Viswanath introduce the media studies framework for health behavior change in Chapter Fifteen. Their chapter is new in the second edition of *Health Behavior and Health Education*; it describes communication theories that are especially relevant to public health and health behavior change. Four perspectives on the effects of media are introduced: the knowledge gap hypothesis, agenda setting, cultivation studies, and risk communication. The authors then present applications of media studies to health in three areas: the day-to-day impact of media on health, heart disease prevention using media communication, and media communication for advocacy and policy change aimed at prevention of alcohol use among adolescents.

Part Four concludes with a summary, comparison, and critique of organizational and community interventions in health promotion and education. Chapter Sixteen discusses parallel elements in concepts and strategies, and converging applications of community and group intervention models of health behavior change.

An understanding of theory, research, and practice in communities, systems, and organizations will be critical to wide improvement of health in the future. This part of *Health Behavior and Health Education* provides a diverse set of frameworks and applications for consideration by both researchers and practitioners.

CHAPTER TWELVE

IMPROVING HEALTH THROUGH COMMUNITY ORGANIZATION AND COMMUNITY BUILDING

Meredith Minkler
Nina Wallerstein

Although a number of new approaches and change strategies have been developed and adopted by health education professionals in recent years, the principles and methods loosely referred to as community organization remain a central method of practice. For the purposes of this chapter, *community organization* is defined as the process by which community groups are helped to identify common problems or goals, mobilize resources, and in other ways, develop and implement strategies for reaching the goals they collectively have set. The newer and related concept of *community building* will be seen, as Walter (forthcoming) suggests, not as a method so much as an orientation to the ways in which people who identify themselves as members of a shared community engage together in the process of community change.

Implicit in both these definitions is the concept of empowerment, viewed as an enabling process through which individuals or communities take control over their lives and their environment (Rappaport, 1984). Indeed Murray Ross, widely regarded as the father of community-organizing practice, argued early on that community organization could not be said to have taken place unless community competence or problem-solving ability had been increased in the process (Ross, 1955). Strict definitions of community organization also suggest that the needs or problems around which community groups are organized must of necessity be identified by the community itself and not by an outside organization or change agent. Thus, although a health education professional may borrow some principles and methods from community organization to help mount, say, an AIDS-related organizing effort in the community, he or she cannot be said to be doing community organization in the pure sense unless the community itself has identified AIDS as a problem area it wishes to address.

Community organization is important in health education in part because it reflects one of the field's most fundamental principles, that of "starting where the people are." The health education professional who begins with the community's felt needs, rather than with a personal or agency-dictated agenda, will be far more likely to experience success in the change process and to foster real community ownership of programs and actions than will the person who imposes an agenda from outside. Community organizing also is important in light of evidence that social involvement and participation can themselves be significant psychosocial factors in improving perceived control, individual coping capacity, health behaviors, and health status (Cohen and Syme, 1985; Eng, Briscoe, and Cunningham, 1990). Finally, the rediscovery today of the importance of community to individuals and the heavy accent that governmental agencies, foundations, and the like are placing on community partnerships and community-based health initiatives suggest the need for further refining of the theory, methods, and measurement techniques in this area.

In this chapter, key concepts and principles of community organization and community building will be examined for their relevance to health education and related disciplines. Following a brief historical look at the field and the process of community organization and the emergence of community-building practice, the concept of community will be examined, and several models of community organization and community building presented. Key theoretical and conceptual bases of community organization and community building then will be explored, and two case studies presented and analyzed to demonstrate the relevance of these models in practice settings.

Community Organization and Community Building in Historical Perspective

The term community organization was coined by American social workers in the late 1800s in reference to their efforts to coordinate services for newly arrived immigrants and the poor (Garvin and Cox, 1995). As Garvin and Cox point out, however, although community organization typically is portrayed as having been born of the settlement house movement, several important milestones reached in fields other than social work should by rights be included in any history of community organization practice. Prominent among these milestones are (1) the post-

Reconstruction organizing by African Americans who were trying to salvage newly won rights that were rapidly slipping away, (2) the Populist movement, which began as an agrarian revolution and became a multisectoral coalition and a major political force, and (3) the labor movement of the 1930s and 1940s, which taught the value of forming coalitions around issues, the importance of full-time professional organizers, and the use of conflict as a means of bringing about change (Garvin and Cox, 1995).

Within the field of social work, early approaches to community organization stressed collaboration and the use of consensus and cooperation as communities were helped to self-identify and to increase their problem-solving ability (Garvin and Cox, 1995; Ross, 1955). By the 1950s, however, a new brand of community organization was gaining popularity, which stressed confrontation and conflict strategies for social change. Most closely identified with Saul Alinsky (1969, 1972), this *social action organizing* emphasized redressing power imbalances by creating dissatisfaction with the status quo among the disenfranchised, building communitywide identification, and helping community members devise winnable goals and nonviolent conflict strategies as means to bring about change.

From the late 1950s onward, strategies and tactics of community organization increasingly were applied to the achievement of broader social change objectives, through the civil rights movement, followed by the women's movement, the gay rights movement, the antiwar organizing during the Vietnam War, and the disability rights movement. The 1980s and early to mid-1990s also witnessed the adaptation and development of new community organization tactics and strategies, in areas as diverse as the AIDS crisis and the New Right's organizing to ban abortions. The effective use of personal computer technology also has greatly increased, with groups across the political spectrum going on-line to build community and to identify and organize supporters on a mass scale.

In the health field, a major new emphasis on community participation, begun in the 1970s, culminated in the World Health Organization's 1986 adoption of a new approach to health promotion that stressed increasing people's control over the determinants of their health, high-level public participation, and intersectoral cooperation (World Health Organization, 1986). Reflecting this new approach, the WHO-initiated Healthy Cities movement emerged and quickly grew to involve more than one thousand healthy cities and communities worldwide. It aims to create sustainable environments and processes through which governmental and nongovernmental sectors work in partnership to create healthy public policies, achieve high-level participation in community-driven projects, and ultimately, reduce inequities and disparities between groups (Duhl, 1993; Tsouros, 1995).

Finally, alongside these developments has been a growing appreciation of the importance of facilitating community *building*, conceptualized as a process that people in a community engage in themselves, rather than solely community *organizing*, viewed typically from the vantage point of the outside organizer (Walter, forthcoming). The community-building orientation is reflected in efforts such as the Black Women's Health Project, a network of close to one hundred groups in the United States and in several Third World countries, which stresses empowerment through self-help and consciousness raising for social change (Avery, 1990). Community-building projects like this one are strength based and grounded in feminist notions of *power to* and *power with*, rather than the more masculine concept of *power over* frequently encountered in traditional organizing (French, 1986). These projects further borrow from feminist organizing an accent on the process of practice (Hyde, 1990) and on organizing as holistic, involving both rational and nonrational elements of human experience (Gutierrez and Lewis, 1995). Although theoretical work and practical applications and research in the area of community building remain in their infancy, community-building practice may become an increasingly important complement to more traditional notions of community organization in the years ahead.

Following a look at the concept of community and at several models of community organization and community-building practice, the key principles and concepts underlying these approaches will be examined in more detail.

The Concept of Community

Integral to a discussion of community organization and community-building practice is an examination of the underlying concept of community. Although typically thought of as geographically based, communities may also be nongeographical, based on shared interests or characteristics such as ethnicity, sexual orientation, or occupation rather than locality (Fellin, 1995). Communities, indeed, have been defined as (1) *functional spatial units* meeting basic needs for sustenance, (2) *units of patterned social interaction*, and (3) *symbolic units of collective identity* (Hunter, 1975). Eng and Parker (1994) add a fourth political definition, identifying communities as social units, that is people coming together to act politically to make changes.

Two sets of theories are relevant for understanding the concept of community. The first of these, the *ecological system perspective*, is particularly useful in the study of autonomous geographical communities, focusing as it does on population characteristics such as size, density, and heterogeneity; the physical environment; the social organization or structure of the community; and the technological forces affecting it. In contrast, the *social systems perspective* focuses primarily on the formal organizations that operate within a given community, exploring the interactions of community subsystems (economic, political, and the like) both horizontally within the community and vertically as they relate to other, extracommunity systems (Fellin, 1995). Warren's classic approach to community (1963) clearly fits within the latter perspective, envisioning communities as entities that change their structure and function to accommodate various social, political, and economic developments. Alinsky's view of communities as reflecting the social problems and processes of an urban society (Reitzes and Reitzes, 1980) provides a similarly good example of a social systems perspective.

Clearly, the perspective on community that a researcher or practitioner adopts will influence his or her view of the appropriate domains and functions of the community organization process. Community development specialists (for example, agricultural extension workers and Peace Corps volunteers) thus have tended to focus over the years on helping people identify with and bring about changes within the geographical community, implicitly defining the latter as a unit unto itself (Khinduka, 1975). By contrast, proponents of a broader approach, typified by Alinsky (1972) and other social action organizers, have encouraged organizing around issues such as public housing and unemployment, in recognition of the tremendous impact these larger socioeconomic issues have on local communities. Similarly, though communities are rich in diversity with multiple interacting subcommunities, whether one *views* the community as more or less heterogeneous will determine the strategies employed and often the types of organizing goals.

Finally, as Rivera and Erlich (1995) have suggested, an appreciation of the unique characteristics of communities of color should be a major consideration in thinking about organizing in such communities. In African American communities, for example, Cornel West (1993) argues that market exploitation has led to a shattering of the religious and civic organizations that have historically buffered these communities from hopelessness and nihilism. He calls for community change through recreating a sense of agency and political resistance based on "subversive memory—the best of one's past without romantic nostalgia" (West, 1993). A view of community that incorporates such a perspective would support building on preexisting social networks rather than creating new structures and would emphasize self-determination and empowerment (Rivera and Erlich, 1995).

The different models of community organization and community building described in the next sections illustrate how alternative assumptions about the nature and meaning of community heavily shape the way community organization and community building are conceptualized and practiced.

Models of Community Organization

Although community organization frequently is treated as though it were a singular model of practice, several typologies have been developed on the premise that community organization is in fact made up of various alternative change models. The best known of these typologies is Rothman's (Rothman and Tropman, 1987) categorization of community organization as consisting of three distinct models of practice: locality development, social planning, and social action. Briefly, *locality development* is seen as heavily process oriented, stressing consensus and cooperation and aimed at building group identity and a sense of community. By contrast, *social planning* is viewed as heavily task oriented, stressing rational-empirical problem solving—usually by an outside expert—as a means of problem solving. Finally, the *social action model* may be seen as both task and process oriented. It is concerned with increasing the community's problem-solving ability and with achieving concrete changes to redress imbalances of power and privilege between an oppressed or disadvantaged group and the larger society. Originally arguing that most community-organizing efforts tended to fall in one or the other of these categories, Rothman more recently has suggested that many professionals use a "mixing and phasing" of two or more of the models (Rothman and Tropman, 1987), rather than relying solely or principally on any one. The heart health community trials and PATCH (Planned Community Action Toward Health) interventions, for example, have mixed social planning with elements of locality development (Farquhar and others, 1984; Centers for Disease Control, 1992; Bracht and Kingsbury, 1990), while organizers in the Alinsky tradition have mixed social action and locality development in their community actions (Marquez, 1990; Wechsler, 1990; Guillory, Willie, and Duran, 1988).

Rothman's typology has remained, for more than twenty years, the dominant framework within which community organization has been examined and understood, and as such, it has had a significant impact on practice (Walter, forthcoming). Despite its continued widespread application, however, the typology and its underlying assumptions have a number of important limitations. Use of the term *locality development,* for example, may be unnecessarily restrictive, discouraging consideration of organizing along nongeographical lines. Second, inclusion of a model (social planning) that often relies heavily on outside technical experts and need not increase the problem-solving ability of the community appears to contradict one of the most basic criteria of effective organizing. Finally, as Walter (forthcoming) has argued, the fact that this typology is problem based and organizer centered, rather than strength based and community centered, constitutes a philosophical and practical limitation that may be particularly problematic as organizing occurs increasingly in multicultural contexts.

In part in reaction to the perceived limitations of the Rothman typology, Walter (forthcoming) and others (Gardner, 1991; Himmelman, 1992; Labonte, 1994; Wallerstein and Sanchez-Merki, 1994; Wolfe, 1993) have suggested newer models of collaborative empowerment and community-building practice that provide important alternative approaches. These models can be seen partially as descendants of the community development model in their emphases on self-help and collaboration. Yet they extend beyond the community development tradition that is externally driven and may implicitly accept the status quo. They take their parentage instead from community-driven development, in which community concerns direct the organizing in a process that creates healthy and more equal power relations (Labonte, 1993; Purdey, Adhikari, Robinson, and Cox, 1994) (see Figure 12.1).

The newer community-building model emphasizes community strengths, not out of nostalgia for the "good old days" but because a diversity of groups and systems can identify these shared values and nurture the development of shared goals (Gardner, 1991). Himmelman's collaborative empowerment model (1992), for example, includes many of the steps or activities stressed in more traditional organizing (for example, clarifying a community's purpose and vision, examining what others have done, and building a community's power base), but puts its heaviest accent on enabling communities to play the lead role in change, so that real empowerment rather than merely "community betterment" is achieved. McKnight's notion of "community regeneration" (1987) has at its heart enabling people to recognize and contribute their "gifts," the totality of which represent the building blocks or assets of a community and which enable the community to care for its members.

Along similar lines, Walter's (forthcoming) community-building practice approach is described not as a method but as "a way of orienting one's self in community" that places community "at the center of practice." Walter's concept of community building attempts to "balance and blend" such elements of community as historicity, identity, and autonomy with the dimensions of community development, community planning, community action, community consciousness, and "the commons" (the latter encompassing the relationship between a community and its broader environment). As such, the community-building approach contrasts significantly with more traditional notions of community organization practice that are "community based" but not necessarily of and by the community (Walter, forthcoming; Wolfe, 1993).

Lying midway between older models of community organizing and newer concepts of community building are models that incorporate some elements of

FIGURE 12.1. COMMUNITY ORGANIZATION AND COMMUNITY-BUILDING TYPOLOGY.

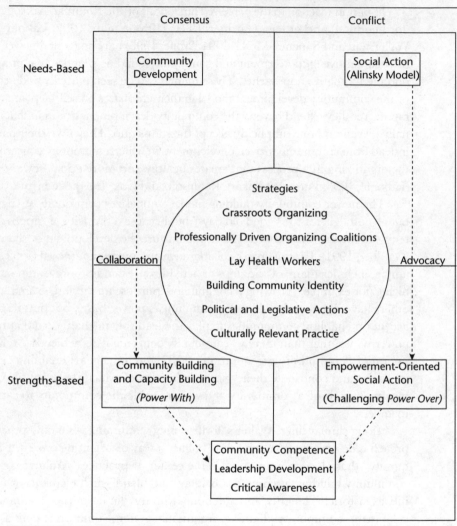

cach while putting the greatest accent on culturally relevant practice. Best known among these approaches is Braithwaite and colleagues' Community Organization and Development (COD) model for health promotion in communities of color (Braithwaite and others, 1989; Braithwaite, Bianchi, and Taylor, 1994). Although written from the perspective of the outside organizer and admonishing that outsider to engage in such initial steps as getting to know the community and its ecology through participatory ethnography and gaining entrée and credibility, the central thrust of the COD model involves facilitating the development and effective functioning of a community-dominated and -controlled coalition board. The board in turn undertakes its own community assessment, sets policy, facilitates leadership development, and on the basis of bottom-up planning and community problem solving, designs culturally relevant interventions. The COD model, in short, appears to move from initial reliance on more traditional community organizing to an incorporation of many of the principles of community-building practice, while stressing throughout the cultural context within which both organizing and community building take place.

Finally, alternately defined as a model of community organization practice and as a strategy or method used across models is coalition building. Increasingly popular in the health field in areas as diverse as chronic disease, drugs and alcohol, violence, and the fight against budget cuts (Goodman, Burdine, Meehan, and McLeroy, 1993; Wolfe, 1993), coalitions have attracted heavy public- and private-sector funding but have only begun to be studied in a systematic fashion (see Chapter Fourteen).

In sum, several models of community organizing and community building have surfaced within the last decade to complement a long history of earlier organizing approaches. Figure 12.1 integrates new perspectives with the older models, presenting a typology that incorporates both needs- and strengths-based approaches. Along the needs-based axis, community development, primarily as a consensus model, is contrasted with Alinsky's social action conflict-based model. The newer strength-based models contrast a community-building and capacity-building approach to an empowerment-oriented social action approach. The two strength-based approaches are spanned by concepts such as community competence, leadership development, and critical awareness. Empowerment, though a separate quadrant on the figure, is also a concept that can be, and ideally is, realized within the three other models of organizing. Collaboration straddles the needs- and strengths-based quadrants as primarily a consensus strategy, and advocacy does the same as primarily a conflict strategy.

In the middle circle are several strategies of organizing, such as grassroots organizing and coalition building. None of these falls into one or another of the quadrants. Rather, each may incorporate multiple tendencies or models depending on the starting place, and the dynamics of an ever-changing social context.

Key Concepts in Community Organization and Community-Building Practice

Even though no single unified model of community organization or community building exists, some key concepts are central to affecting and measuring change on the community level. The concept of participation and relevance was discussed at the beginning of the chapter. Several additional concepts and principles—empowerment and critical consciousness, community competence, and issue selection—are presented in the next sections (see Table 12.1).

Empowerment and Critical Consciousness

The term empowerment has been justifiably criticized as a "catch-all phrase" in social science (Rappaport, 1984); it nevertheless represents a central tenet of com-

TABLE 12.1. COMMUNITY ORGANIZATION AND COMMUNITY BUILDING.

Concept	Definition	Application
Participation and relevance	Community organizing "starts where the people are" and engages community members as equals.	Community members create their own agenda based on felt needs, shared power, and awareness of resources.
Empowerment	Social action process for people to gain mastery over their lives and the lives of their communities.	Community members assume greater power or expand their power from within to create desired changes.
Critical consciousness	Consciousness based on reflection and action in making change.	Community members engage in dialogue that links root causes and community actions.
Community competence	Community ability to engage in effective problem solving.	Community members work to identify problems, create consensus, and agree on change strategies to reach goals.
Issue selection	Identification of winnable and specific targets of change that unify and build community strength.	Community members identify issues through community participation, decide on targets as part of a larger strategy.

munity organization and community-building practice. Within the public health field, *empowerment,* or *community empowerment,* has been variously defined, as communities' achieving equity (Katz 1984), as communities' having the capacity to identify problems and solutions (Braithwaite and others, 1989; Cottrell, 1983), and as communities' fostering participatory self-competence in the political life of the community (Florin and Wandersman, 1990; Kieffer, 1984).

Though many limit their definition of empowerment to a narrow individual focus—so that it is similar in meaning to self-esteem or self-confidence—for community organizing and community building, the following broader definition is most useful: empowerment is a social action process through which individuals, communities, and organizations gain mastery over their lives in the context of changing their social and political environment to improve equity and quality of life (Rappaport, 1984; Wallerstein, 1992).

Such a definition highlights issues of power and the ability to create change on a personal, interpersonal, and political level (Gutierrez and Lewis, 1995). Labonte addresses power as a social relationship with contradictory elements (Bernstein and others, 1994; Labonte, 1990). Power from within and power with (the collective aspect of power from within) are moral, spiritual sources of power that can be constantly expanding as people empower themselves. Power over has a material base of domination through force or ideological hegemony. People without power cannot gain against exploitation without others' losing their historical authority. Empowerment therefore means taking power or transforming the power relations from one group to another.

For health educators, these contradictory elements raise issues about our own practice. Many professionals have higher status positions than community members. Can people in positions of dominance or privilege derived from culture, gender, race, or class empower others? Or must people empower themselves? If empowerment includes the dimension of transferring power to others, professionals may need to let go of their power, to make it more available to others. In Labonte's words, "Empowerment . . . is a fascinating dynamic of power given and taken all at once, a dialectical dance between consensus and conflict, professional expertise and lay wisdom, hierarchic institutions and community circles" (Bernstein and others, 1994).

The processes and outcomes of empowerment need to accommodate a view of the change process that includes the interaction of individuals, individuals in relation to others and communities, and the changes in the social structure itself. For individuals, empowerment challenges the perceived or real powerlessness that comes from the injuries to health of poverty, chronic stressors, and lack of control and few resources, or what Len Syme has termed lack of "control over destiny" (Syme, 1988). Individuals may experience enhanced psychological empowerment, which includes increased political efficacy and motivation to act (Zimmerman, 1990) and enhanced social support.

As individuals engage in community-organizing efforts, community empowerment outcomes can include increased sense of community; greater participatory processes and community competence; and outcomes in the form of actual changes in policies, transformed conditions, or increased resources that may reduce inequities. As communities become empowered and better able to engage in collective problem solving, key health and social indicators may reflect this, with rates of alcoholism, divorce, suicide, and other social problems beginning to decline. Moreover, the empowered community that works effectively for change can bring about changes in some of the very problems that contributed to its ill health in the first place (Israel, 1985; Minkler, 1992).

The link between individual- and community-level empowerment is strengthened through the development of critical consciousness, or *conscientization*, a concept that comes from Brazilian educator Paulo Freire (1970, 1973). Freire developed a methodology for teaching illiterate peasants to read by teaching them to "read" their political and social reality. His work has been a catalyst worldwide during the last three decades for programs in adult education, health, and community development (Hope and Timmel, 1984; Minkler and Cox, 1980; Wallerstein and Bernstein, 1994; Wallerstein and Weinger, 1992).

Freire's central premise is that the purpose of education should be liberatory, to transform the status quo in the classroom and in people's lives. He asks whether education reinforces powerlessness by treating people as objects who receive knowledge or whether education enables people to engage in active dialogue and to challenge the conditions that keep them powerless. Freire proposes a dialogical problem-posing process, with equality and mutual respect, between learner-teachers and teacher-learners. Problem posing contains a listening-dialogue-action cycle that enables all participants to engage in continuous reflection and action. Through structured dialogue, group participants listen for the issues contained in their own experiences, discuss common problems, look for root causes and interconnections among the "problems behind the problem-as-symptom," and devise strategies to transform their reality (Freire, 1970, 1973).

Conscientization is the consciousness that comes through the social analysis of conditions and peoples' role in changing those conditions. This kind of awareness enables community groups to analyze moments and open spaces to enact change or to understand those *limit-situations* that may prohibit change (Barndt, 1989). Conscientization is a key ingredient to maintaining a broader vision and sustaining community-organizing efforts over time and is one of the links between individual psychological empowerment and community empowerment.

Community Competence

Closely related to the concept of empowerment is the notion of *community competence*, or problem-solving ability, as a central goal and outcome of community organization practice. The "competent community" is defined by Cottrell (1983) as "one in which the various component parts of the community are able to collaborate effectively on identifying the problems and needs of the community; can achieve a working consensus on goals and priorities; can agree on ways and means to implement the agreed upon goals; can collaborate effectively in the required actions."

Important recent refinements in our thinking about community competence have come with lay health worker programs, which have incorporated community development and an emphasis on lay health workers themselves, instead of assessing only their impact on clients (Eng and Parker, 1994; Ovrebo, Ryan, Jackson, and Hutchinson, 1994). A major challenge has been to find measurement variables that encompass community competence and capacity change and are not simply aggregates of measures on individuals or service providers. Leadership development also represents a key aspect of developing competent communities. In particular, the development of leaders able to fulfill the roles of animator (stimulating people to think critically and to identify problems and new solutions) and facilitator (providing a process through which the group can discuss its own content in the most productive possible way) is key to building group competence and effectiveness (Hope and Timmel, 1984).

Cottrell (1983) and others (Eng and Parker, 1994; Fellin, 1995) have tended to apply the concept of community competence primarily to geographical communities, yet its relevance to nongeographical communities also is apparent. Indeed, whether the community is a neighborhood in the South Bronx, a union local in Ohio, or people with HIV or AIDS working together for change, increasing the community's capacity for collective problem identification and problem solving is of paramount importance if the community is to effectively reach both its current and future goals.

Many principles and concepts basic to health education have relevance for increasing community competence. In addition to the concept of empowerment, Israel (1985) has noted that key approaches within social network theory and social support may be usefully applied in the development of competent communities. Social network techniques by which one can "map" the web of social ties in which individuals are embedded may be employed to help identify natural helpers or leaders within a community; to help these natural leaders in turn identify their own networks; to identify high-risk groups within the community; and to involve network members in undertaking their own community assessment and actions necessary to strengthen networks within the community. A number of network assessment tools are available for mapping personal and community networks (McCallister and Fischer, 1978; Heitzmann and Kaplan, 1988) and other community assets (McKnight and Kretzmann, 1992) and may usefully be employed by health education professionals.

Issue Selection

One of the most important steps in community organization practice involves the effective differentiation between *problems,* or things that are troubling, and *issues,* or problems the community feels strongly about. As Miller (1985) suggests, a good issue must meet several important criteria: it must be *winnable,* to ensure that working on the campaign does not simply reinforce people's fatalistic attitudes and beliefs. It must be simple and *specific,* so that any member of the group can explain it clearly in a sentence or two. It must *unite members* of the group, and it must *involve them in a meaningful way* in achieving problem resolution. It should *affect lots of people,* should *build up the community or organization* (giving people leadership experience, increased visibility, and so on), and finally, it should be *part of a larger plan or strategy.* A variety of methods familiar to health education professionals can be used to help a community group acquire the data needed for issue selection. Among those most popular currently is the focus group, through which a moderator, using a predetermined discussion guide or series of questions, elicits input from a small group of community members to determine their qualitative perceptions of key issues or concerns facing the community (Stewart and Shamdasani, 1990). As is the case with other face-to-face data collection processes, the value of focus groups depends upon how they are developed and run. They can be empowering for members and a valuable information source or of little relevance to the community and its issue selection efforts.

Nominal Group Process (NGP), a structured technique that allows a large number of people to have input in issue selection and related activities (Delbecq, Van de Ven, and Gustafson, 1975), door-to-door surveys, and other data collection instruments also can be useful in assessing felt needs and in increasing a sense of participation. Too often, however, community members are merely invited to express their relative agreement with the outside professionals' preconceived notion of what the problems of significance in the community really are. Surveys and other methods are useful for issue selection only to the extent that they enable the discovery of the real issues of concern to the community.

Even when organizers genuinely attempt to "start where the people are," they may lack access to the "hidden discourse" in a community and misinterpret an

apparent community apathy due to their own lack of cultural competence, lack
of access to key stakeholders or cultural translators, or lack of self-reflection on
the problematic nature of the power dynamics between themselves and community members (Scott, 1990). They may have access to community discourse, yet
find community resistance and organizing strategies that challenge their own level
of comfort. They may have a working relationship with community leaders, yet
find the group has chosen issues that are too broad to be winnable. In the case of
issue selection, the organizer has the responsibility to pose questions to refocus the
group on specific targets.

Further, as Labonte (1994) has suggested, the community's selection of an
issue may reflect racism, sexism, homophobia, or other discriminatory attitudes
(as when communities in California, Oregon, and Colorado organized to put
anti–gay rights ballot initiatives on their state or local ballots). In cases like these,
the health education practitioner's commitment to starting where the people are
and to community self-determination must be tempered by a concern with the
paramount principle of social justice in the larger community, whose interests are
not served by the parochial and prejudicial concerns and actions of one subgroup
(Minkler, 1994).

An approach to issue selection that has proven especially helpful in overcoming some of these difficulties involves the use of Freire's dialogical problem-posing
method (1970, 1973). As noted earlier, part of the Freirian approach engages participants in identifying their core generative themes, those themes that elicit social
and emotional involvement and therefore high-level motivation to participate.
Community development approaches worldwide have adopted Freire's educational strategies to identify the core issues for starting organizing efforts (Arnold
and others, 1991; Hope and Timmel, 1984). Community organizers in the United
States also have adopted strategies from organizational development, creating
strategic action plans to prioritize issues by available resources, appropriate timelines, and barriers to reaching goals (French and Bell, 1990). Politically minded
organizers have included an analysis of the power brokers, allies, and resisters
when choosing an issue that may be feasible to win (Staples, 1984; Feldblum,
Wallerstein, Varela, and Collins, 1994).

As suggested, on the one hand, issue selection processes, undertaken thoughtfully, can contribute to community empowerment and serve as a positive force for
social change. On the other hand, calls increasingly have been made for "a new
process of community organizing—one relying less on issue-based mobilization
and more on community education, leadership development and support, and
building local sustainable organizations" (Traynor, 1993). Community-building
practice increasingly is being looked to as this "new process of community organizing," one that as we have seen, is less concerned with community issue selection

than with the identification, nurturing, and celebration of community strengths and the creation of a context, by people in the community, for the sharing of those strengths (McKnight, 1987; Walter, forthcoming).

Measurement and Evaluation Issues

A major limitation of most community-organizing and community-building efforts to date has been the failure to adequately address evaluation processes and outcomes. This failure typically stems from several sources, among them severe funding constraints and lack of skills for building a meaningful evaluation component into the organizing effort. As Connell and others (1995) have pointed out, the continually evolving nature of community-organizing and community-based initiatives, complex contextual issues, and the fact that initiatives often seek change on multiple levels make many traditional evaluation approaches inappropriate or ill suited to the organizing endeavors. Similarly, many standard evaluation approaches focus on long-term change in health and social indicators and may miss the shorter-term system-level impacts with which community organizing is heavily concerned. Among these latter effects are improvements in organizational collaboration, increased levels of community involvement and action, and the promotion of healthier public policies or environmental conditions.

The lack of formal evaluations coupled with the failure of many engaged in community projects to publish their results has made it difficult to amass a literature of "successful" and "unsuccessful" organizing efforts and the hallmarks of each. Although some characteristics of successful community collaborations have been identified (for example, shared vision, strong leadership, and an accent on process and not merely task achievement) (Connell and others, 1995), much remains to be examined and assessed. The careful evaluation and documentation of both successful and unsuccessful community-organizing projects must be a vital part of a new database.

Fortunately, the late 1980s and early to mid-1990s have brought important steps forward in evaluation of community organizing and related areas. Key among these steps was the convening of a roundtable on community initiatives for children and families, which developed the publication *New Approaches to Evaluating Community Initiatives* (Connell and others, 1995). This collection of essays explores dilemmas commonly faced in the design, measurement, and interpretation of community initiatives, as well as a variety of options and strategies for evaluators working with such projects. A special issue of *Health Education Research* on community coalitions (Goodman, Burdine, Meehan, and McLeroy, 1993) included several articles that addressed measurement and evaluation issues. A two-part issue of *Health Education Quarterly,* entitled *Community Empowerment, Participatory Education and Health* (Wallerstein and Bernstein, 1994), further added to the literature with both concepts and case studies that dealt in part with evaluation and measurement issues.

Within the latter collection, Eng and Parker's development and testing of a scale for measuring community competence (1994) represents a particularly important contribution, offering readers an effective new tool for measuring a key dimension of community-organizing efforts. Similarly, Israel, Checkoway, Schulz, and Zimmerman's development, validation, and application of a scale for measuring perceptions of individual, organizational, and community control (1994) provides a critical missing piece in the evaluation literature to date and one well suited to evaluating community organization outcomes.

Still another useful evaluation resource is the self-reflection workbook developed in New Mexico to evaluate community organizing and community building in the context of creating healthier communities (Maldrud, Polacsek, and Wallerstein, forthcoming). The workbook focuses on such changes in community processes as levels of grassroots participation and such changes in short-term system-level outcomes as the development of new programs as a result of the organizing experience. As previously noted, it is these middle-level outcomes rather than long-term changes in self-rated health and other health or social indicators that are often most important in documenting community competence and empowerment.

A final recent contribution to the literature in this area lies in the publication of Fetterman, Kaftarian, and Wandersman's comprehensive volume *Empowerment Evaluation* (1996). Empowerment evaluation is defined as "an interactive and iterative process by which the community, in collaboration with the support team, identifies its own health issues, decides how to address them, monitors progress toward its goals and uses the information to adapt and sustain the initiative" (Fawcett and others, 1996). Although some of the evaluation approaches (for example, of HIV prevention initiatives) fit a social-planning rather than a true community-organizing approach to practice, most have immediate relevance for health education professionals concerned with the evaluation of community organization efforts.

The availability of new theoretical contributions and practical tools that lend themselves to evaluation of community organization fails, of course, to solve the problem of insufficient funding and low commitment to carrying out high-quality evaluative research. Yet the increased attention of both foundation and governmental funders to evaluation and measurement issues in community organization and community-based initiatives is encouraging. If translated into increased funding, this increased attention, together with the availability of new measurement tools and processes, could spur major advances in the evaluation and documentation of community organization and community building in the years ahead.

Applications of Community Organization and Community Building

The next section of this chapter describes two applications of the concepts and methods of community organizing and community building. The first case study is the Tenderloin Senior Organizing Project (TSOP), a community organization effort involving elderly residents of San Francisco's Tenderloin district. The second case study discusses the Adolescent Social Action Program (ASAP), a youth-centered experiential prevention program in communities throughout New Mexico.

Case Study: The Tenderloin Senior Organizing Project

For the low-income elderly in single-room occupancy (SRO) hotels in the United States, poor health, social isolation, and powerlessness often are intimately connected. This case study describes a community organization effort to address these interrelated problems by fostering social support and social action organizing among elderly residents of San Francisco's Tenderloin District.

Of the many health and social problems facing elders in the Tenderloin, poor nutrition and clinical depression have been among the most prevalent and important. A survey conducted in the early 1980s thus suggested that at least 40 percent of Tenderloin elders were malnourished or seriously undernourished (Wechlser and Minkler, 1986), and high rates of suicide, a problem drinking rate of 20 percent (Arean, 1994), and related health and social indicators suggest that clinical depression also is a frequent fact of life for elders in this neighborhood (Minkler, 1996).

Poverty, social isolation, physical illness and disability, and social stressors such as fear of crime if one ventures outdoors are among the factors contributing to the high rates of both malnutrition and clinical depression observed (Minkler, forthcoming). Finally, the social marginalization of people in neighborhoods like the Tenderloin, and their classification by some as undeserving poor, place them at high risk for dependency on stigmatizing and miserly health and social programs (for example, food stamps, Medicaid, and Supplemental Security Income [SSI])—programs that are frequent targets of budget cuts in times of fiscal retrenchment.

Originally known as the Tenderloin Senior Outreach Project, TSOP was established in 1979 by graduate students and faculty at the University of California,

Berkeley, School of Public Health with the dual goals of (1) improving physical and mental health among Tenderloin residents by reducing their social isolation and providing relevant health education and (2) facilitating, through dialogue and participation, a process that encouraged residents to work together to identify common problems and to seek solutions to these shared problems and concerns.

Student volunteers began in a single Tenderloin hotel, encouraging resident interaction and eventually forming an informal group that met weekly and included a core of twelve residents and two outside facilitators. As levels of trust and rapport increased, group members began to share personal concerns regarding such issues as fear of crime, loneliness, rent increases, and their own sense of powerlessness. Student facilitators used a combination of organizing and educational approaches to help residents select an initial issue on which they wanted to focus (crime and safety) and to foster group solidarity and social action organizing. A modified Freirian problem-posing process thus was used to help residents engage in dialogue about shared problems and their causes and to generate potential action plans. In addition, Alinsky's admonitions (1972) to create dissatisfaction with the status quo and help people identify specific winnable issues were among the community organization precepts followed, as were the emphases of McKnight (1987, 1993) and Miller (1993) on identifying and building on community strengths. Finally, drawing on social support theory that stresses the importance of social interaction opportunities, the student facilitators attempted to create a group atmosphere conducive to meeting the purely social needs of residents as well as the more political and task-oriented concerns of some group members (Minkler, 1992).

As the first hotel group evolved into an established entity, seven additional groups were organized in other Tenderloin hotels. In all but one of these, empowerment was facilitated through decreased reliance on outside facilitators and broader resident participation in discussion and decision making occurred. A second trend observed in the groups, one critical to TSOP's evolution, was the realization among residents of the need to look beyond hotel boundaries and work with residents of other hotels and community groups on shared problems. TSOP residents in several hotels thus identified crime and safety as their key area of concern and formed an interhotel coalition to begin work on this problem. The coalition in turn started the Safehouse Project, recruiting during its first year forty-eight neighborhood businesses and agencies that agreed to display colorful posters indicating that they had become places of refuge for residents in time of emergency. Through this and other actions (for example, convincing the mayor to increase the number of beat patrol officers in the neighborhood), the coalition was credited with helping to bring about an 18 percent drop in crime during its first year of operation and a 26 percent drop by the end of year two ("Safehouses Now Easing the Fears of Elderly Residents," 1982). Concurrent changes in individual health

and social behavior also were seen, with increased feelings of self-efficacy and social support leading some residents to quit smoking or cut down on problem drinking, and others to demonstrate dramatic improvements in their mental health and
self-esteem (Minkler, forthcoming).

Encouraged by the success of the Safehouse Project, TSOP members turned
their attention to the problem of undernutrition and poor food access, establishing mini-markets in three hotels and a cooperative breakfast program in a fourth
and creating and widely disseminating a "no cook cookbook" for residents not allowed to cook in their rooms (Minkler, 1992). Alongside these and other tangible
projects, TSOP engaged in significant leadership training, through one-on-one
and small-group activities and a leadership training conference and later by arranging for about twenty indigenous leaders to participate in four-day intensive
organizer training workshops with other organizers around the country.

As Tenderloin residents became increasingly willing and able to take control
of this project, TSOP staff and volunteers played a less visible role, serving primarily as resource persons and sounding boards for residents' ideas and strategy
discussions. Indeed, TSOP changed the "O" in its name from "Outreach" to "Organizing" in 1988, to reflect this change in orientation, and increasingly defined
its role as one of facilitating community empowerment by drawing out the competence, self-confidence, and leadership skills of elderly residents (Miller, 1993).

TSOP's key mechanism of action also changed over time from health educator–facilitated support groups to resident-run tenant associations. Prior to its
closing in 1995, TSOP had helped organize sixteen autonomous tenant associations and trained more than two hundred indigenous leaders. Their victories included getting hot water turned on in a building that had gone without for ten
years; winning back rent for residents of a building whose elevator had been "out
of service" for five months; making one hotel wheelchair accessible; getting a vending machine selling nutritious foods in another; and getting security guards, trash
pickup, and other discontinued services reinstated in still other residences. Although small in and of themselves, each of these victories contributed both to the
health and safety of residents and to their feelings of empowerment, self-esteem,
and community competence (Minkler, 1996).

TSOP was not without problems, including resident burnout on some issues
residents had earlier decided to tackle, occasional power conflicts within groups,
and leadership turnover as a consequence of illness, transiency, and other problems. Project evaluation also proved difficult because many residents harbored an
understandable distrust of outside researchers and because project staff were committed to avoiding data-gathering activities that might confuse residents about
TSOP's true mission. A comprehensive external evaluation recently was completed, however. It explored residents' perceptions of individual and community

control through informal interviews with a variety of key nonresidents and structured interviews with 150 residents of both TSOP and comparison non-TSOP buildings. That evaluation was unable to document specific improvements in physical health that could be directly linked to the project. However, significant increases in sense of control (making decisions that affect one's life), social interaction, morale, perceived safety, and perceived ability to improve one's housing conditions were among the outcomes demonstrated (Shaw, 1995).

Although TSOP was forced to close its doors in mid-1995 as a consequence of severe funding constraints, a number of tenant organizations that TSOP helped get underway continue to organize in the Tenderloin. A detailed replication manual also has been produced and disseminated, and known TSOP replication projects include one currently involving nine SRO hotels in Vancouver, British Columbia. In this way, it is hoped that the TSOP model will continue to make a difference in the lives of people for whom organizing and creating a sense of community can be an important route to improved health and quality of life.

Case Study: The Adolescent Social Action Program

Youths today are confronted with multiple risks in their lives: fears about the future, lack of employment opportunities, media targeting by the alcohol and tobacco industries, family and community violence, and social norms of peer pressure to engage in risky behaviors. This case study illustrates how a university-community partnership is working with youths to address the interconnectedness of personal choices and social conditions through a mix of empowerment education and community-organizing strategies.

The Adolescent Social Action Program (ASAP) is a youth-centered experiential prevention program that has involved a collaboration between the University of New Mexico, the university hospital, the county detention center, and over thirty multi-ethnic schools and communities throughout New Mexico since 1982. Originally known as the Alcohol and Substance Abuse Prevention Program, ASAP has several major goals: to reduce excess morbidity and mortality among youths who live in high-risk environments, to encourage these youths to make healthier choices in their lives, and to empower them to take an active political and social role to improve their neighborhoods and communities.

The ASAP program consists of a seven-week experience for small groups of youths who are brought into the hospital and detention center setting to interview and interact with patients and jail residents who have problems related to drug and alcohol abuse, interpersonal violence, and other risky behaviors (Wallerstein and Bernstein, 1988). Follow-up school and community-based organizing activities extend the length of the intervention to one semester, with a structured booster session at the end. At the heart of the program is Freire's educational empowerment approach (Wallerstein and Sanchez-Merki, 1994). Through Freirian problemposing structured dialogue led by university health professional students trained as facilitators, the youths discuss the patients' and jail residents' life stories and their own experiences and lives, examining the consequences of their actions and how they might make healthier choices for themselves and their communities. Unlike "scared-straight" programs, which have been proven to be ineffective (Rogers and Mewborn, 1976; Job, 1988), ASAP also incorporates protection-motivation theory directed at increasing students' threat appraisal and coping self-efficacy for behavioral change (Rogers, 1984; Stainback and Rogers, 1983). The integration of behavioral and social change is especially important for youths of color who face poverty, discrimination, and unemployment and who therefore are overrepresented in injury and mortality statistics.

Employing Freirian empowerment education, ASAP incorporates a listening-dialogue-action model that links educational processes to community organizing. During the structured curriculum in the hospital and detention center, the predominant model is the development of critical consciousness toward the goals of leadership development and community building as the youths develop empathy with each other and with the communities they belong to in their neighborhoods and schools. After listening to the patient and detainee stories, the youths begin to dialogue critically about their own lives and their relationships to their communities. Active participation is a key tenet of ASAP in the issues youths bring to the dialogue and in their choice of follow-up activities.

As the seven-week curriculum ends, the ASAP program typically has offered youths two possibilities: to enter a peer education component or to work in social action. The peer education program allows them to continue the educational model with younger elementary students. The social action model extends into community organizing, and the youths are encouraged to devise their own prevention projects for their school site with the aid of project staff. This approach has encouraged them to explore existing social and legal policies, the current prevention strategies for risky behaviors, and ways to change alcohol norms in their own communities.

Early examples of ASAP social action projects include youth panel discussions at the ASAP Summer Institutes, local booths at school fiestas, and red-ribbon rallies. Issue selection has been added more recently, with youths connecting to citywide organizing and developing their own long-term initiatives, such as the production of videotapes and photonovellas. The ASAP videos, including a recent music video, and the series of photonovellas have been conceptualized, written, and produced by groups of youths, who learned the necessary technical skills and developed the issues they wanted to examine about their neighborhoods and society. These products have been distributed widely in the local schools and community centers as aids to other educational and organizing endeavors that promote youth problem solving and community competence.

Certain issues, such as gang activity, have demanded larger neighborhood and citywide attention. The Albuquerque South East Community Gang Task Force provides youths with the opportunity to act as advisory committee board members and task force members. Street Reach is a gang prevention project in which ASAP youth have shared the health information and coping strategies they have learned through ASAP. At the New Mexico State Fair in 1994, ASAP youth helped plan and participated in the presentation "A Day Without Alcohol Is Fair." Youths participated in A Day Without Colors by directing activities and running the ASAP booth at Albuquerque's Civic Plaza. ASAP youths have been involved in a local youth-produced television program on teenagers. They have helped cook and serve Thanksgiving dinner at a local community center.

Some core issues about the limits of community organizing exist within a program such as ASAP. The first issue is the extent of the responsibility for organizing that youths can assume. ASAP youths depend on adults to mentor them and to facilitate the logistics of organizing; middle school youths, in particular, need parental permission and transportation to organizing events. The hope is, however, that they will develop a belief in group action, a belief in social responsibility, and a belief in themselves as leaders who can make a difference. The second issue is that the school is the starting place for the program, which raises questions about youths' base for organizing. Unfortunately, many youths today identify with their school, their neighborhood, or their gang and will not work across these boundaries. Broader organizing must take these polarized subcommunities into account, bridging the differences and building a community of youths who can have citywide policy impact. The third organizing issue is that the majority of funding for ASAP is categorical—aimed at alcohol and other drug use prevention. Despite the potential this has to narrow the issues, in practice alcohol and drugs have been a prominent concern for teenagers, and youths have been able to choose projects within the broad range of adolescent risky behaviors. One photonovella, for example, delved into the difficulties in adolescent relationships.

In sum, ASAP presents a comprehensive model that combines elements of empowerment education, critical consciousness, leadership development, community building, and high-level participation with some of the elements of traditional community organizing. Though its immediate starting place is not community organization, the ASAP model is one example of how to combine specific program principles with an overarching social change agenda.

Conclusion

The continued pivotal role of community organization in health education practice reflects not only its time-tested efficacy but also its high degree of philosophical fit with the most fundamental principles of effective community health education. Community organization stresses the principle of relevance or starting where the people are, the principle of participation, and the importance of creating environments in which individuals and communities can become empowered as they increase their community competence and problem-solving ability. Similarly, newer conceptualizations of community building stress many of the same principles, within an overall approach that focuses on community growth and change from the inside, through increased group identification; discovery, nurturing, and mapping of community assets; and creation of critical consciousness—all toward the end of building stronger and more caring communities.

The San Francisco–based TSOP project is an example of an effort in which a relatively "pure" application of community-organizing principles and methods by health educators was undertaken with considerable success. Far more frequently, however, health and social service professionals are employed by an agency with specific agendas and often with categorical funding. The practitioner in this setting may find that he or she cannot undertake community organizing in the strictest sense of the term because an outside group, rather than the community itself, has identified the specific health problem(s) to be addressed. Yet professionals in such situations can apply with effectiveness many of the core principles and approaches of community organization and community-building practice. They thus can elicit high-level community participation and, further, can strive to build leadership skills and increase community competence as an integral part of the overall health education project. Further, as demonstrated by the ASAP case study, although the overall problem area (for example, alcohol and substance abuse) may initially have been identified by an outside group or agency, the health education professional, using community-organizing and community-building skills and approaches, can help communities identify within this designated framework the specific issues of greatest relevance to them.

Most importantly, professionals can challenge themselves to examine their own dynamic of power with their professional colleagues and members of the community, to understand the complexities of working in partnership toward the goals of community ownership of the projects undertaken and increased empowerment and community competence. In sum, both community organization and newer conceptualizations of community-building practice have essential messages for health education professionals in a wide variety of settings and may hold particular relevance in the changing sociopolitical climate of the mid-1990s and beyond.

References

Alinsky, S. D. *Reveille for Radicals.* Chicago: University of Chicago Press, 1969.

Alinsky, S. D. *Rules for Radicals.* New York: Random House, 1972.

Arean, P. "Implications and Service Use of Mental Disorders in Older Medical Patients." Paper presented at the 8th annual meeting of the National Institute of Mental Health Conference on Psychiatric Disorders in the General Health Care Sector, Washington, D.C., Nov. 1994.

Arnold, R., and others. *Educating for a Change.* Toronto: Between the Lines and Doris Marshall Institute for Education and Action, 1991.

Avery, B. "Breathing Life into Ourselves: The Evolution of the Black Women's Health Project." In E. White (ed.), *The Black Women's Health Book.* Seattle, Wash.: Seal Press, 1990.

Barndt, D. *Naming the Moment: Political Analysis for Action.* Toronto: Jesuit Center for Social Faith and Justice, 1989.

Bernstein, E., and others. "Empowerment Forum: A Dialogue Between Guest Editorial Board Members." *Health Education Quarterly,* 1994, *21*(3), 281–294.

Bracht, N., and Kingsbury, L. "Community Organization Principles in Health Promotion: A Five-Stage Model." In N. Bracht (ed.), *Health Promotion at the Community Level.* Thousand Oaks, Calif.: Sage, 1990.

Braithwaite, R. L., Bianchi, C., and Taylor, S. E. "Ethnographic Approach to Community Organization and Health Empowerment." *Health Education Quarterly,* 1994, *21*(3), 407–419.

Braithwaite, R. L., and others. "Community Organization and Development for Health Promotion Within an Urban Black Community: A Conceptual Model." *Health Education,* 1989, *2*(5), 56–60.

Centers for Disease Control, National Center for Chronic Disease Prevention and Health Promotion. "PATCH: Planned Approach to Community Health." *Journal of Health Education,* 1992, *23*(3), 129–192.

Cohen, S., and Syme, S. L. (eds.). *Social Support and Health.* Orlando, Fla.: Academic Press, 1985.

Connell, J. P., and others (eds.). *New Approaches to Evaluating Community Initiatives: Concepts, Methods and Contexts.* Washington, D.C.: Aspen Institute, 1995.

Cottrell, L. S., Jr. "The Competent Community." In R. Warren and L. Lyon (eds.), *New Perspectives on the American Community.* Florence, Ky.: Dorsey Press, 1983.

Delbecq, A., Van de Ven, A. H., and Gustafson, D. H. *Group Techniques for Program Planning: A Guide to Nominal Group and Delphi Processes.* Glenview, Ill.: Scott, Foresman, 1975.

Duhl, L. "Conditions for Healthy Cities: Diversity, Game Boards and Social Entrepreneurs." *Environment and Urbanization,* 1993, *5*(2), 112–124.

Eng, E., Briscoe, J., and Cunningham, A. "The Effect of Participation in State Projects on Immunization." *Social Science and Medicine,* 1990, *30*(12), 1349–1358.

Eng, E., and Parker, E. "Measuring Community Competence in the Mississippi Delta: The Interface Between Program Evaluation and Empowerment." *Health Education Quarterly,* 1994, *21*(2), 199–220.

Farquhar, J. W., and others. "The Stanford Five City Project: An Overview." In J. D. Matarazzo and others (eds.), *Behavioral Health: A Handbook of Health Enhancement and Disease Prevention.* New York: Wiley, 1984.

Fawcett, S. B., and others. "Empowering Community Health Initiatives Through Evaluation." In D. Fetterman, S. Kaftarian, and A. Wandersman (eds.), *Empowerment Evaluation.* Thousand Oaks, Calif.: Sage, 1996.

Feldblum, M., Wallerstein, N., Varela, F., and Collins, G. (eds.). *Community Organizing: An Experience for Building Healthier Communities.* (3rd ed.) Albuquerque. N.M.: New Mexico Department of Health, Public Health Division, 1994.

Fellin, P. "Understanding American Communities." In J. Rothman, J. L. Erlich, and J. E. Tropman (eds.), *Strategies of Community Organization.* (5th ed.) Itasca, Ill.: Peacock, 1995.

Fetterman, D., Kaftarian, S., and Wandersman, A. (eds.). *Empowerment Evaluation.* Thousand Oaks, Calif.: Sage, 1996.

Florin, P., and Wandersman, A. "An Introduction to Citizen Participation, Voluntary Organizations, and Community Development: Insights for Empowerment Through Research." *American Journal of Community Psychology,* 1990, *18*(1), 41–54.

Freire, P. *Pedagogy of the Oppressed.* New York: Seabury Press, 1970.

Freire, P. *Education for Critical Consciousness.* New York: Seabury Press, 1973.

French, M. *Beyond Power: On Women, Men And Morals.* London: Abacus, 1986.

French, W., and Bell, C. *Organization Development: Behavioral Science Interventions for Organization Improvement.* (2nd ed.) Englewood Cliffs, N.J.: Prentice Hall, 1990.

Gardner, J. *Building Community.* Washington, D.C.: Independent Sector Leadership Studies Program, 1991.

Garvin, C. D., and Cox, F. M. "A History of Community Organizing Since the Civil War with Special Reference to Oppressed Communities." In J. Rothman, J. L. Erlich, and J. E. Tropman (eds.), *Strategies of Community Organization.* (5th ed.) Itasca, Ill.: Peacock, 1995.

Goodman, R. M., Burdine, J., Meehan, E., and McLeroy, K. R. "Coalitions." *Health Education Research,* 1993, *8*(3), 313–314.

Guillory, B., Willie, E., Jr., and Duran, E. "Analysis of a Community Organizing Case Study: Alkali Lake." *Journal of Rural Community Psychology,* 1988, *9*(1), 27–35.

Gutierrez, L., and Lewis, E. "A Feminist Perspective on Organizing with Women of Color." In F. Rivera and J. Erlich (eds.), *Community Organizing in a Diverse Society.* (2nd ed.) Needham Heights, Mass.: Allyn & Bacon, 1995.

Heitzmann, C. A., and Kaplan, R. M. "Assessment of Methods for Measuring Social Support." *Health Psychology,* 1988, *7*(1), 75–109.

Himmelman, A. T. "Communities Working Collaboratively for a Change." Unpublished manuscript, July 1992.

Hope, A., and Timmel, S. *Training for Transformation: A Handbook for Community Workers.* Gweru, Zimbabwe: Mambo Press, 1984.

Hunter, A. "The Loss of Community: An Empirical Test Through Replication." *American Sociology Review,* 1975, *40*(5), 537–552.

Hyde, C. "A Feminist Model for Macro Practice." *Administration in Social Work,* 1990, *13,* 145–181.

Israel, B. A. "Social Networks and Social Support: Implications for Natural Helper and Community Level Interventions." *Health Education Quarterly,* 1985, *12*(1), 65–80.

Israel, B. A., Checkoway, B., Schulz, A., and Zimmerman, M. A. "Health Education and Community Empowerment: Conceptualizing and Measuring Perceptions of Individual, Organizational, and Community Control." *Health Education Quarterly,* 1994, *21*(2), 149–170.

Job, R. "Effective and Ineffective Use of Fear in Health Promotion Campaigns." *American Journal of Public Health,* 1988, *78,* 163–167.

Katz, R. "Empowerment and Synergy: Expanding the Community's Healing Resources." *Prevention in Human Services,* 1984, *3,* 201–226.

Khinduka, S. K. "Community Development: Potentials and Limitations." In R. M. Kramer and H. Specht (eds.), *Readings in Community Organization Practice.* (2nd ed.) Englewood Cliffs, N.J.: Prentice Hall, 1975.

Kieffer, C. "Citizen Empowerment: A Developmental Perspective." *Prevention in Human Services,* 1984, *3*(2–3; special issue: *Studies in Empowerment: Steps Toward Understanding and Action*), 9–36.

Labonte, R. "Empowerment: Notes on Professional and Community Dimensions." *Canadian Review of Social Policy,* 1990, *26,* 1–12.

Labonte, R. "Community Development and Partnerships." *Canadian Journal of Public Health,* 1993, *84*(4), 237–240.

Labonte, R. "Health Promotion and Empowerment: Reflections on Professional Practice." *Health Education Quarterly,* 1994, *21*(2), 253–268.

Maldrud, K., Polacsck, M., and Wallerstein, N. *A Workbook for Participatory Evaluation of Coalitions.* Albuquerque: University of New Mexico and New Mexico Partnership for Healthier Communities, forthcoming.

Marquez, B. "Organizing the Mexican American Community in Texas: The Legacy of Saul Alinsky." *Policy Studies Review,* Winter 1990, pp. 355–373.

McCallister, L., and Fischer, C. S. "A Procedure for Surveying Personal Networks." *Sociological Methods and Research,* 1978, *7,* 131–149.

McKnight, J. L. "Regenerating Community." *Social Policy,* Winter 1987, pp. 54–58.

McKnight, J. L. "Local Social Community Development and Economic Development Issues." Paper presented at the annual meeting of the American Public Health Association, San Francisco, Oct. 27, 1993.

McKnight, J. L., and Kretzmann, J. P. *Mapping Community Capacity.* Evanston, Ill.: Center for Urban Affairs and Policy Research, Northwestern University, 1992.

Miller, M. "Turning Problems into Actionable Issues." Unpublished manuscript, Organize Training Center, San Francisco, 1985.

Miller, M. "The Tenderloin Senior Organizing Project." In *A Journey to Justice.* Presbyterian Committee on the Self Development of People. Report of the Special Task Force. Louisville, Ky.: Presbyterian Church of the USA, 1993.

Minkler, M. "Community Organizing Among the Elderly Poor in the U.S.: A Case Study." *International Journal of Health Services,* 1992, *22,* 303–316.

Minkler, M. "Ten Commitments for Community Health Education." *Health Education Research,* 1994, *9*(4), 527–534.

Minkler, M. "Empowerment of the Elderly in San Francisco's Tenderloin District." In B. Amick and R. Rudd (eds.), *Society and Health: Case Studies.* Cambridge, Mass.: Harvard University Press, 1996.

Minkler, M., and Cox, K. "Creating Critical Consciousness in Health: Applications of Freire's Philosophy and Methods to the Health Care Setting." *International Journal of Health Services,* 1980, *10*(2), 311–322.

Ovrebo, B., Ryan, M., Jackson, K., and Hutchinson, K. "The Homeless Prenatal Program: A Model for Empowering Homeless Pregnant Women." *Health Education Quarterly,* 1994, *21*(2), 187–198.

Purdey, A., Adhikari, G., Robinson, S., and Cox, P. "Participatory Health Development in Rural Nepal: Clarifying the Process of Community Empowerment." *Health Education Quarterly,* 1994, *21*(3), 329–344.

Rappaport, J. "Studies in Empowerment: Introduction to the Issue." *Prevention in Human Services,* 1984, *3*(2–3), 1–7.

Reitzes, D. C., and Reitzes, D. C. "Saul Alinsky's Contribution to Community Development." *Journal of the Community Development Society,* 1980, *11*(2), 39–52.

Rivera, F., and Erlich, J. "An Option Assessment Framework for Organizing in Emerging Minority Communities." In J. Tropman and others (eds.), *Tactics and Techniques of Community Intervention.* (3rd ed.) Itasca, Ill.: Peacock, 1995.

Rogers, R. W. "Changing Health-Related Attitudes and Behavior: The Role of Preventive Health Psychology." In R. McGlyn, J. Maddox, C. Stoltenberg, and R. Harvey (eds.), *Interfaces in Psychology.* Lubbock: Texas Tech University Press, 1984.

Rogers, R. W., and Mewborn, C. R. "Fear Appeals and Attitude Change: Effects of a Threat's Noxiousness, Probability of Occurrence, and the Efficacy of Coping Responses." *Journal of Personality and Social Psychology,* 1976, *34,* 54–61.

Ross, M. *Community Organization: Theory and Principles.* New York: HarperCollins, 1955.

Rothman, J., and Tropman, J. E. "Models of Community Organization and Macro Practice: Their Mixing and Phasing." In F. M. Cox, J. L. Erlich, J. Rothman, and J. E. Tropman (eds.), *Strategies of Community Organization.* (4th ed.) Itasca, Ill.: Peacock, 1987.

"Safehouses Now Easing the Fears of Elderly Residents." *Los Angeles Times,* Nov. 21, 1982, p. 1.

Scott, J. *Domination and the Arts of Resistance: Hidden Transcripts.* New Haven, Conn.: Yale University Press, 1990.

Shaw, F. "Tenderloin Senior Organizing Project Evaluation." Unpublished report for the California Wellness Foundation, Woodland Hills, Calif., Nov. 1995.

Stainback, R., and Rogers, R. W. "Identifying Effective Components of Alcohol Abuse Prevention Programs: Effect of Fear Appeals, Message Style, and Source Expertise." *The International Journal of the Addictions,* 1983, *18*(3), 393–405.

Staples, L. *Roots to Power: A Manual for Grassroots Organizing.* New York: Praeger, 1984.

Stewart, D., and Shamdasani, P. *Focus Groups: Theory and Practice.* Thousand Oaks, Calif.: Sage, 1990.

Syme, S. L. "Social Epidemiology and the Work Environment." *International Journal of Health Services,* 1988, *18*(4), 635–645.

Traynor, B. "Community Development and Community Organizing." *Shelterforce,* Mar.-Apr. 1993, n.p.

Tsouros, A. "The WHO Healthy Cities Project: State of the Art and Future Plans." *Health Promotion International,* 1995, *10*(2), 133–141.

Wallerstein, N. "Powerlessness, Empowerment, and Health: Implications for Health Promotion Programs." *American Journal of Health Promotion,* 1992, *6,* 197–205.

Wallerstein, N., and Bernstein, E. "Empowerment Education: Freire's Ideas Adapted to Health Education." *Health Education Quarterly,* 1988, *15,* 379–394.

Wallerstein, N., and Bernstein, E. (eds.). *Health Education Quarterly,* 1994, *21* (entire issue 2 and 3: *Community Empowerment, Participatory Education and Health*).

Wallerstein, N., and Sanchez-Merki, V. "Freirian Praxis in Health Education: Research Results from an Adolescent Prevention Program." *Health Education Research*, 1994, *9*(1), 105–118.

Wallerstein, N., and Weinger, M. "Health and Safety Education for Worker Empowerment." *American Journal of Industrial Medicine*, 1992, *22*(5), 619–635.

Walter, C. "Community Building Practice." In M. Minkler (ed.), *Community Organizing and Community Building to Improve Health*. New Brunswick, N.J.: Rutgers University Press, forthcoming.

Warren, R. *The Community in America*. Skokie, Ill.: Rand McNally, 1963.

Wechsler, R. "Harnessing People Power: A Community-Based Approach to Preventing Alcohol and Drug Abuse." *Western City*, June 1990, pp. 1–4.

Wechsler, R., and Minkler, M. "A Community Oriented Approach to Health Promotion: The Tenderloin Senior Outreach Project." In K. Dychtwald (ed.), *Wellness and Health Promotion for the Elderly*. Rockville, Md.: Aspen Systems, 1986.

West, C. *Race Matters*. Boston: Beacon Press, 1993.

Wolfe, T. "Coalition Building: Is This Really Empowerment?" Presentation to the annual meeting of the American Public Health Association, San Francisco, Nov. 17, 1993.

World Health Organization. *Ottawa Charter for Health Promotion*. Copenhagen: World Health Organization, 1986.

Zimmerman, M. A. "Taking Aim on Empowerment Research: On the Distinction Between Individual and Psychological Conceptions." *American Journal of Community Psychology*, 1990, *18*, 169–177.

CHAPTER THIRTEEN

DIFFUSION OF INNOVATIONS

Brian Oldenburg
Deborah M. Hardcastle
Gerjo Kok

While considerable effort and resources are devoted to developing innovations, less attention is usually given to developing effective methods for their diffusion. This chapter provides a conceptual framework for understanding the process of diffusion and its various stages, an overview of key methodological and research issues, and some applications of diffusion theory to health promotion and education innovations.

According to Orlandi and colleagues (Orlandi, Landers, Weston, and Haley, 1990), many health promotion innovations fail because of "the gap that is frequently left unfilled between the point where innovation-development ends and diffusion planning begins." The assumption has often been made that widespread adoption and uptake of an innovation occur automatically. There is now ample evidence, however, that even users' initial attempts at implementation do not usually lead to sustained use of an effective health education program and that uptake by other users beyond the innovation development stage is usually poorer still. For example, in a project involving a smoking cessation program designed for administration by Australian physicians to their patients, and beyond the re-

The authors wish to thank Margot Ffrench for her contribution to the final draft of this chapter.

search and development phase, Copeman, Swannell, Pincus, and Woodhead (1989) found that after one year, less than 5 percent of the thirty-eight physicians who had attended the initial workshop had counseled smokers and kept records of their progress. In addition, while a total of 121 smokers were counseled, they constituted only 7 percent of all patients who smoked.

In another example, the success that was experienced in the United States with HIV risk reduction programs during the first ten years of the epidemic, due to effective diffusion of campaign messages, has not continued. Lapses and relapses have been reported in the gay male population, and there has been limited diffusion to other population groups exhibiting HIV risk behaviors (Kelly, Murphy, Silkema, and Kalichman, 1993).

Description of Key Terms

Rogers (1983) defines an *innovation* as "an idea, practice or object that is perceived as new by an individual or other unit of adoption." *Diffusion* is defined as "the process by which an innovation is communicated through certain channels over time among the members of a social system" (Rogers, 1983). Effective diffusion involves more than program dissemination at an individual level; it involves the implementation of strategies through various settings and systems, using a variety of formal or informal media and communication channels (Basch, 1984).

Historically, the study of diffusion of innovations evolved from rural sociology, and some of the earliest applications included research directed at understanding how new agricultural techniques spread among farmers. Since that time, diffusion theory as applied to health has been used to study the uptake of behaviors such as family planning, the use of new tests and technologies by health professionals, and the uptake of new pharmaceutical agents (Rogers and Shoemaker, 1971; Rogers, 1983).

Among contemporary examples of diffusion at a variety of levels is the success of widely disseminated efforts aimed at getting smokers to quit. This success has been encouraged by a variety of mass media strategies, social pressures, quit smoking programs, and smoking control policies or regulations and has resulted in a significant decline in reported national rates of current smoking in many developed countries over the past twenty years, including the United States and Australia (Hill and Borland, 1989). Another example of diffusion is the uptake and adoption of safe sexual practices, including the use of condoms, in the general population (De Vroome and others, 1994), and the reduction of unsafe sex in gay men (Hospers and Kok, 1995).

Diffusion Theory and Practice

Diffusion theory is derived from a body of research that has attempted to identify predictable patterns of program adoption, among a variety of population groups and across a range of innovations (Green, Gottlieb, and Parcel, 1987). These patterns of adoption can be described mathematically, and a number of key theoretical constructs have been identified as important (Rogers, 1983; Green and Anderson, 1986; Green and Lewis, 1986; Green, Gottlieb, and Parcel, 1987). The diffusion process involves attending to the innovation as well as to the channels used to communicate the innovation (*communication channels*) and to the characteristics of the systems or environment in which this process takes place (*diffusion context*).

Based on the statistical properties of the diffusion curve, the five adopter categories identified by Rogers (1983) include innovators, early adopters, early majority adopters, late majority adopters, and laggards. The identification of such categories is the basis for designing and implementing intervention strategies targeted at particular groups of individuals. These strategies can be based on the source of influence to which a particular group is most likely to respond. For example, Green, Gottlieb, and Parcel (1987) suggest that a cognitively oriented intervention might be most appropriate for early adopters, a motivational emphasis might be most effective for the majority adopters, and later adopters might require efforts to overcome barriers.

Rogers (1983) and Zaltman and Duncan (1977) have identified those attributes or characteristics most likely to affect the speed and extent of the diffusion process. These are summarized in Table 13.1.

Given the importance of the characteristics summarized in Table 13.1, practitioners and researchers need to ensure that these features are preempted and dealt with at the innovation development stage, and that in turn, these are then communicated to potential users.

A number of commentators (including Rogers, 1983; Basch, Eveland, and Portnoy, 1986) have drawn attention to the need for diffusion studies to focus on more than just the adoption stage. As Orlandi, Landers, Weston, and Haley (1990) write, "the adoption decision is only one step in a multistep process that ranges from the first phases of innovation development to a point beyond adoption at which the innovation either succeeds or fails in achieving a lasting and meaningful impact."

Furthermore, an innovation needs to be considered in relation to achieving the ideal "fit" between innovation and user. Maximizing this fit requires detailed consideration of the appropriate communication channels to use as well as an understanding of the environment and context in which diffusion is occurring. The environment or context in which the diffusion process occurs is inevitably dynamic

TABLE 13.1. ATTRIBUTES THAT ARE KEY DETERMINANTS OF DIFFUSION'S SPEED AND EXTENT.

Relative advantage	Is the innovation better than what it will replace?
Compatibility	Does the innovation fit with the intended audience?
Complexity	Is the innovation easy to use?
Trialability	Can the innovation be subjected to trial?
Observability	Are the results of the innovation observable and easily measurable?
Impact on social relations	Does the innovation have a disruptive effect on the social environment?
Reversibility	Can the innovation be reversed or discontinued easily?
Communicability	Can the innovation be understood clearly and easily?
Time required	Can the innovation be adopted with a minimal investment in time?
Risk and uncertainty level	Can the innovation be adopted with minimal risk and uncertainty?
Commitment required	Can the innovation be used effectively with only modest commitment?
Modifiability	Can the innovation be updated and modified over time?

and unpredictable rather than static and unidimensional. The aim of diffusion in health promotion and health education is to maximize the exposure and reach of innovations, strategies, or programs for which there is already established evidence of their efficacy and effectiveness. This requires development of the innovation, followed by its dissemination. The stages are defined in the following paragraphs.

Innovation development includes "all the decisions and activities (and their impacts) that occur from the early stage of an idea through to its development and production" (Rogers, 1983). Persons from the user system should play a major role in identifying the relevant target audiences, contributing to further development of the innovation, and in providing information and feedback on its content, design, layout, and presentation. Further development of promotional strategies and product designs are critical features of this stage. A social marketing framework can aid the practitioner in further designing, targeting, refining, and implementing the innovation (Winett, 1995; Lefebvre and Flora, 1988; Manoff, 1985).

Dissemination is defined as "an active approach for knowledge transfer from the resource system to the user system" (Orlandi, Landers, Weston, and Haley, 1990). It involves the identification of communication channels and systems (either formal or informal) that are best used for the diffusion of an innovation to a target audience. For example, dissemination of a program for community-based cholesterol screening (as in the Mount Vernon Cares Project described by Orlandi, Landers, Weston, and Haley, 1990) may require use of both formal channels such as public service announcements and press releases and informal channels such as community announcements at social and recreational events.

Adoption refers to the uptake of the program by the target audience. During this step, the target adopters need to be identified along with any relevant subgroups and their characteristics. The following points generally require attention: the needs of the target adopters, their current attitudes and values, their probable response to the innovation, the factors that will increase the likelihood of adoption, the ways target adopters can be influenced to change their existing practices and adopt the new behavior, the barriers that exist to adoption of the innovation, and the ways those barriers can be overcome.

Implementation refers to the initial use of the program in practice. A major focus here is on improving the self-efficacy and skills of adopters, and encouraging trial of the innovation. A *linkage agent* can play a major role, facilitating the smooth implementation of programs by providing training, troubleshooting problems that arise, and answering any questions (Orlandi, Landers, Weston, and Haley, 1990).

Maintenance refers to the ongoing implementation and continued use of the innovation in practice. Programs may be terminated for many reasons. Encouraging sustained use of the program and addressing reasons for termination (such as the lack of financial incentives for preventive medicine activities) is a challenging task for health professionals.

While diffusion usually takes place through informal systems, deliberately created and organized diffusion systems are of increasing importance. Orlandi, Landers, Weston, and Haley (1990) stress the need for linkage between the "resource system" and the "user system" to bridge the gap between innovation development and program diffusion. That is, the diffusion process should involve a close collaborative partnership between the group or individual who is promoting the program (resource system) and the potential users of the program (user system) (Havelock, 1976; Orlandi, 1986; Orlandi, 1987; Orlandi, Landers, Weston, and Haley, 1990). A number of studies have provided consistent evidence to support the importance of an interorganizational collaboration or linking agent, as mentioned earlier, to enhance the diffusion process (Monahan and Scheirer, 1988; also see Chapter Fourteen).

In a school situation, the linkage might take the form of a liaison group including representatives of the user system, representatives of the resource system, and a change agent facilitating the collaboration. Diffusion of the innovation may be carried out collectively by the members of this liaison group. The critical point is that the innovation development and diffusion-planning processes should be conducted to improve the fit between innovation and user, to attune intervention innovations to practical possibilities and constraints, and to facilitate widespread implementation.

Communication channels are an important component of diffusion theory. As suggested previously, diffusion theorists view communication as a two-way process rather than the mere persuasion of an audience to take action. The *two-step flow of communication,* in which opinion leaders (or credible linking agents) mediate the impact of mass media communications, emphasizes the value of social networks, or interpersonal channels, over and above mass media for innovation adoption decisions (Rogers, 1983). Recent examples of diffusing innovations through schools and other systems or settings illustrate the shift in focus from considering innovation attributes and adopter characteristics to considering communication channels and the diffusion context (Fullan, 1991; Kolbe and Iverson, 1981; Rogers, 1983). Paulussen and his coworkers, for example, have examined the stages in the diffusion of AIDS education curricula in schools in the Netherlands (Paulussen, Kok, and Schaalma, 1994). In this context, *dissemination* refers to the transfer of information about the innovation to potential users (that is, schoolteachers), *adoption* refers to the teachers' intention to use the innovation, *implementation* refers to the actual use of the innovation, and the *continuation* or *maintenance* step covers the long-term use of the program.

Achieving satisfactory diffusion of an innovation (whether at the individual, social, or organizational level) involves change (Parcel, Perry, and Taylor, 1990). In essence, the change principles that underpin the diffusion process at these various levels are no different from those identified for the individual, organizational, or community level. At the level of the individual, family, or small group, uptake and implementation of a health promotion innovation typically involve changes in behaviors or lifestyle practices that will either reduce risk factors or promote health. At the organizational level, such as the workplace, school, or the health care setting, successful uptake of an innovation may require the introduction of particular programs or services, changes in policies or regulations, or changes in the roles and functions of particular personnel. At a broader communitywide or even societal level, the diffusion process can involve the use of the mass media and be supported by governmental policies and legislation as well as by coordination of a variety of other initiatives at the individual and the settings level. Complexity arises in the principles that underpin the diffusion of innovations due to the need to consider change occurring at multiple levels and across many different settings and resulting from the use of many different change strategies. Success requires the application of multiple models and theories in order to develop frameworks with sufficient explanatory power. Most of the theories or models that have been used extensively to understand and describe change at the individual or small-group level, such as Social Cognitive Theory or the Theory of Planned Behavior (Ajzen, 1991), also aid greatly in understanding the change and diffusion process at the organizational level (Parcel, Perry, and Taylor, 1990; Paulussen, Kok, and Schaalma, 1994).

Application to Health Promotion

This section describes three applications of diffusion theory to health promotion, demonstrating key constructs and the application of diffusion theory in both intervention research and explanatory research. Each application involves innovation implementation in a specific type of organization, either a health care setting or a school. The examples address cardiovascular risk reduction counseling, reduction of alcohol consumption, and adoption of AIDS prevention curricula.

Case Study: Development and Dissemination of the Fresh Start Program

The Fresh Start Program was developed as a joint initiative of the Department of Public Health, the University of Sydney, and the National Heart Foundation of Australia (N.S.W. Division), which is the lead nongovernmental agency for promoting cardiovascular health in Australia. The Fresh Start program is a standardized approach that can be used by primary care physicians and other health professionals to reduce patients' risk of cardiovascular disease through lifestyle change. It uses a variety of print- and video-based materials to promote the behavioral changes of smoking cessation, dietary revision, and increased physical activity (Oldenburg, Graham-Clarke, Walker, and Shaw, 1995; Graham-Clarke and Oldenburg, 1994). The program is intended to help individuals achieve long-term lifestyle changes and is based on Social Learning Theory (Bandura, 1986) and an adaptation of the stages of change model (Prochaska and DiClemente, 1992) that identifies the three basic stages: preparation, action, and maintenance (Oldenburg, 1994a, 1994b; Brownell, Marlatt, Lichtenstein, and Wilson, 1986).

Results of an effectiveness trial of the Fresh Start Program indicate that the greatest benefits accrued to "high risk" males and to the least physically active patients, who were more likely than others to change, moving from the *precontemplation* stage toward the *preparation* and *action* stages (Graham-Clarke and Oldenburg, 1994).

Innovation Development and Dissemination. Dissemination of the Fresh Start Program to physicians through the divisions of general practice provided both a means of diffusion and a linking agent through which the program could be made available to a relatively large number of physicians. In Australia, a division of general practice is a geographically based organizational structure made up of, on average, one hundred family physicians. Divisions receive funding from the federal government for training, education, and other program initiatives, and they often receive additional support from and collaborate extensively with universities and a range of community health and other local services. The divisions were a strategic link between the university project team that conducted the evaluation, the Heart Foundation (resource system), and the family physicians (user system). They formed a convenient network through which a relatively large group of primary care physicians could be reached and through which program maintenance could occur.

The three strategies used to disseminate the Fresh Start Program and then evaluated in a randomized experiment included a mailing of a promotional pamphlet, small-group educational workshops, and educational detailing.

Results of Dissemination. Program reach (or the uptake rate) was defined as the proportion of physicians who accepted an invitation to take up use of the Fresh Start Program. As illustrated in Figure 13.1, of all physicians approached, 32 percent agreed to participate in the workshops, 38 percent requested a Fresh Start kit in response to the mailing strategy, and 64 percent agreed to receive detailing. Of the physicians who attended the introductory workshop, 58 percent attended the follow-up workshop. Physicians allocated to the workshop and detailing strategies were more likely to report ongoing use of the program at twelve months (83 percent and 80 percent respectively) than were those who received the mailing alone (42 percent). Although all groups except the detailing division physicians were relatively consistent in their use of the program over time, more physicians reported using the program at twelve months than at four months.

Diffusion Theory Exemplified. This application illustrates the ways in which a variety of models and theories—in particular, diffusion theory and social marketing principles—can be applied to disseminating a preventive medicine program to family physicians. This approach has taken advantage of the way in which family general practice is currently organized in Australia, with the development of divisions of general practice. It demonstrates the importance of clearly identifying the linkages between a number of different organizations and agencies, and by using cluster randomization with divisions as the unit of randomization, shows how rigorous measurement and research design can be used to formally evaluate the effectiveness of different dissemination strategies. The researchers also conducted an economic evaluation to assess the relative costs and benefits of different dissemination strategies.

FIGURE 13.1. INITIAL UPTAKE AND ONGOING USE OF THE FRESH START PROGRAM.

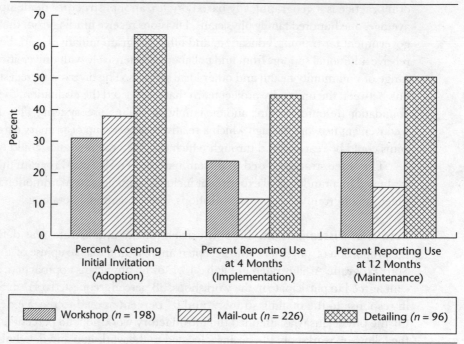

Note: Percentages are based on the total number of initial program invitees.

Case Study: Diffusion Through Primary Health Care of a Brief Intervention Program for Hazardous Alcohol Use: The Drink-Less Experience

Primary care physicians are in an excellent position to conduct brief intervention for hazardous alcohol use, given their high level of contact with the community and their perceived credibility with patients. These facts and the evidence available to support the efficacy of brief intervention in primary health care suggested that there was a need to develop a program that could assist doctors in identifying patients with alcohol-related problems and providing a brief intervention.

Innovation Development and Dissemination. The brief intervention program developed was called Drink-Less and was adapted from materials used previously. Given that the environment in which physicians practice is often busy and hectic, the program was designed to be simple, brief, and easy to use. The basic package consists of a screening questionnaire (AUDIT), scoring template, handycard, and self-help booklet. Accessories included are the program guidelines for the physician and program guidelines for the receptionist, a Drink-Less poster, Drink-Less stickers, and a zip folder.

In order to identify communication channels and systems for the diffusion of the program to physicians, a randomized, controlled dissemination trial was conducted. The trial had two phases—a marketing phase that evaluated three social marketing strategies, and a training and support phase that compared a number of different strategies. All the marketing strategies (direct mail, telephone marketing, and academic detailing) were conducted by consultants (trained research personnel). Each marketing strategy promoted program endorsements from major medical authorities, emphasized the benefits of using the program, and addressed possible barriers to effective program implementation, such as time constraints.

In both the telemarketing and academic detailing strategies, consultants were trained to anticipate and address perceived barriers among physicians (for example, if time was a barrier, the brevity and simplicity of the program were emphasized). There were four training and support conditions: maximal support, minimal support, no support, and a control condition.

Diffusion Theory Exemplified. Results from the marketing phase suggested that the telemarketing and academic detailing strategies were superior to direct mail in enhancing the adoption of the program. However, there was no difference in uptake rates between academic detailing and telemarketing strategies (Hardcastle and others, 1995). Preliminary results for the training and support phase indicate that physicians who received a maximum level of training and support in implementing the program had higher screening and counseling rates than those who received either no support or minimal support. It also appears that initial training in the use of the program may be an important factor in promoting its long-term use. In both phases, the use of a consultant to act as a linkage agent between the resource system (health promotion professionals) and the user system (physicians) was an important aspect. The provision of initial training to both physicians and receptionists was vital to the effective implementation of the innovation in the physician's practice.

In Table 13.1, we summarized the attributes most likely to affect the speed and extent of the diffusion process. Table 13.2 illustrates the way a number of these same attributes were considered as the Drink-Less program was developed.

Another important aspect of the dissemination trial was the ability of the consultant who implemented the marketing strategies to take into account the five adopter categories. For example, for late majority adopters in the telemarketing strategy, a more intensive approach was required, and the marketing sales script was flexible enough to allow the caller to provide the physician with more information and discuss barriers to adoption.

TABLE 13.2. DIFFUSION THEORY CONSIDERED IN DEVELOPING THE DRINK-LESS PROGRAM.

Attribute	Attribute Identified for the Drink-Less Program
Relative advantage	Easier identification of patients' risk of harm from alcohol use, and easier and quicker administration of counseling to patients identified as at risk.
Complexity	Package unobtrusive and simple to use and understand—no intensive manuals to read, only brief guidelines.
Compatibility	Program designed specifically for use by physicians and other health professionals. Endorsed by medical authorities including WHO, the Australian Medical Association, and the Royal Australian College of General Practitioners.
Impact on social relations	• Between doctors and patients: overall positive patient perceptions of the program; physicians more aware of the alcohol issue when caring for the at-risk patient
	• Between physicians and other practice staff: despite increased workload due to the program, physician support by practice staff (such as receptionists) facilitated program's overall implementation.
	• Between physicians and other health professionals: the program has the potential to improve communication between physicians and other health professionals, such as drug and alcohol counselors, and to provide an assessment "standard."
Reversibility	Physician may choose to revert to previous practice—program easily terminated.
Communicability	Program easily communicated to practice staff and other health professionals.
Time required	Program simple and designed to be administered quickly.
Risk and uncertainty level	No risk in the use of the program.
Commitment required	The physician can choose to screen for a certain time period only.
Modifiability	The overall program and its individual components can be easily generalized to other settings and for use by other health professionals.

Case Study: Diffusion of AIDS Education Curricula in Dutch Schools

Paulussen, Kok, and Schaalma (1994, 1995) have described the steps involved in the diffusion of AIDS education curricula via schoolteachers in Dutch schools. They have identified the steps leading from the initial development of the innovation to an increase in teachers' awareness and knowledge and to the uptake and implementation of four nationally disseminated AIDS curricula. Their work describes the application of an extended model of planned behavior (Ajzen, 1991; Bandura, 1986; de Vries and others, 1994) as an organizing schema for a measuring instrument that helped improve their understanding of teachers' preparedness to take up and use various AIDS curricula.

When the extent of diffusion of classroom AIDS education was examined, the rates were very similar to those reported for most externally developed curricula. That is, while about 50 percent of teachers received curricula, only 25 percent actively adopted and implemented curriculum content, and only 5 to 10 percent maintained use of the curricula to any great extent.

Acquisition of knowledge about the AIDS programs was mainly determined by the extent of the diffusion networks between teachers within schools. Teachers' intentions to provide AIDS education were determined, in turn, by a range of psychosocial, attitudinal, and ecological factors. Adoption of a specific curriculum was, above all, related to its perceived instrumentality by teachers and to their having observed colleagues' use of the AIDS curricula (that is, modeling).

One of the most striking results of this research was that teachers' innovation decision making was not significantly affected by the perceived importance and feasibility of student learning outcomes. These results are congruent with much other research on the uptake of educational innovations, indicating that teachers are more concerned with procedural content and the perceived feedback from their colleagues and students than they are with specific student outcomes (compare Clark and Peterson, 1986; Borko, Livingston, and Shavelson, 1990; Hall and Hord, 1987).

Future Directions and Research Challenges

With an increasing focus on the importance of socioenvironmental and ecological factors as determinants of both the rate of diffusion and the rates of adoption, implementation, and maintenance, a key question is the extent to which these determinants are specific to particular settings. We have learned a lot in recent years about the dissemination of health curricula within the school setting. *Environmental turbulence,* for example, has been noted by Smith and colleagues as being very important in the school environment (Smith, Steckler, McCormick, and McLeroy, 1995). And this factor is also likely to be an important determinant of diffusion in other settings, such as the workplace. Indeed, where such strategies as governmental legislation and policies are being used to diffuse an innovation, turbulence in the organizational environment is likely to be quite critical.

However, other determinants of curriculum adoption, implementation, and maintenance in schools are more setting specific (such as whether students' knowledge of health behavior is examined on standardized state and national tests). The extent to which determinants related to leadership and training that have importance for disseminating health curricula to schools are relevant to diffusion of innovations in other settings is not well researched at this point in time (Smith, Steckler, McCormick, and McLeroy, 1995). Indeed, the extent to which the research in the primary medical care setting is generalizable to other settings is also not clear. For example, clearly identified factors are now known to be necessary for increasing the uptake and maintenance of preventive medicine by physicians. Elford and others (1994) have called this a "sustaining office system in prevention," with its key components being (1) a practice coordinator for prevention, (2) clear clinical prevention-related job descriptions, (3) an information management system that reinforces prevention, and (4) a practice feedback and problem-solving strategy.

Basch, Eveland, and Portnoy (1986) have identified and compared many barriers to and enhancers of diffusion of specific health promotion innovations in the health care, workplace, and school settings. It is important to bear in mind, though, that an innovation needs to be seen as such by the potential adopter, and that the essence of an innovation is information and knowledge. Although many innovations, particularly those in health promotion, have a substantial product component, most complex innovations for promoting health also consist of procedures, regulations, and practice. Of course, this is why many of the principles involved in marketing, particularly social marketing, have been so usefully applied to disseminating innovations. Activating a change process at a personal, organizational, or communitywide level, rather than relying solely on passive diffusion, becomes a major challenge for practitioners and researchers alike.

Recent applications of diffusion theory demonstrate the importance of linking relevant theories to large-scale efforts aimed at reducing communitywide death and disability. Howze and Redman (1992), for example, report how diffusion of innovations and other social science theories have been employed by a statewide coalition, the Health Promotion and Education Council of Virginia, which has worked through legislative action and opinion leaders, created information-exchange relationships, and used advocacy, to increase the impact of effective health promotion practice. With the increasing emphasis in most developed countries on linking health promotion strategies and interventions to health outcomes and other well-defined goals and targets, well-organized and large-scale communitywide efforts aimed at diffusion through multiple levels will become much more common.

In many areas of health promotion, the research and evaluation effort has not kept up with the demand. For example, a recent audit of thirteen leading public health and health promotion journals for the year 1994 has shown that very few empirical papers surveyed were relevant to the stages of innovation development (6 percent), diffusion (1 percent), and institutionalization (4 percent) (Oldenburg, Ffrench, Sallis, and Owen, 1996). Basch, Eveland, and Portnoy (1986) have proposed a useful framework for evaluation of the diffusion process that requires explicitly identifying the rates of adoption, implementation, and maintenance of an innovation while also measuring these elements at a variety of levels—including individual, group, setting, community, and state and national levels. As identified by Basch, Eveland, and Portnoy (1986), rigorous, controlled research designs are still unusual in this type of research. In any case, it is important to consider the pros and cons of experimental, quasi-experimental, and case study designs for evaluation of diffusion of an innovation, as in many instances, an experimental design is neither acceptable or feasible. The type and intensity of measurement is also a key consideration, particularly, if it is important to assess the diffusion of an innovation unobtrusively and not reactively. Use of multiple data sources and triangulation of measures are especially relevant in the evaluation of program diffusion. Cost-benefit measurement is particularly critical in the evaluation of different dissemination strategies and methods. Such evaluation can often yield valuable information that can then be used to further develop strategies and methods that enhance the likelihood of substantial diffusion. For example, when the various strategies used to disseminate the Fresh Start Program were subjected to an economic evaluation, the workshop method was shown to be the most expensive. It involved much more of the physician's time in terms of travel and participation than did educational detailing.

Conclusion

An improved understanding of how new methods, strategies, practices, and innovations are spread is critical for improving the practice of health promotion and for ensuring that this practice is based upon the best available research evidence. Given that we now know that successful diffusion is more the exception than the rule, there is an irrefutable need for more diffusion research. Such research requires innovative approaches to study design and measurement. This is most challenging, however, because rigorous research designs are usually difficult to implement on a large scale, measurement can be intrusive and reactive, and control over contextual factors is usually poor. Moreover, such intervention studies are, by their very nature, very large and can be very costly and take a number of years to implement and evaluate. Development of innovations and their diffusion will inevitably be enhanced by good quality program implementation by practitioners and by the application of multiple theories and models.

References

Ajzen, I. "The Theory of Planned Behavior." *Organizational Behavior and Human Decision Processes,* 1991, *50,* 179–211.

Bandura, A. *Social Foundations of Thought and Action: A Social Cognitive Theory.* Englewood Cliffs, N.J.: Prentice Hall, 1986.

Basch, C. E. "Research on Disseminating and Implementing Health Education Programs in Schools." *Journal of School Health,* 1984, *54,* 57–66.

Basch, C. E., Eveland, J. D., and Portnoy, B. "Diffusions Systems for Education and Learning About Health." *Family and Community Health,* 1986, *9,* 1–26.

Borko, H., Livingston, C., and Shavelson, R. J. "Teachers' Thinking About Instruction." *Remedial and Special Education,* 1990, *11,* 40–49.

Brownell, K. D., Marlatt, G. A., Lichtenstein, E. R., and Wilson, G. T. "Understanding and Preventing Relapse." *American Psychologist,* 1986, *41,* 765–782.

Clark, C. M., and Peterson, P. L. "Teachers' Thought Processes." In M. C. Wittrock (ed.), *Third Handbook of Research on Teaching.* New York: Macmillan, 1986.

Copeman, R., Swannell, R., Pincus, D., and Woodhead, K. "Utilization of the 'Smokescreen' Cessation Programme by General Practitioners and Their Patients." *Medical Journal of Australia,* 1989, *151,* 83–87.

de Vries, H., and others. "A Dutch Social Influence Smoking Prevention Approach for Vocational School Students." *Health Education Research,* 1994, *9,* 365–374.

De Vroome, E. M., and others. "Increase in Safe Sex Among the Young and Non-Monogamous: Knowledge, Attitudes and Behavior Regarding Safe Sex and Condom Use in the Netherlands from 1987 to 1993." *Patient Education and Counseling,* 1994, *24,* 179–288.

Elford, R. W., and others. "Putting Prevention into Practice." *Health Reports,* 1994, *6*(1), 142–153.

Fullan, M. G. *The New Meaning of Educational Change.* New York: Teachers College Press, 1991.

Graham-Clarke, P., and Oldenburg, B. F. "The Effectiveness of a General Practice Based Physical Activity Intervention on Patient Physical Activity Status." *Behavior Change,* 1994, *11*(3), 132–143.

Green, L. W., and Anderson, C. *Community Health.* (5th ed.) St. Louis, Mo.: Mosby-Year Book, 1986.

Green, L. W., Gottlieb, N. H., and Parcel, G. S. "Diffusion Theory Extended and Applied." In W. B. Ward (ed.), *Advances in Health Education and Promotion.* Greenwich, Conn.: JAI Press, 1987.

Green, L. W., and Lewis, F. M. *Measurement and Evaluation in Health Education and Health Promotion.* Mountain View, Calif.: Mayfield, 1986.

Hall, G. E., and Hord, S. M. *Change in Schools: Facilitating the Process.* Albany: State University of New York Press, 1987.

Hardcastle D. M., and others. "A Controlled Trial to Examine the Dissemination of an Early Intervention Program for Hazardous and Harmful Alcohol Consumption in General Practice." Paper presented in Symposium 20, *Effective Dissemination of Health Promotion Programs,* at the 16th annual meeting of the Society of Behavioral Medicine, San Diego, Mar. 22–25, 1995.

Havelock, R. G. *Planning for Innovation Through Dissemination and Utilization of Knowledge.* Ann Arbor: Center for Research on Utilization of Scientific Knowledge, University of Michigan, 1976.

Hill, D., and Borland, R. "Are Doctors Doing Enough to Stop Their Patients Smoking?" *Medical Journal of Australia,* 1989, *150,* 413–414.

Hospers H. J., and Kok, G. "Determinants of Safe and Risk-Taking Sexual Behavior Among Gay Men: A Review." *AIDS Education and Prevention,* 1995, *7*(1), 74–96.

Howze, E. H., and Redman, L. J. "The Uses of Theory in Health Advocacy: Policies and Programs." *Health Education Quarterly,* 1992, *19*(3; special issue: *Roles and Uses of Theory in Health Education Practice*), 369–383.

Kelly, J. A., Murphy, D. A., Silkema, K. J., and Kalichman, S. C. "Psychological Interventions to Prevent HIV Infection Are Urgently Needed." *American Psychologist,* 1993, *48,* 1023–1034.

Kolbe, L. J., and Iverson, D. C. "Implementing Comprehensive Health Education: Educational Innovations and Social Change." *Health Educational Quarterly,* 1981, *8,* 57–80.

Lefebvre R. C., and Flora J. A. "Social Marketing and Public Health Interventions." *Health Education Quarterly,* 1988, *15*(3), 299–315.

Manoff, R. K. *Social Marketing: New Imperative for Public Health.* New York: Praeger, 1985.

Monahan, J. I., and Scheirer, M. A. "The Role of Linking Agents in the Diffusion of Health Promotion Programs." *Health Education Quarterly,* 1988, *15*(4), 417–433.

Oldenburg, B. F. "Health Promotion and Disease Prevention in the Primary Health Care Setting: Setting the Scene." *Behavior Change,* 1994a, *11,* 129–131.

Oldenburg, B. F. "Promoting Health: Integrating the Clinical and Public Health Approaches." *International Review of Health Psychology,* 1994b, *3,* 121–143.

Oldenburg, B. F., Ffrench, M. L., Sallis, J. F., and Owen, N. "Translating Health Promotion Research into Practice." Paper presented to the Fourth International Congress for Behavioral Medicine, Washington, D.C., March 13–16, 1996.

Oldenburg, B. F., Graham-Clark, P., Walker, S., and Shaw, J. "Modification of Health Behaviour and Lifestyle Mediated by Physicians." In K. Orth-Gomer and N. Schneiderman (eds.), *Behavioral Medicine Approaches to Cardiovascular Disease Prevention.* Hillsdale, N.J.: Erlbaum, 1995.

Orlandi, M. A. "The Diffusion and Adoption of Worksite Health Promotion Innovations: An Analysis of Barriers." *Preventive Medicine,* 1986, *15,* 522–536.

Orlandi, M. A. "Promoting Health and Preventing Disease in Health Care Settings: An Analysis of Barriers." *Preventive Medicine,* 1987, *16,* 119–130.

Orlandi, M. A., Landers, C., Weston, R., and Haley, N. "Diffusion of Health Promotion Innovations." In K. Glanz, F. M. Lewis, and B. K. Rimer (eds.), *Health Behavior and Health Education: Theory, Research, and Practice.* San Francisco: Jossey-Bass, 1990.

Parcel, G. S., Perry, C. L., and Taylor, W. C. "Beyond Demonstration: Diffusion of Health Promotion Innovations." In N. Bracht (ed.), *Health Promotion at the Community Level.* Thousand Oaks, Calif.: Sage, 1990.

Paulussen, T. G., Kok, G., and Schaalma, H. P. "Antecedents to Adoption of Classroom-Based AIDS Education in Secondary Schools." *Health Education Research,* 1994, *9,* 485–496.

Paulussen, T. G., Kok, G., Schaalma, H. P., and Parcel, G. S. "Diffusion of AIDS Curricula Among Dutch Secondary School Teachers." *Health Education Quarterly,* 1995, *22,* 227–243.

Prochaska, J. O., and DiClemente, C. C. "Stages of Change in the Modification of Problem Behaviors." *Progress in Behavior Modification,* 1992, *28,* 183–218.

Rogers, E. M. *Diffusion of Innovations.* (3rd ed.) New York: Free Press, 1983.

Rogers, E. M., and Shoemaker, F. *Communication of Innovations: A Cross-Cultural Approach.* New York: Free Press, 1971.

Smith, D., Steckler, A., McCormick, L., and McLeroy, K. R. "Lessons Learned About Disseminating Health Curricula to Schools." *Journal of Health Education,* 1995, *26*(1), 37–43.

Winett, R. A. "A Framework for Health Promotion and Disease Prevention Programs." *American Psychologist,* 1995, *50*(5), 341–350.

Zaltman, G., and Duncan, R. *Strategies for Planned Change.* New York: Wiley, 1977.

CHAPTER FOURTEEN

MOBILIZING ORGANIZATIONS FOR HEALTH ENHANCEMENT

Theories of Organizational Change

Robert M. Goodman
Allan Steckler
Michelle C. Kegler

Organizational theory is like an oriental box puzzle. When the key is found and the box unlocked, another box is revealed within that requires a different key. In the smaller box is another box, and another still, each requiring a separate key. Organizational theory, like the box puzzle, can be penetrated on many levels.

Organizations are layered. Their strata range from the organization embedded in its surrounding environment at the broadest level, to the organizational structure, to the management within, to work groups, and to each individual member. Change may be influenced at each of these strata (Harrison, 1987; Kaluzny and Hernandez, 1988), and health promotion strategies directed at several levels simultaneously may be most durable in producing the desired results (McLeroy, Bibeau, Steckler, and Glanz, 1988). The practitioner who understands the ecology of organizations and who can apply appropriate strategies has powerful tools for stimulating change.

Because organizations may be influenced at the many levels their ecology comprises, no single theory is sufficient for explaining how and why organizations change. In this chapter, we analyze three theories of organizational change: stage theory, organizational development theory, and interorganizational relations theory. These theories were selected for several reasons. First, they illustrate how theory can be directed at different organizational levels. Second, they suggest specific intervention strategies. Thus, the practitioner can translate these theories into prescriptions for action. Third, the strategies that extend from these theories are directed at levels of the organization at which health promotion may be most influential. Fourth, the strategies can be used simultaneously, thus creating synergistic results.

Two cases are presented in this chapter to illustrate how the theories may be used together and at the different organizational strata. Before these applications are presented, the origins and elements of each theory are described.

Stage Theory of Organizational Change

Stage theory of organizational change explains how organizations innovate new goals, programs, technologies, and ideas (Kaluzny and Hernandez, 1988). (It is not related to Prochaska and DiClemente's stages of change; see Chapter Four.) Stage theory is so named because organizations, as they innovate, pass through a series of steps or stages. Each stage requires a unique set of strategies if the innovation is to grow and to mature. Strategies that are effective at one stage may be misapplied at the next, thereby disabling the innovation. Therefore, the skillful application of stage theory requires an accurate assessment of an innovation's current stage of development and the selection of strategies appropriate for that stage.

History

Stage theory emerges from two research traditions. The first extends from the work of Lewin, who developed one of the earliest stage models (Lewin, 1951). Lewin's model, which emphasizes factors resisting change efforts, has three stages: (1) unfreezing of past behaviors and attitudes; (2) moving by exposure to new information, attitudes, and theories; and (3) refreezing through processes of reinforcement, confirmation, and support for the change.

The second influence on the development of stage theory is diffusion of innovation theory. (See Chapter Thirteen for further analysis of diffusion theory.) In the 1950s, diffusion theory focused on how individuals such as farmers, teachers, and physicians adopted innovations (Rogers, 1983). In the 1960s, innovation theorists realized that individuals often adopt innovations as members of organizations, and that such individuals seldom adopt an innovation until it is first accepted by the organization.

Modern Stage Theory

Beyer and Trice (1978) have developed a comprehensive, well-defined, and contemporary model of stage theory that consists of seven stages:

1. *Sensing of unsatisfied demands on the system.* Some part of the system receives information indicating a problem or potential problem.
2. *Search for possible responses.* Elements in the system try to find alternative solutions.
3. *Evaluation of alternatives.* The various alternatives are compared.
4. *Decision to adopt a course of action.* An alternative is chosen from among those evaluated. Operative goals and means are specified; that is, a strategy is adopted.
5. *Initiation of action within the system.* A policy or other directive for implementing the change is formulated. Resources necessary for implementation are acquired.
6. *Implementation of the change.* Resources are allocated for implementation. The innovation is carried out.
7. *Institutionalization of the change.* The innovation part of routine organizational operations.

How Stage Theory Operates

How innovations "move" from one stage to the next is still an open question. Most studies measure the dynamics within stages, but only a few suggest what mechanisms might lead from one stage to the next (Steckler and others, 1992).

In their study of innovations in schools, Huberman and Miles (1984) demonstrated that different actors play leading roles at different innovation stages: senior-level administrators are important at the problem definition and early adoption stages, midlevel administrators such as curriculum coordinators and principals are important actors at the adoption and early implementation stages, teachers are instrumental at the implementation stage, and senior-level administrators once again play a key role at the institutionalization stage. The Huberman and Miles study suggests that decisions to adopt and to institutionalize are essentially political, therefore administrators take a leading role at these times. Implementation appears to be a more technical enterprise and involves professional skills like teaching ability more than administrative and political skills.

Future Challenges

Stage theory holds promise for guiding the practitioner's efforts to nurture health promotion programs, but greater consensus about the optimal number of stages within the model is desirable. Currently, the number of stages varies depending on whose model is employed. Clearer definition of the stages will lead to greater precision of strategies for each stage. Second, the completeness of stage models has been questioned. To date, no models extend beyond institutionalization. Yet evidence indicates that beyond institutionalization is renewal, a stage during which well-established programs evolve to meet changing demands (Goodman and Steckler, 1989). Third, those factors known to enable a program's development at each stage should be expanded. As additional factors are identified as important at each developmental stage, both researchers and practitioners will find a greater array of strategies for enhancing program development.

Organizational Development Theory

Organizational development (OD) is defined as the application of behavioral sciences to improve organizational effectiveness. It has the dual goals of improving organizational performance and the quality of work life. These goals generally are accomplished through interventions directed at organizational processes and structures and at worker behaviors (Brown and Covey, 1987). The interventions often are stimulated by an OD consultant who is engaged by management and who implements a set of strategies to help the organization diagnose, evaluate, and address its perceived concerns.

History

The theory of organizational development is rooted in the human relations perspective that emerged in the 1930s. Prior to the 1930s, organizational effectiveness was equated with structural efficiencies, such as establishing precise lines of authority (Weber, 1964). In the 1920s and 1930s, research that became known as the Hawthorne studies demonstrated that increasing the attention paid to workers also increased productivity (Roethlisberger and Dickson, 1939). These studies resulted in an expanded view of organizational effectiveness as influenced largely by worker motivation.

Developments in social science in the late 1940s and 1950s provided the theoretical and philosophical basis for management that is worker concerned (Margulis and Adams, 1982). Paramount here is Lewin's scientific and humanizing influence on the field of organizational behavior. In emphasizing practical applications, Lewin's *action research* converted organizations into vibrant laboratories for scientific and self-discovery (Cooperrider and Srivastva, 1987). His stage model of unfreezing, moving, and refreezing is the basis for action research and the precursor of most contemporary organizational change theories.

Like Lewin, Argyris (1957) rejected classical bureaucracy, arguing that individual needs must be fulfilled in the contexts of work and organization. MacGregor (1960) also rejected bureaucratic organization, which he termed Theory X, a set of axioms that held that managers must exert control if workers are to comply with organizational goals. MacGregor proposed an alternative, Theory Y, which held that work is natural to human activity and that workers will readily fulfill management's requirements given a supportive environment. Likert (1961) added that managers served as "linking pins" among semiautonomous work groups into which the individual worker was integrated.

Typology

By the 1960s, the term organizational development had emerged in the literature. OD was characterized by interventions aimed at either an organization's design and technologies or its human processes. Today, greater emphasis is directed at environmental influences and how the norms and values of entire organizations are transformed (Brown and Covey, 1987). Also, increased attention has been devoted to the development of OD theory. Porras and Robertson (1987) describe a typology, depicted in Figure 14.1, in which organizational change theories are categorized into two main branches: change process theories and change implementation theories (summarized in the following sections).

Change Process Theories. Change process theories specify the underlying dynamics of change. That is, they define the causal relationships among variables that the practitioner may influence, mediator variables or intermediate stages of the change process, and moderator variables or other influences on intended outcomes. Porras and Robertson (1987) note that few such theories exist and those that do have not been integrated into a coherent explanation of the change process.

Implementation Theories. In contrast to change process theories, implementation theories are relatively well defined. They concern the activities that practitioners employ to ensure that change is successful. Implementation theory is actually an umbrella term for three levels of theories: strategy, procedure, and technique. *Strategy theories* provide broad perspectives for implementing change but generally do not specify guidelines for intervening. Strategy theories describe rather than prescribe: they describe how organizational and other factors may contribute to change but offer few prescriptions for affecting change. *Procedure theories* identify the sequence of actions for producing change that is missing from strategy theories. Thus, procedure theories are more prescriptive than strategy theories. *Technique theories* consist of a set of activities that practitioners may employ at each step derived from a procedure theory. These activities enable the change process to move from one step to the next.

FIGURE 14.1. TYPOLOGY OF ORGANIZATIONAL CHANGE THEORY.

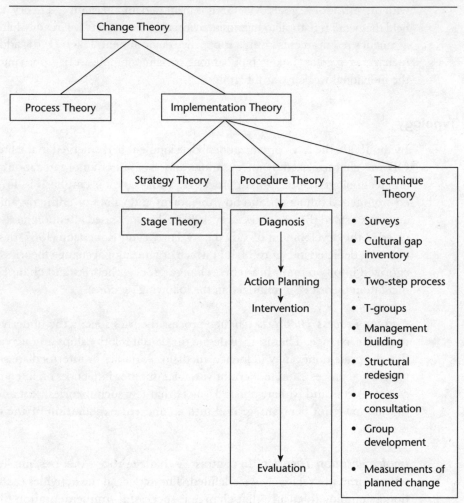

Source: Adapted from Porras and Robertson, 1987.

An Expanded View of Implementation Theory. Porras and Robertson (1987) analyze the steps common to several prominent implementation theories. They conclude that the four steps of diagnosis, action planning, intervention, and evaluation are the core steps for affecting change. These steps (described in the following paragraphs) are analogous to the model for action research first developed by Lewin (Argyris, Putnam, and Smith, 1985).

Implementation theory step 1: diagnosis. Diagnosis can be equated with Lewin's unfreezing stage. Diagnosis aids an organization in identifying problems or gaps that may impede its functioning. The diagnosis is often conducted by an outside consultant who helps the organization identify its most salient problems. The most traditional diagnostic technique is a formal survey of organizational members (Sommer, 1987). A more recent technique examines cultural gaps between management and work groups in order to reduce such gaps (Kilmann, 1986). Variables commonly studied include environmental factors; the organization's mission, goals, policies, procedures, structures, technologies, and physical setting; social and interpersonal factors; desired outcomes (Porras and Robertson, 1987); and readiness to take action (Weisbord, 1988).

Implementation theory step 2: action planning. Diagnosis is often followed by action planning or the development of strategies or interventions for addressing the diagnosed problems. Porras and Robertson (1987) describe a two-step process for selecting interventions. In the first step, several possible interventions are identified based on the gaps or problem areas that are diagnosed. In the second step, the number of interventions is narrowed based on three criteria: the organization's readiness to adopt a proposed strategy (for example, sufficiency of resources, time commitment, and administrative support), the availability of *leverage points* (that is, where and how to intervene within the organization), and the skill of the OD practitioner in applying the chosen interventions. The two-step process contains the essential ingredients of action planning: the practitioner and members of the organization assess the feasibility of different strategies for change. By so doing, the practitioner raises the organization's commitment to the chosen course of action.

Implementation theory step 3: OD interventions. The literature is richest in describing OD interventions. Lewin is credited with the development of T-groups, originally used to encourage managers to become more aware of their interpersonal style and impact. Other interventions include management building (Lippitt, 1961), structural redesign, process consultation (Schein, 1969), and group development (Bradford, 1978). In *process consultation,* the consultant helps members of the organization identify problems, questions, and barriers to a desired change, and then works with the organization to address these potential impediments

(Lippitt, Langseth, and Mossop, 1985). The consultant usually does not offer specific solutions but rather facilitates problem solving among members. Face-to-face contact and group interaction are integral to this approach. Process consultation is employed in the two applications described later.

Implementation theory step 4: evaluation. The final step in implementation theory is evaluation, which assesses the planned change effort. Several evaluation techniques measure planned change in organizations. An essential feature of evaluation is that the organization takes stock of its progress in moving to a new state and determines whether additional alterations are needed (Goodman and Wandersman, 1994). Evaluation often allows the changes in an organization to settle, or refreeze.

Future Challenges

Organizational development can benefit from refinements in both theory and practice. First, change process theories require greater development; they are not yet well defined.

Second, although more developed than change process theories, implementation theories of change require further refinement. To illustrate, Weisbord (1988) questions Lewin's premise that frozen organizations can become unfrozen. This question challenges one of the basic concerns of implementation theory: Under which conditions are implementation theories of change applied to best advantage? Today, most organizations dwell in uncertain environments, and implementation theories of change must account for the effects of such variable conditions on the change process (Brown and Covey, 1987).

Third, several scholars question whether OD interventions are truly effective (Cooperrider and Srivastva, 1987). To date, most OD research has been based on case studies, and few studies have tested OD strategies in randomized controlled trials. Additional research that uses experimental designs is necessary to demonstrate the effectiveness of OD interventions.

Finally, most OD interventions are not specific to the stage of development of the organizations at which they are directed. Although the two cases presented in this chapter are quite distinctive, the first being experimental and the second being a multiple case study, they both demonstrate how OD strategies may be tailored to fit an organization's stage of development.

Interorganizational Relations Theory

Interorganizational relations (IOR) is a branch of organizational theory that focuses on how organizations work together. With the increasing complexity of health and social issues, economic and political factors, and other environmental demands like increased competition, organizations began to link their efforts to create more comprehensive and effective responses. Examples of interorganizational linkages range from grassroots coalitions of community organizations formed to combat substance abuse (Davis, 1991) to multihospital systems that reduce competition and provide flexibility in the face of accelerated changes in technology (Zuckerman, Kaluzny, and Ricketts, 1995). Because such interorganizational relationships are hard to form and maintain, they often require facilitation by skilled consultants.

History

Focus on IORs grew out of organizational theory in the 1960s as more attention was devoted to the impact of the environment on organizational behavior. Researchers became interested in how organizations decreased uncertainty in the environment by working together. Early research focused on single organizations and their relationships with other organizations, but over time, the field evolved to focus on networks of organizations and multimember organizations such as coalitions and alliances (Whetten, 1981).

Until recently, research on IORs concentrated on factors that influence an organization's decision to enter into a collaborative relationship and was based largely on an assessment of the benefits versus the costs of the relationship (Gray, 1989). Major benefits of collaboration include access to new information, ideas, materials, and other resources; potential to minimize duplication of services and to use existing resources more efficiently; potential to maximize power and influence by combining forces; ability to address issues beyond a single organization's domain; and shared responsibility across organizations for complex or controversial issues (Alter and Hage, 1993; Butterfoss, Goodman, and Wandersman, 1993).

Potential costs associated with an organization's participation in collaborative relationships include diversion of an organization's resources to the IOR; dilution of an organization's position or focus on issues that are central to its mission; incompatibility with a policy or position taken by the IOR; and delays in taking action due to the often slow and cumbersome process of reaching consensus by which IORs frequently operate (Alter and Hage, 1993). Other factors that are important in forming IORs include recognition of interdependence and the need for coordination; acknowledgment that an organizational goal is more likely to be attained through collaboration; clear and mutually shared goals; similar organizational interests and values; a positive attitude toward cooperation and norms for collaboration; successful previous experience in working together; resources such as time, staff, and expertise for maintaining a coordinated process; awareness of potential partners and geographical proximity; and mandates from a powerful outside force such as a funding agency or regulating body (Gray, 1989; D'Aunno and Zuckerman, 1987; Alter and Hage, 1993).

Development of IORs as Informed by Stage Theory. Recently, researchers have shifted their focus from factors contributing to the formation of IORs to their continued development and maintenance. Stage theory has been used to explain the ongoing development of these collaborative relationships. For example, Gray (1989) outlines three stages of the collaborative process: *problem setting* for developing a common definition of the problem, identification of stakeholders, and a commitment to collaborate; *direction setting* for setting the agenda, exploring options, establishing ground rules, organizing subgroups, and reaching agreement; and *implementation* for building external support, establishing structures to sustain collective activities, and monitoring the agreement.

Alter and Hage (1993) propose a three-stage model of network development as a continuum from informal to formal linkages. The three stages are *exchange or obligational networks,* composed of loosely linked organizations devoted to resource exchange with few joint activities and maintained by individuals who coordinate and integrate tasks across organizations; *action or promotional networks* of organizations that share and pool resources to accomplish concerted action but whose interorganizational activities tend to be peripheral to member organizations' goals; and *systemic networks* of organizations that have long-term formal links to abet the joint production of goods or services.

Florin, Mitchell, and Stevenson (1993) articulate a model for the development of community coalitions based on the stages of initiating mobilization, establishing organizational structure, building capacity for action, planning for action, implementing activities, and refining and institutionalizing the activities and the coalition itself. They note that diagnosing a coalition's current stage of development is important in determining the appropriate type of training and technical assistance to provide at any given time.

Evolution of IORs as Informed by Organizational Development Theory. The work by Florin, Mitchell, and Stevenson (1993) suggests that the organizational development concepts discussed earlier apply to interorganizational development. As previously mentioned, organizational development largely focuses on enhancing structure and processes. The formation of IOR structure and processes is based on contingency theory of organizations, which postulates that organizational design reflects the degree of complexity of the environment in which the organization operates (Shortell and Kaluzny, 1988). Alter and Hage (1993) apply the principles of contingency theory to interorganizational designs. They have developed a model for understanding the structure and operational processes of

IORs as contingent on selected characteristics of the environment and the nature of the work to be undertaken. The structure and operational processes, in turn, influence the level of conflict between the participating organizations and the perceived effectiveness of the network in producing desired outcomes. For instance, Alter and Hage assert that the degree of external control, an environmental factor, influences the structure of the IOR. To illustrate, if an interorganizational network is dependent on a single funding source, Alter and Hage postulate that the resulting structure will tend to be highly centralized, that is, dominated by a single organization or small group of organizations, because centralized structures enhance the funding agency's ability to regulate work objectives and to control costs.

Another illustration of IOR structure as contingent on the environment is the way it changes depending on whether the IOR's actual work is voluntary or mandated. According to the Alter and Hage model, IORs that engage in mandated work will be high in centrality to ensure accountability. Alter and Hage postulate that the higher the level of external control, the greater the amount of disharmony and conflict in the IOR network and the lower the perceived effectiveness of the network. Where funding comes from multiple sources and the work is voluntary, the resulting networks are more likely to use group or interagency committees for coordination. Such group methods of coordination occur when networks are less regulated and when the IOR has more choice in selecting the nature of the work that it performs. In some cases, the funder may desire and promote increased coordination through group methods, an organizational development strategy. Additionally, the infusion of new resources from multiple sources may facilitate a more intensive coordinating process that results in less conflict and greater perceived effectiveness.

According to the Alter and Hage model, IOR structure and processes are influenced not only by patterns of funding and external mandates, but also by the level of demand or *task volume* of the service that the IOR provides. When task volume is high, the Alter and Hage model predicts that the size of the network will be larger, the IOR structure will be more complex, and the degree to which member organizations connect will be low in order to control workflow. In contrast, when task volume is low, group methods of coordination rather than strict adherence to rules and protocols become the norm. Moreover, Alter and Hage predict that the level of conflict will be lower where group methods of coordination predominate. Because environmental factors like task volume, external mandates, and funding patterns influence the structure and processes of IORs, organizational development techniques applied at the appropriate stage of IOR development can help ensure that the IOR produces functional structures and processes with minimal conflict and maximum perceived effectiveness.

Future Challenges

Interorganizational relations theory has the potential to provide valuable insights into the effective use of interorganizational arrangements like multi-agency networks and community coalitions, thus improving practitioners' facilitation of operation. The field, however, is relatively new and several challenges remain.

First, a taxonomy of IORs is needed. Many types of IORs exist, and throughout their evolution they are likely to be influenced by different factors. For example, a network formed to serve as an integrated service delivery system is quite different from a coalition formed to support passage of a local smoking control ordinance. These differences have implications for IOR structure, process, and outcomes. Second, greater understanding of the stages through which IORs develop is desirable. For instance, existing models have little consistency in the number of stages: Florin, Mitchell, and Stevenson (1993) propose seven stages, Butterfoss, Goodman, and Wandersman (1993) propose four, and Alter and Hage (1993) propose three. Third, more research is needed on the factors that influence IOR functioning at each stage. The Alter and Hage model (1993) is one of the first to explain how external control and technology influence structure, operational processes, and outcomes. But empirical support for the model is limited. A final remaining challenge for IOR theory is the selection and definition of IOR outcomes. Alter and Hage (1993) discuss four approaches to measuring IOR effectiveness including the extent to which goals are met, needed resources are acquired, smooth internal functioning is exhibited, and all constituents are minimally satisfied.

Table 14.1 summarizes the organizational change concepts discussed in this chapter.

Applications of Organizational Change Theories

The following sections illustrate how organizational change theories have been applied by researchers and practitioners to understand and influence health promotion efforts in school and community settings. The first example describes a program of research to integrate tobacco use prevention into public schools. The second is an analysis of interorganizational relationships in a multisectoral project to reduce tobacco use statewide.

Application: Integrating Tobacco Use Prevention into School Systems

Each year, cigarette smoking is responsible for over 390,000 deaths and is reported to be the leading preventable cause of death and disability in the United States

TABLE 14.1. SUMMARY OF ORGANIZATIONAL CHANGE CONCEPTS.

Concept	Definition	Application
Stages	Steps that organizations pass through as they change.	Help organizations move through all the stages; do not stop at adoption.
Problem definition[a] (awareness stage)	Problems recognized and analyzed; solutions sought and evaluated.	Involve management and other personnel in awareness-raising activities.
Initiation of action[a] (adoption stage)	Policy or directive formulated; resources for beginning change allocated.	Provide process consultation to inform decision makers and implementers of what adoption involves.
Implementation of change[a]	Innovation is implemented, reactions occur, and role changes occur.	Provide training, technical assistance, and problem-solving aid.
Institutionalization of change[a]	Policy or program becomes entrenched in the organization; new goals and values are internalized.	Identify high-level champion, work to overcome obstacles to institutionalization, and create structures for integration.
Organizational development	An approach that tries to improve the quality of work life.	Identify aspects of work life (through organizational diagnosis) that positively and negatively affect workers.
Action research	Four steps for improving organizations: diagnosis, action planning, intervention, and evaluation; also known as procedure theory.	Based on organizational diagnosis, develop and implement a plan for change.
Organizational development interventions	Specific techniques, such as T-groups, used to help improve organizations.	Use techniques such as surveys, cultural inventories, T-groups, and process consultation.
Interorganizational relations	How organizations collaborate to solve problems of mutual interest.	Determine which organizations in a community are concerned about a given health problem.
Stages of interorganizational collaboration	Steps that organizations go through as they attempt to collaborate.	Develop strategies (for example, process evaluation of coalition effectiveness) to help collaborating organizations overcome barriers at each stage.

[a]Glanz and Rimer, 1995.

(U.S. Public Health Service, 1989). Health curricula with effective smoking pre-vention components can help prevent up to 60 percent of adolescents from smok-ing (Perry, Murray, and Klepp, 1987). Yet the rate of tobacco use among adolescents generally has remained constant over the past decade (Johnston, O'Malley, and Bachman, 1991). Due primarily to a failure of dissemination and effective imple-mentation, effective school health curricula reach only a small portion of adoles-cents in the United States (Parcel, Perry, and Taylor, 1990).

In 1987, the National Cancer Institute funded a large-scale project to test the effectiveness of strategies for disseminating health curricula (NCI Grant no. RO1 CA45997). The five-year study, the North Carolina School Health and Tobacco Education Project, was designed to assess and influence schools' curriculum awareness, adoption, implementation, and institutionalization. Of the 140 school districts in North Carolina, 28 were randomly selected and subsequently contacted about participating in the study. After 22 districts agreed to participate, they were randomly assigned to either an experimental or control condition (Goodman, Smith, Dawson, and Steckler, 1991). The treatment group received intensive in-tervention strategies and the control districts received just enough attention to re-tain them in the study. In order to give schools a program choice, three curricula were used.

Four-Stage Model. Stage theory informed the interventions for disseminating the health curricula to schools. Different intervention strategies were employed at each of four stages: awareness, adoption, implementation, and institutionalization. Furthermore, organizational development theory was the basis for the strategies used during the adoption, implementation, and institutionalization stages.

Awareness stage. Because senior-level administrators are most influential in de-cisions to adopt new programs (Huberman and Miles, 1984), the project directed its initial strategies at increasing administrator awareness and concern for tobacco use prevention. Two intervention strategies were employed. The first was incor-porated into an annual weeklong conference to which school districts sent teams of administrators and teachers. At this conference, awareness and adoption of the eight components of comprehensive school health were emphasized (Girven and Cottrell, 1987). The second awareness strategy was a site visit by members of the research team with senior administrators of the school districts that were asked to participate in the project (Goodman, Smith, Dawson, and Steckler, 1991).

Both awareness interventions were evaluated. The evaluation of the statewide conference included pre- and posttest measures of administrator and teacher awareness and concern for tobacco use prevention among adolescents (Smith and others, 1991; Steckler and others, 1992). The statewide conference was successful in increasing teachers' and administrators' awareness and concern about comprehensive school health. Evaluation of the individual site visits indicated that administrators' awareness of and concern over tobacco use prevention increased when the research team identified a local intermediary who could help establish legitimacy for the research project and when the investigators were able to arrange for more than one meeting with the district administrators in order to continue discussions about the project (Goodman, Smith, Dawson, and Steckler, 1991).

Adoption stage. Once a school district's administrators agreed to participate, the research team offered each school district a choice of one of three curricula; both experimental and control districts were given this choice. Additionally, the experimental districts were exposed to the organizational development technique of process consultation, in which an outside agent works with organizational personnel to identify problems, questions, and barriers and then helps them resolve the identified concerns by facilitating desired changes (Schein, 1969). For experimental districts, the process consultation consisted of a three-hour workshop with district personnel, at least one follow-up meeting, and telephone contacts. In contrast, the researchers mailed written material about the three curricula to the control districts, instructing them to write to the project indicating which curriculum they wanted to adopt.

The adoption stage was evaluated in several ways. Whether a school district actually adopted one of the study curricula was signified by a letter of agreement between the district and the project indicating which of the three curricula had been selected, when it would be taught, and which teachers would teach it. The time of adoption was signified by the number of weeks that elapsed between the process consultation or receipt of written materials and the signing of the letter of agreement. Case studies of the adoption process were conducted in a sample of experimental and control districts. The average length of time of adoption was fifteen weeks with no significant difference between experimental and control districts in time or in the number of districts that adopted. The decision to adopt was influenced by the degree to which a teacher or health supervisor championed the curriculum and by the active support of the champion by a central office administrator (Goodman, Tenney, Smith, and Steckler, 1992).

Implementation stage. The main implementation intervention was intensive training for teachers in using the adopted curriculum. Three-part training was employed: a pretraining consultation meeting with experimental districts to plan for the upcoming teacher training; a training workshop conducted by nationally recognized specialists in each of the three study curricula and lasting from two to four days, depending on the curriculum adopted; and a posttraining consultation with teachers and administrators about one month after the workshop, intended to boost skills and help each district plan for curriculum implementation (Smith,

McCormick, Steckler, and McLeroy, 1993). The control districts received the adopted curriculum in the mail, but no training was conducted.

Evaluation results indicated that more experimental than control district teachers taught the adopted curricula and that they taught more lessons than control district teachers. The study also found that school districts with an active health coordinator and a supportive administrator had greater implementation of the curricula (Smith, McCormick, Steckler, and McLeroy, 1993). Moreover, larger school districts were more likely to implement one of the three study curricula than were smaller districts. The researchers surmised that larger districts had more resources available to support implementation activities (McCormick, Steckler, and McLeroy, 1995).

Institutionalization stage. After a school district had taught one of the study curricula for one school year, the researchers employed a process consultation for institutionalization that consisted of the dissemination of a guidebook to program champions (for instance, school health coordinators) on how to institutionalize curricula; consultative meetings with these champions; and a two-hour meeting with superintendents, assistant superintendents, middle school coordinators, health coordinators, principals, teachers who had taught the curriculum, and teachers who might teach it in the future. The main purpose of this meeting was to assess experiences with the adopted curriculum and to determine necessary steps to maintain and increase its use in the future.

The study produced no difference in institutionalization between experimental and control districts. In both conditions, institutionalization was moderate to low due to a number of factors. The process consultation for institutionalization was a weak intervention. There was "turbulence" in the school environment: for example, teacher and administrator turnover, change in school format from junior high to middle schools, and inadequate overall funding. Finally, there was a lack of strong leadership for health among school administrators, the combining of health instruction with physical education or science, inadequate K–12 planning for health instruction or comprehensive school health, and lack of training for teachers beyond that provided by the research project (Smith, Steckler, McCormick, and McLeroy, 1995).

Organizational Change Theories. *Project strengths.* By using an experimental design, the health curriculum dissemination project randomized intervention and control school districts. Thus, the effectiveness of the strategies was compared across two similar groups of which only one received an intervention, and the bias that often influences retrospective explanations for a program's outcomes was reduced.

Perhaps the project's most important contribution is that stage and OD theories were intertwined, and the related strategies were directed at multiple organizational levels. The application of process consultation illustrates how OD techniques can be applied to specific stages of organizational change. At the adoption stage, the project had to overcome three major impediments: the project was sponsored by outsiders who were trying to influence schools to adopt one of three new health curricula; school personnel had limited knowledge about the curricula being offered and the requirements for instruction; and tobacco use prevention was not a priority in schools.

At the implementation stage, process consultation was combined with training to help prepare teachers for using the curriculum that their district had adopted. The combination of process consultation and traditional training proved effective in leading to greater implementation among experimental school districts. At the institutionalization stage, process consultation focused on the political skills of individuals such as school health coordinators who championed the program. Skill development centered on building coalitions of program advocates, to entrench the program within the school system.

In addition to contouring OD techniques to fit specific stages, the curriculum dissemination study intervened at different organizational levels. For instance, the on-site visits were directed exclusively at district-level administrators and were focused on increasing their awareness of tobacco use prevention among youths and their concern for addressing the problem in their school district. The process consultation for adoption included administrators and teachers; the administrators were from both the district and building levels. The training and consultation for implementation were primarily at the teacher level. At the institutionalization stage, the focus was once again on administrators.

Project weaknesses. Despite the curriculum dissemination project's strengths in conceptualization and design, it also illustrates areas in which the application of theory can be improved. For instance, in both the on-site awareness visits and the process consultation for adoption, the research team had a preplanned agenda, for example, getting schools to recognize the need for tobacco use prevention curricula, getting them to participate in the project, and getting them to adopt one of the three study curricula. The traditional approach to OD is less directed in that the consultant is more generally interested in identifying gaps between actual and desired practice. At the awareness stage in particular, process consultation strategies could have been used more effectively than they were to help each school assess its own needs.

At the institutionalization stage, focusing on the political and organizational skills of the program champion and holding a one-meeting process consultation for adoption proved to be a weak intervention. Institutionalization is a process that occurs over a number of organizational cycles (school years in this case). To be effective, institutionalization interventions need to be multifaceted and to occur over several cycles.

In actuality, the curriculum dissemination study did not adhere to the action research model. Action research extends from procedure theory (Figure 14.1) and therefore outlines the steps along which change occurs. Stage theory, as applied in this project, functioned as a strategy theory. That is, it provided broad parameters for influencing change at each stage even though not in itself identifying specific activities. Process consultation at the adoption and institutionalization stages is an application of technique theory. The study, therefore, was missing the middle layer, procedure theory, which should be sandwiched between strategy and techniques. Had the action research model been more closely followed, the research team would have included a more detailed diagnosis of each school system, followed by action planning, an intervention such as process consultation, and finally, an evaluation of the change effort.

Application: Interorganizational Relationships in Project ASSIST

The American Stop Smoking Intervention Study, Project ASSIST, is a seven-year project funded by the National Cancer Institute in partnership with the American Cancer Society (Shopland, 1993). The goals of Project ASSIST are to accelerate the decline in overall smoking prevalence and to reduce tobacco use among adolescents (Malek and Enright, 1995). The project relies heavily on partnerships among organizations at different levels of government and across other organizations in local communities. In North Carolina, one of seventeen participating states, Project ASSIST operates through a statewide coalition and ten local-community coalitions. In a multiple case study of these ten local North Carolina Project ASSIST coalitions, Kegler (1995) describes the evolution of the coalitions from their formation through the first year of implementation. Using the stages of coalition development (Florin, Mitchell, and Stevenson, 1993), this study illustrates key tasks associated with each stage and the application of concepts from organizational development and interorganizational relations theory.

Stage 1: initiating mobilization. According to Florin, Mitchell, and Stevenson (1993), the tasks associated with the initial mobilization stage include actively engaging participants and key community sectors. The local North Carolina ASSIST coalitions were successful in recruiting organizations and individuals. Average coalition size was twenty-seven active members and forty-three total members. Many of the coalitions had a difficult time creating a diverse and representative membership, however. Of the members representing organizations, 51 percent represented a health organization, 19 percent represented the education sector, and 13 percent represented the voluntary sector. The other community sectors (criminal justice, communication, economic, political, recreational, religious, social welfare, and community groups) accounted for less than 10 percent of the members. In addition, the members tended to be white (88 percent), female (72 percent), and well-educated (88 percent college graduates). The North Carolina Project ASSIST coalitions are not unique in this respect (Florin, Mitchell, and Stevenson, 1993; Rogers and others, 1993).

Lack of diversity of membership actually may facilitate mobilization. IOR theory suggests that collaboration among organizations is more likely when there are mutually shared goals, similar organizational interests, norms for collaboration, successful previous experience in working together, and awareness of potential partners (Gray, 1989; D'Aunno and Zuckerman, 1987). Early in coalition formation, health professionals from several organizations formed the core of each coalition. Core participants usually knew each other prior to Project ASSIST and had worked together on numerous other projects. Additionally, their organizations were interested in similar issues and had mutually shared goals.

For some other organizations, the costs of participation were too high. For instance, several chose not to join a coalition because they did not want to jeopardize financial or political support from tobacco interests. In a survey of the coalition membership, 16 percent of those representing organizations listed problems that could best be categorized as political. Yet only a small percentage of the active members (8 percent) felt that the costs of membership were higher than the benefits for their organization. When asked to name the benefits of membership for their organization, members mentioned the opportunity to build new relationships (15 percent) and access to new information, ideas, and materials (12 percent). Other benefits included increased coordination, visibility for the organization, resources to support smoke-free policies, a vehicle for meaningful community involvement, and help in meeting organizational goals (Kegler, 1995).

Stage 2: establishing organizational structure and functioning. This stage focuses on establishing a structure for task forces and addressing issues related to effective group functioning. In ASSIST, the typical coalition structure consisted of an advisory board, a coordinating committee, and several action teams that corresponded to the Project ASSIST channels of worksites, community groups, community environment, schools, and health care. The majority of the coalitions developed bylaws, which had several important uses, most notably preventing members from expecting coalition staff to take formal leadership positions. Many of the bylaws also specified that organizational members must replace themselves when they leave the coalition, and many barred individuals and organizations with conflicts of interest from membership. Mechanisms for communication, decision making, and leadership development were also addressed.

Stage 3: building capacity for action. One of the tasks associated with this stage is the establishment of interorganizational linkages among community sectors. By bringing organizations from multiple community sectors together to form Project ASSIST coalitions, organizations that had never worked together in the past were able to form new relationships. A survey of the coalition members found that for 66 percent of them, linkages with other organizations had increased due to coalition participation (Kegler, 1995).

A second dimension of building capacity for action is the orientation of coalition members. Florin, Mitchell, and Stevenson (1993) recommend the creation of an *enabling system,* an intermediary organization that supports multiple community coalitions. The components of the system include training, consultation, information and referral, recognition of achievement, and creation of linkages among coalitions. The staff from the state-level Project ASSIST office functioned as an enabling system for this project. They played a major role in orienting both local health department staff and coalition members to tobacco control issues and strategies. They helped organize a statewide conference that highlighted successful interventions, structured the statewide coalition meetings to include a training component and time for networking, and organized retreats for local coalition staff and members. In addition, the state staff served as process consultants thus employing an organizational development strategy. A state consultant was assigned to work with each local coalition, attending meetings, meeting with coalition leadership and staff, and identifying problems and recommending solutions. The consultants also facilitated regional meetings for staff working with coalitions at the local level.

Stage 4: planning for action. This stage involves assessing needs, articulating goals and objectives, and selecting intervention strategies. The assessment in Project ASSIST consisted of a site analysis relying heavily on key informant interviews. These interviews, conducted by coalition members and staff, served several purposes: to actively involve the coalition members, to establish new linkages among organizations, and to obtain information for developing annual action plans. The coalitions differed in level of member involvement. Two of the ten had functioning task forces at the time of plan development, and these task forces generated intervention ideas and wrote their own action plans. Four of the coalitions had only minimal member input into the action plan. In these coalitions, the staff wrote the plan to meet the deadline imposed by the state health department and the National Cancer Institute.

The Alter and Hage (1993) model predicts that IORs that engage in mandated work, such as the production of an annual action plan, will be high in centrality to ensure accountability. Because Project ASSIST operates through contracts (the National Cancer Institute contracts with state health departments and the state health departments contract with local health departments) some of the work is mandated and "deliverables" and deadlines occasionally interfere with the natural evolution of the coalitions. This was evident in development of the action plans. In some coalitions, staff were forced to sacrifice member involvement in developing the plans in order to meet deadlines, thus giving the impression that local health departments were dominating the coalitions. As stated previously, the Alter and Hage model predicts that networks dominated by a single organization or a small group of organizations will have higher levels of conflict and lower levels of perceived effectiveness. An obvious solution is for funders to relax deadlines to accommodate differences in the pace of coalition development. Another solution is to train staff in techniques for balancing the pressures of deadlines with the sometimes slow and cumbersome process of coalition decision making.

Stage 5: implementing activities. This stage includes the involvement of key organizations and community members in the implementation of the action plans. The local Project ASSIST coalitions implemented a variety of activities including arranging youth buying operations and merchant education campaigns (Cohen, Stanley, Martin, and Goldstein, 1995), supporting public and private smoking-control policies (Bearman, Goldstein, and Bryan, 1995), training health care providers in smoking cessation (Malek and Enright, 1995), developing and disseminating smoking cessation resource guides, and conducting communitywide "quit to win" campaigns.

The coalitions relied heavily on interorganizational relationships in implementing many of these activities. One of the more interesting examples of the importance of partnerships was the youth buying operation, which sent youths to purchase cigarettes from vending machines and merchants to assess the extent of illegal tobacco sales to minors. The health department in one community was reluctant to be a visible partner in the project, fearing a political backlash if it supported a smoking-control ordinance. The coalition was still able to conduct the youth buying operation by recruiting a youth council to take on the project. That council rather than the coalition or health department became the focus of media attention.

Relationships formed through the coalitions also were critical in passing local smoking-control ordinances before a deadline imposed by a preemptive state-level "smokers rights" law. Health departments were limited to providing health statistics and information on environmental tobacco smoke, but coalition organizations were free to lobby and contact public officials about smoking-control ordinances. The partnerships between health departments and organizations represented in the coalitions contributed to the passage of eighty-nine city and county smoking-control regulations (Bearman, Goldstein, and Bryan, 1995).

Stages 6 and 7: refining and institutionalizing. These stages involve using evaluation data to refine programs, identify gaps for additional programming, and ultimately, integrate programs into organizational missions (Florin, Mitchell, and Stevenson, 1993). Although it is too early to know how these stages will progress in Project ASSIST, it is clear that success will depend on the coalitions' ability to sustain effective relationships among their member organizations.

Conclusion

Organizational change is important to health promotion researchers and practitioners for several reasons: (1) often new health promotion programs are created and implemented within organizations, for example, a worksite might create a new physical fitness program for employees; (2) frequently organizations adopt and implement new health promotion policies, for example, a hospital or school might adopt a policy banning smoking in its facilities; (3) usually, health promotion practitioners work within organizations that must change and adapt if the practitioner is to successfully create and implement new programs, services, and policies; and (4) increasingly, health promotion organizations collaborate with other organizations in the community in order to reach goals no single organization can accomplish alone. In all of these instances, the practitioner who understands principles of organizational change and who has tools and skills for analyzing and facilitating such change likely will be more successful than his or her counterpart who does not possess such knowledge.

Organizational change theories like those presented in this chapter, however, have not often been applied (or if applied have not been reported) as foundations for health promotion or public health programs (see Chapter Two). We can only speculate why this might be so. Perhaps it is because individual change theories and strategies are better developed than organizational theories. Health education and health promotion are dominated by and heavily reliant on well-developed social-psychological theories of individual change. Perhaps it is because health promotion researchers and practitioners want to believe in free will—that individuals are masters of their fate and will adopt health-promoting behaviors if they have the right knowledge, values, skills, beliefs, help, and support. Perhaps it is because considering organizational factors introduces a whole new level of complexity in the needs assessment, program planning, implementation, and evaluation process, a level that researchers and practitioners are unwilling to consider due to the time and cost that would be involved. Perhaps it is due to the lack of attention to organizational change in the graduate programs where researchers and practitioners are trained. Curricula tend to be very full, and it is uncommon to find courses or even sections of courses devoted to careful examination of the role that organizations play in health promotion.

This chapter has indicated the importance of organizational change to health promotion researchers and practitioners and offered some concepts and tools for successfully guiding organizational change. Three theories of organizational change were analyzed: stage theory, organizational development theory, and interorganizational relationship theory. The theories were applied to two distinct cases. The first application, a randomized experimental study, illustrated how OD techniques may be used to intervene at different stages of an innovation's development. The second application, a case study, illustrated how attention to stages can inform and describe the development of complex interorganizational arrangements like the ASSIST coalitions. In the first case, organizational change was influenced by university researchers, individuals employed outside of the innovating organization. In the second case, change was influenced by staff from the state health department as representatives of the lead agency in organizing the ASSIST coalitions. Taken together, these applications illustrate that health promotion specialists can stimulate organizational change from either inside or outside a targeted organization.

Whether directing change strategies from within or outside an organization, health practitioners are presented with unique challenges. As in the first application, schools may not view health promotion as a priority issue. As in the second application, governmental and community organizations may not see the relevance of interorganizational alliances for health promotion. Organizational change theories suggest strategies to mediate such challenges. The theories discussed in this chapter, when applied effectively, can influence change.

References

Alter, C., and Hage, J. *Organizations Working Together.* Thousand Oaks, Calif.: Sage, 1993.

Argyris, C. *Personality and Organization.* New York: McGraw-Hill, 1957.

Argyris, C., Putnam, R., and Smith, D. M. *Action Science: Concepts, Methods, and Skills for Research and Intervention.* San Francisco: Jossey-Bass, 1985.

Bearman, N., Goldstein, A., and Bryan, D. "Legislating Clean Air: Politics, Preemption, and the Health of the Public." *North Carolina Medical Journal,* 1995, *56*(1), 14–19.

Beyer, J. M., and Trice, H. M. *Implementing Change: Alcoholism Policies in Work Organizations.* New York: Free Press, 1978.

Bradford, L. P. (ed.). *Group Development.* (2nd ed.) La Jolla, Calif.: University Associates, 1978.

Brown, L. D., and Covey, J. G. "Development Organizations and Organization Development: Toward an Expanded Paradigm for Organization Development." In R. W. Woodman and W. A. Pasmore (eds.), *Research in Organizational Change and Development.* Vol. 1. Greenwich, Conn.: JAI Press, 1987.

Butterfoss, F. D., Goodman, R., and Wandersman, A. "Community Coalitions for Prevention and Health Promotion." *Health Education Research: Theory and Practice,* 1993, *8* (3), 315–330.

Cohen, J., Stanley, L., Martin, J., and Goldstein, A. "Illegal Sales of Cigarettes to Minors in North Carolina." *North Carolina Medical Journal,* 1995, *56*(1), 59–63.

Cooperrider, D. L., and Srivastva, S. "Appreciative Inquiry in Organizational Life." In R. W. Woodman and W. A. Pasmore (eds.), *Research in Organizational Change and Development.* Vol. 1. Greenwich, Conn.: JAI Press, 1987.

D'Aunno, T., and Zuckerman, H. "A Life-Cycle Model of Organizational Federations: The Case of Hospitals." *Academy of Management Review,* 1987, *12*(3), 534–545.

Davis, D. J. "A Systems Approach to the Prevention of Alcohol and Other Drug Problems." *Family Resource Coalition,* 1991, *10,* 3.

Florin, P., Mitchell, R., and Stevenson, J. "Identifying Technical Assistance Needs in Community Coalitions: A Developmental Approach." *Health Education Research,* 1993, *8,* 417–432.

Girven, J. T., and Cottrell, R. "The Impact of the Seaside Health Education Conference on Middle School Health Programs in Oregon." *Health Education,* 1987, *18*(5), 78–82.

Glanz, K., and Rimer, B. K. *Theory at a Glance: A Guide for Health Promotion Practice.* NIH publication no. 95–3896. Bethesda, Md.: National Institutes of Health, National Cancer Institute, 1995.

Goodman, R. M., Smith, D. W., Dawson, L., and Steckler, A. "Recruiting School Districts into a Dissemination Study." *Health Education Research: Theory and Practice,* 1991, *6,* 373–385.

Goodman, R. M., and Steckler, A. "A Framework for Assessing Program Institutionalization." *Knowledge in Society: The International Journal of Knowledge Transfer,* 1989, *2*(1), 52–66.

Goodman, R. M., Tenney, M., Smith, D. W., and Steckler, A. "The Adoption Process for Health Curriculum Innovations in Schools: A Case Study." *Journal of Health Education,* 1992, *23*(4), 215–220.

Goodman, R. M., and Wandersman, A. "FORECAST: A Formative Approach to Evaluating the CSAP Community Partnerships." *Journal of Community Psychology,* 1994 (CSAP special issue), 6–25.

Gray, B. *Collaborating: Finding Common Ground For Multiparty Problems.* San Francisco: Jossey-Bass, 1989.

Harrison, M. I. *Diagnosing Organizations: Methods, Models, and Processes..* Thousand Oaks, Calif.: Sage, 1987.

Huberman, A. M., and Miles, M. B. *Innovation Up Close: How School Improvement Works.* New York: Plenum, 1984.

Johnston, L., O'Malley, P. M., and Bachman, J. G. *Drug Use Among American High School Seniors, College Students and Young Adults: 1975–1990.* Washington, D.C.: U.S. Department of Health and Human Services, National Institute for Drug Abuse, 1991.

Kaluzny, A. D., and Hernandez, S. R. "Organization Change and Innovation." In S. M. Shortell and A. D. Kaluzny (eds.), *Health Care Management: A Text in Organization Theory and Behavior.* (2nd ed.) New York: Wiley, 1988.

Kegler, M. "Community Coalitions for Tobacco Control: Factors Influencing Implementation." Unpublished doctoral dissertation, University of North Carolina at Chapel Hill, 1995.

Kilmann, R. H. "Five Steps for Closing Culture-Gaps." In R. H. Kilmann, M. J. Saxton, R. Serpa, and Associates (eds.), *Gaining Control of the Corporate Culture.* San Francisco: Jossey-Bass, 1986.

Lewin, K. "Field Theory and Learning." In K. Lewin, *Field Theory in Social Science: Select Theoretical Papers* (D. Cartwright, ed.). New York: HarperCollins, 1951. (Originally published 1942.)

Likert, R. A. *New Patterns of Management.* New York: McGraw-Hill, 1961.

Lippitt, G. L. (ed.). *Leadership in Action.* Fairfax, Va.: National Training Laboratories, 1961.

Lippitt, G. L., Langseth, P., and Mossop, J. *Implementing Organizational Change: A Practical Guide to Managing Change Efforts.* San Francisco: Jossey-Bass, 1985.

MacGregor, D. *The Human Side of Enterprise.* New York: McGraw-Hill, 1960.

Malek, S., and Enright, T. "North Carolina Project ASSIST: A Call to Action." *North Carolina Medical Journal,* 1995, *56*(1), 56–58.

Margulis, N., and Adams, J. "Introduction to Organizational Development." In N. Margulis and J. Adams (eds.), *Organizational Development in Health Care Organizations.* Reading, Mass.: Addison-Wesley, 1982.

McCormick, L. K., Steckler, A., and McLeroy, K. R. "Diffusion of Innovations in Schools: A Study of Adoption and Implementation of School-Based Tobacco Prevention Curricula." *American Journal of Health Promotion,* 1995, *9*(3), 210–219.

McLeroy, K. R., Bibeau, D., Steckler, A., and Glanz, K. "An Ecological Perspective on Health Promotion Programs." *Health Education Quarterly,* 1988, *15*, 351–377.

Parcel, G. S., Perry, C. L., and Taylor, W. C. "Beyond Demonstration: Diffusion of Health Promotion Innovations." In N. Bracht (ed.), *Health Promotion at the Community Level.* Thousand Oaks, Calif.: Sage, 1990.

Perry, C. L., Murray, D. M., and Klepp, K. I. "Predictors of Adolescent Smoking and Implications for Prevention." *Morbidity and Mortality Weekly Report,* 1987, *36*(45), 41–45.

Porras, J. I., and Robertson, P. J. "Organization Development Theory: A Typology and Evaluation." In R. W. Woodman and W. A. Pasmore (eds.), *Research in Organizational Change and Development.* Vol 1. Greenwich, Conn.: JAI Press, 1987.

Roethlisberger, F. J., and Dickson, W. J. *Management and the Worker.* Cambridge, Mass.: Harvard University Press, 1939.

Rogers, E. M. *Diffusion of Innovations.* (3rd ed.) New York: Free Press, 1983.

Rogers, T., and others. "Characteristics and Participant Perceptions of Tobacco Control Coalitions in California." *Health Education Research,* 1993, *8*(3), 345–357.

Schein, E. H. *Process Consultation: Its Role in Organization Development.* Reading, Mass.: Addison-Wesley, 1969.

Shopland, D. "Smoking Control in the 1990's: A National Cancer Institute Model for Change." *American Journal of Public Health,* 1993, *83*(9), 1208–1210.

Shortell, S. M. and Kaluzny, A. D. "Organization Theory and Health Care Management." In S. M. Shortell and A. D. Kaluzny (eds.), *Health Care Management; A Text in Organization Theory and Behavior.* (2nd ed.) New York: Wiley, 1988.

Smith, D. W., McCormick, L. K., Steckler, A., and McLeroy, K. R. "Teachers' Use of Health Curricula: Implementation of Growing Healthy, Project SMART, and the Teenage Health Teaching Modules." *Journal of School Health,* 1993, *63*(8), 349–354.

Smith, D. W., Steckler, A., McCormick, L. K., and McLeroy, K. R. "Lessons Learned About Disseminating Health Curricula to Schools." *Journal of Health Education,* 1995, *26*, 37–43.

Smith, D. W., and others. "Promoting Comprehensive School Health Programs Through Summer Health Promotion Conferences." *Journal of School Health,* 1991, *61*(2), 69–74.

Sommer, R. "An Experimental Investigation of the Action Research Approach." *Journal of Applied Behavioral Science,* 1987, *23*(2), 185–199.

Steckler, A., and others. "Measuring the Diffusion of Innovative Health Promotion Programs." *American Journal of Health Promotion*, 1992, *6*(3), 214–224.

U.S. Public Health Service. Office of the Surgeon General. *Reducing the Health Consequences of Smoking: 25 Years of Progress. A Report of the Surgeon General.* DHHS publication no. 89–8411. Washington, D.C.: U.S. Department of Health and Human Services, Public Health Service, Centers for Disease Control, Office of Smoking and Health, 1989.

Weber, M. *The Theory of Social and Economic Organization.* New York: Free Press, 1964.

Weisbord, M. R. "Towards a New Practice Theory of OD: Notes on Snapshooting and Moviemaking." In R. W. Woodman and W. A. Pasmore (eds.), *Research in Organizational Change and Development.* Vol. 2. Greenwich, Conn.: JAI Press, 1988.

Whetten, D. "Interorganizational Relations: A Review of the Field." *Journal of Higher Education,* 1981, *52*(1), 1–28.

Zuckerman, H., Kaluzny, A. D., and Ricketts, T. "Strategic Alliances: A Worldwide Phenomenon Comes to Health Care." In A. D. Kaluzny, H. Zuckerman, and T. Ricketts (eds.), *Partners for the Dance: Forming Strategic Alliances in Health Care,* Ann Arbor, Mich.: Health Administration Press, 1995.

CHAPTER FIFTEEN

COMMUNICATION THEORY AND HEALTH BEHAVIOR CHANGE

The Media Studies Framework

John R. Finnegan, Jr.
K. Viswanath

The word *communication* comes from the Latin "to make common to many" or "to give to another as a partaker" (*Oxford English Dictionary*, 1986). It incorporates at least three complex ideas: (1) the conveying or exchanging of intangible elements such as information, ideas, and meaning; (2) a union or relationship implying mutual revelation, discovery, and effects; and (3) a recognition that these processes occur at all levels of human experience. The word entered common English usage at about the same time that printing technology emerged in fifteenth-century Europe and made possible the growth and diffusion of knowledge on a heretofore unattained scale.

Today, we define human communication as the production and exchange of information and meaning by use of signs and symbols (Gerbner, 1983). It involves processes of encoding, transmission, reception (decoding), and synthesis of information and meaning. As political psychologist Harold D. Lasswell (1948) put it, to study an act of communication is to pose the question: "Who Says What In Which Channel To Whom With What Effect?" Thus, Lasswell identified some key components of communication study: the sender (who encodes and transmits), the content or message (communication substance), the channel (the medium through which content is transmitted), the receiver or audience (who decodes communication to derive meaning), and effect (some measurable outcome of the process).

Due to the centrality of communication in human affairs, its study as an empirical, critical, and applied phenomenon is claimed by many fields, public health included. Public health is influenced particularly by applied communication perspectives. That is, how do communication processes at all levels of human experience contribute to, or detract from, health behavior change? Second, how can communication strategies be used in a planned way to influence health behavior change?

The purpose of this chapter is to describe communication theories especially relevant to public health and health behavior, to review and critique their application in the study of health behavior effects, and finally to provide examples of how communication theory informs health behavior change interventions. For reasons that will become clear shortly, we emphasize communication theory in a media studies context applied to public health.

Organization of Communication Studies

Communication scholar George Gerbner (1983) has described a widely accepted framework for communication studies that includes three main branches. The first is the study of how signs and symbols combine into *codes* to create messages that convey meaning in a variety of social contexts. This branch is frequently described as *semiotics,* the science of symbols, signs and codes. From an applied perspective, this branch of communication studies is often concerned with the construction of *meaning.* How do signs, symbols, and codes combine to construct reality—that is, influence us to think about things in some ways and constrain us from thinking about them in other ways? Language, for example, is a code that may be analyzed by its constituent signs and symbols to understand how meaning is constructed. There are also aural and visual codes that communicate meaning as well (consider, for example, how a slow-motion film sequence enhances meaning, increasing communication of beauty and grace, for example).

Gerbner describes the second branch of communication studies as the study of behavior and interaction through exposure to messages. Here the emphasis is on measuring, explaining, and predicting communication effects on cognitions, beliefs, attitudes, and public opinion. This branch is strongly influenced by the fields of psychology and social psychology.

The third branch is the study of how communication is organized through large-scale social institutions and systems and the history, regulation, and policy-making impact of those institutions and systems.

Within each branch, communication study may be further broken down to examine effects at various levels of human experience on a micro-to-macro continuum. At the level of the individual, for example, we may study how a person processes information about health and converts it into action. At the interpersonal level (dyadic), we may examine how two people interact and influence one another in regard to some health behavior outcome. At the group or organizational level, we may examine how formal or informal communication among many people influences health behavior change including, perhaps, the effective delivery of a health service. Finally, at the level of the community, society, or culture, we may examine how communication contributes to health behavior change within the constraints of social structure.

It is important to recognize that just as there is no single unifying theory that explains and predicts all human behavior, there is also no theory that explains and predicts all communication effects. Theories tend to diverge along the levels of analysis just described and also according to effects relevant to each discipline that studies communication. Some view this as symptomatic of fragmentation in our understanding of communication. Others view it as a healthy theoretical diversity, necessary to an understanding of human activity in many complex dimensions (Finnegan and Viswanath, 1989). In either case, current trends in communication research increasingly seek to connect and to integrate effects across levels of analysis from the micro to the macro (Hawkins, Weimann, and Pingree, 1988).

All three branches and each level of study are important to understanding health behavior change. Public health's applied emphasis means that its approach to human communication is necessarily eclectic. Most chapters in this book illustrate this diversity in their treatments of health behavior change theories. Whether studied in individual, group, or community contexts, most health behavior change theories implicate critical roles and effects of communication. It is not the aim of this chapter to repeat these insights, but to carry the discussion of communication and health behavior change into an area of growing interest in public health: mass communication and its research framework, media studies.

The reasons for this emphasis are several. First, as communication scholars Clarke and Evans (1983) have described, a media studies framework cuts across Gerbner's three branches of communication theory as well as across the micro to macro levels of analysis. It "consists in the study of media by which information and entertainment are delivered in society, the conditions and processes by which this content is shaped, and the effects that content and form exert on individuals . . . groups," communities, societies and cultures. Above all, communication in this context is "distinguished . . . by its social complexity and self-conscious organization and use of technological instruments to extend and preserve symbolic exchange in time and space." These processes can have important effects on public health, in light of the mass media's ubiquity and their role as primary sources of our information about health and most other human activities.

Second, communication effects on health behavior may be studied in this framework from the perspective of day-to-day interactions and also of planned use of mass communication to influence health behavior. Third, the community-based intervention to influence health behavior change has gained currency in public health during the past twenty years. This approach recognizes the need to seek change in health behavior across multiple levels of human experience—from the individual to the community (Rogers and Storey, 1987). Interventions are planned, multistrategy efforts that seek different dimensions of change that will lead to population shifts in health outcomes (see especially Chapters Seventeen and Eighteen for a fuller treatment of this approach). Mass communication has become a key part of this approach whether the object of change is to build the community's agenda for prevention, to change public policy, or to educate individuals about specific health behavior changes. Media institutions play a crucial role in health behavior change because they are key gatekeepers for disseminating information in social systems and because, as socializing agents, they have a powerful impact in legitimizing behavioral norms.

Major Study Areas

There is a widespread popular and academic perception that media are powerful, particularly that they play strong roles in promoting, discouraging, or even inhibiting healthy behaviors. If we are to understand the nature of these roles, we must evaluate how, where, and with whom media interact and with what consequences.

Two areas of research are germane. One deals with message production itself. It asks the question, What are the social and organizational factors in media work that may impinge on the creation of media messages influencing behavioral change? Here, we are interested particularly in message production: the creation of news, information, advertising, and entertainment. In Lasswell's terms (1948), these are the *sender* and *channel* characteristics that form media work and content. The second area of research asks, What are the consequences of media exposure on individuals, groups, institutions, and social systems? This question has been traditionally studied as *media effects*. Here, we are interested in some of the major media effects hypotheses and their relevance to health behavior change.

Media Message Production

Mass media organizations are bureaucracies in which tasks are specialized and routinized to enhance efficiency in creating news, advertising, and entertainment. For example, journalists seek established or official sources routinely to gather information that is used to create "news" (Sigal, 1973, 1987). The criteria for using sources are usually straightforward: sources should be credible, available, and able to supply reliable information. Sources thus essentially subsidize the process of gathering information (Gandy, 1982). Sources may be established spokespersons for governmental agencies, businesses, or other powerful groups and elites in the social system (Hilgartner and Bosk, 1988). Journalists routinize their news-gathering process to insure predictability in an idiosyncratic world. However, reliance on a regular supply of information from established sources means that groups without social power are less likely to gain access to news making and, therefore, have less influence.

News becomes a product of the interaction of sources and media professionals. Sources perform the key role of identifying social problems and bringing them to the attention of the media. Whether representing campaigns, governmental agencies, advocacy groups, or other interests, sources compete for media and therefore also for public attention, seeking to define and to increase the public profile of an issue or problem.

For example, the U.S. Surgeon General's office, a major official source of public health information, regularly releases reports on the status of smoking and its effects on health in the United States. From year to year, the report's emphasis differs, identifying specific aspects of the smoking problem the Public Health Service wishes to bring to the attention of news media and the general public (for example, the increasing prevalence of smoking among young women). Despite their dependency on such official sources, media professionals also enjoy some autonomy in defining a problem, particularly in the ways they construct news stories. The definition of a social problem is crucial to how the public understands it, the actions individuals or communities are likely to take to ameliorate the problem, the attention given the problem by different groups, and the knowledge acquired by them (Viswanath, Finnegan, Hannan, and Luepker, 1991).

Media Effects

The consequences of media dissemination of images, ideas, themes, and stories are commonly discussed under the rubric of media effects (Bryant and Zillman, 1994). At first blush, the term would seem to imply unidirectional study of the effect of media on some outcome (knowledge, opinion, attitude, or behavior, for instance) among individuals, groups, institutions, or communities largely regarded as passive (McLeod, Kosicki, and Pan, 1991). However, media effects research is varied and also looks at effects flowing in the opposite direction—from audiences to media. Moreover, strong traditions in media effects research regard audiences not as passive recipients of impact but as active seekers and users of information (Blumler and Katz, 1974).

Media studies, like other social and behavioral sciences, also vary in the unit of analysis employed, from the individual to community and social systems. Table 15.1 provides an overview of this variety in media studies and effects research. Major theories and concepts are organized by level of analysis. At each level, a few key studies and also the disciplinary origin and relationship to other fields are given.

At the individual level of analysis, media studies emphasize effects on motivations, cognitions, involvement, attitudes, and behaviors as a result of exposure to media messages. A long-standing interest has been the relationship between individuals' knowledge, attitudes, and behaviors. Important theories drawn from psychology and social psychology include hierarchies of effects, persuasion, and social cognitive theories. They have been traditions in media effects research, dominating the field for much of this century.

Specifically, researchers have looked at *learning hierarchies,* in which knowledge change affects attitudes, which in turn affect behavior (K-A-B). Others have noted different hierarchies: *dissonance attribution,* in which behavioral change affects attitude change, which in turn affects knowledge (B-A-K), and the *low-involvement hierarchy,* in which knowledge change affects behavior, which in turn affects attitudes (K-B-A). More recently, researchers have suggested that there are not three distinct hierarchies of effects but a single continuum (Chaffee and Roser, 1986). The order of effects will depend on where individuals or groups are positioned at the start with respect to some outcome.

Early persuasion studies by Hovland and colleagues at Yale (1953) were controlled experiments testing various conditions under which opinion or attitude change would occur in the context of such variables as source credibility, fear, organization of arguments, the role of group membership in resisting or accepting communication, and personality differences. This line of research continues today, with an emphasis on cognitive processing of information leading to persuasion (Perloff, 1993).

Since the 1960s, media effects research has changed its dominant focus from attitude change to the cognitive impact of mediated information (Beniger and Gusek, 1995) and has also emphasized community and social systems levels of analysis. The latter happened partly because of Latin American scholars' interest in developing new approaches to the use of mass communication in guided social change projects in developing countries (Lee, 1980). Units of observation in this macro-level perspective have included populations in diverse community settings, groups, organizations, social institutions, and large-scale social systems including communities and nation-states. This perspective has an obvious connection to public health, in which guided social change and community-based health

TABLE 15.1. SELECTED COMMUNICATION THEORIES AND LEVELS OF ANALYSIS.

Level of Analysis	Theory or Concept	Major Studies and Reviews	Disciplinary Origin
Individual	Hierarchies of effects	Ray and others (1973) McGuire (1984) Chaffee and Roser (1986)	Psychology Social psychology
	Persuasion theories	Hovland, Janis, and Kelley (1953) Roloff and Miller (1980) Petty and Cacioppo (1981) McGuire (1985) Perloff (1993)	Psychology Social psychology
	Social Cognitive Theory	Bandura (1994)	Social psychology
Organization	News gatekeeping	Donohue, Tichenor, and Olien (1975) Shoemaker (1991)	Sociology of organizations
	Reporter-source relations	Sigal (1973, 1987)	Sociology
	Media work routines	Roshco (1975) Tuchman (1978)	Sociology
	Media message systems	Gerbner, Gross, Morgan, and Signorelli (1980) Turow (1992)	Sociology of organizations
Communities and social systems	Diffusion of innovations	Rogers ([1962] 1995)	Sociology Social psychology
	Knowledge gap	Tichenor, Donohue, and Olien (1980) Gaziano (1983) Viswanath and Finnegan (1995)	Sociology Structural functionalism Social conflict
Mass society and culture	Cultivation studies	Gerbner, Gross, Morgan, and Signorelli (1994)	Sociology of mass society
Cross-level analysis	Agenda setting	McCombs and Shaw (1972) Kosicki (1993)	Sociology Psychology Political science
	Definition, framing of social problems	Iyengar and Kinder (1987) Entman (1993) Gamson and Modigliani (1987) Hilgartner and Bosk (1988)	Sociology Psychology
	Risk communication	Weinstein (1984) Sandman (1987) Slovic, Fischoff, and Lichtenstein (1991) Glanz and Yang (1996)	Sociology Psychology

interventions have become ideal settings for testing macro-social applications of communication strategies.

Because of their relevance to public health efforts to guide social and behavioral change, this chapter reviews and critiques in greater detail four of the media effects perspectives listed in Table 15.1: the knowledge gap, agenda setting, cultivation studies, and risk communication.

The Knowledge Gap. Conventional wisdom long held that persistent social problems could be resolved through public education. To paraphrase the film *Field of Dreams,* the assumption was that "if you tell them, they will know." However, studies examining public knowledge on a variety of topics and issues have shown that "they" do not always know. Moreover, knowledge and information turned out not to be equally distributed across populations. Studies have shown that people with more formal education learn and know more about many issues than do people with less formal education (Hyman and Sheatsley, 1947; Mosteller and Moynihan, 1972).

These findings were formally presented as the knowledge gap hypothesis by Minnesota researchers Tichenor, Donohue, and Olien (1970). They proposed that an increasing flow of information into a social system (from a campaign, for example) is more likely to benefit groups of higher socioeconomic status (SES) than those of lower SES. Increasing the information available in the system, then, would only exacerbate already existing differences between these groups. The researchers supported this proposition with studies of several topics including health. The disturbing implications were, of course, that public campaigns would only perpetuate inequities. Because these results called into question the entire basis of guided social change efforts, they attracted the attention of scholars and policy makers.

As a media studies perspective, knowledge gap research arises from a longstanding sociological tradition emphasizing how the structure and organization of communities and societies function as means of social control and conflict management. This tradition has also long viewed the mass media as important institutions of social control and conflict management. This hypothesis has advanced our idea of media effects in at least two important ways. It contradicted conventional wisdom that social interventions are a simple panacea for resolving social problems. It also suggested that media have differential impact on audiences—impact that is importantly mediated by the social structural conditions in which audiences live. The knowledge gap hypothesis was thus one of the first hypotheses in media studies to draw attention to the role of environment in media effects on individuals (Viswanath and Finnegan, 1995).

Fortunately, subsequent studies found that knowledge gaps were not intractable. Researchers discovered a variety of contingent and contributory conditions that could affect knowledge gaps and also present opportunities for applications in public health campaigns (Table 15.2): content domains, channel influence, social conflict and community mobilization, community structure, and individual motivational factors (Donohue, Tichenor, and Olien, 1975; Ettema and Kline, 1977; Gaziano, 1983; Viswanath and Finnegan, 1995).

Content and channel factors. Although studies have found SES-based knowledge gaps in the content domain of health, others have suggested that as a general topic, health may appeal broadly to all SES groups (Ettema, Brown, and Luepker, 1983; Snyder, 1990; Yows, Salmon, Hawkins, and Love, 1991; Zandpour and Fellow, 1992). That is, audiences may be more involved in the topic because, a priori, it affects everyone in some way. This aspect, however, does not account for other factors influencing knowledge gaps. For example, studies of channel influence show that people who obtain their news from print media are usually more knowledgeable than those who receive it from other media (Viswanath and Finnegan, 1995). There is, of course, a slight tendency for readers of newspapers to have more formal education than nonreaders. Television has the potential to be a knowledge equalizer if it could overcome several critical barriers: its inveterate orientation to entertainment largely devoid of educational content and the high cost of television production and delivery, especially through the new technologies of cable and digital satellite broadcasting (Shinghi and Mody, 1976; Gunter, 1987). An additional modifiable aspect of channel influence has to do with the link between media and interpersonal communication. Tichenor, Donohue, and Olien (1980) have suggested, for example, that interpersonal discussion is helpful in narrowing knowledge gaps because it may reinforce information received in mass media channels.

Social conflict and mobilization. Media studies have also shown that where social conflict or community mobilization occurs, significant knowledge gaps are less likely to be found (Donohue, Tichenor, and Olien, 1975). Social conflict, an engine of social change, appears to increase public awareness of issues, encouraging greater interpersonal communication. Mobilization of community groups, institutions, and advocates to address a public problem has a similar effect, even when overt conflict is not present (Gaziano, 1983).

Community structure and pluralism. An important though largely nonmodifiable factor affecting knowledge gaps is the structure of communities themselves. Large communities are characterized by greater specialization in interest groups, services, and institutions including government, business, the media, and other organized centers of power. The potential for conflict is higher in these pluralistic communities because of such diversity and specialization. Small towns are less specialized and differentiated across all these sectors. Knowledge gaps are influenced by such social characteristics. For example, knowledge gaps are more likely

TABLE 15.2. KNOWLEDGE GAP CONCEPTS, DEFINITIONS, AND APPLICATIONS.

Concept	Definition	Application
Knowledge gap	Difference in measured knowledge between groups of differing socioeconomic status (SES) over time.	Potential unintended consequence of public health interventions and may increase SES-based differences over time.
Knowledge	Factual and interpretive information leading to understanding or useful for taking informed action.	Communicative factual and interpretive information about causes and prevention of disease and about skills for health improvement.
Information flow	Degree of availability of information on an issue or topic in a social system such as a community.	Increase community opportunities (through multiple media and other channels) to encounter health information and knowledge.
Socioeconomic status	Population units or subunits characterized by differing education, income, wealth, or occupation.	Emphasize information of interest and use to differing SES groups; emphasize channel strategies designed to reach especially low SES groups.
Social structure/ pluralism	Differentiation and interdependence among community subsystems including social institutions, organizations, interest groups, and other centers of power and influence that maintain the social system; often influenced by size of the community (the larger the community, the greater the differentiation).	Highly differentiated communities increase competition for public attention to health information. The level of communication activity required is often more intensive than would be needed in a smaller, less differentiated community, and public health resources seldom permit public health education to dominate the information flow. Emphasize targeting of media and other strategies to reach groups of interest.
Social conflict	Opposition or disagreement over an issue or problem, often representing a struggle for power and influence between social groups or leaders.	Controversy attracts media attention especially in highly differentiated communities; tends to increase public interest and may lead to equalizing topic information across SES groups.
Mobilization	Organized activity seeking to focus community power and influence to address a problem or issue.	Media publicity about a public health issue is frequently driven by the actions of social groups and leaders, increases public attention, and may lead to equalizing information across SES groups.
Motivation	Factors influencing individuals to attend to and act upon information and knowledge (for example, personal interest, involvement, self-efficacy).	Emphasize strategies to increase motivational factors that support acquiring and acting upon information and knowledge.

in larger more complex communities and less likely in smaller less pluralistic communities (Donohue, Tichenor, and Olien, 1975; Shinghi and Mody, 1976; Ettema, Brown, and Luepker, 1983; Gaziano, 1988). However, some recent studies, particularly in health communication, have reported findings counter to this: gaps were more likely to be found in smaller communities (Viswanath and others, 1994). It has been suggested that in certain domains, such as health, the greater availability of diverse sources may work to the advantage of residents of larger communities (Viswanath and Finnegan, 1995).

Motivational factors. An important set of modifiable factors affecting knowledge gaps was proposed by Ettema and Kline (1977). They argued that gaps between higher and lower SES groups were not necessarily due to the effects of less formal education or economic deprivation but to differential levels of motivation, interest, and salience in specific topics. They shifted the focus in knowledge gap studies to the role of variables of individual difference. Support for this alternative explanation appeared in several studies reporting that the association between knowledge and individual variables such as interest, salience, motivation, and involvement was greater than the association between knowledge and education (Ettema, Brown, and Luepker, 1983; Zandpour and Fellow, 1992; Fredin, Monnett, and Kosicki, 1994). Contrary evidence has been reported by other studies (Griffin, 1990; Snyder, 1990; Viswanath, 1990; Yows, Salmon, Hawkins, and Love, 1991; McLeod and Perse, 1994). Viswanath and colleagues (1993), in a study of a dietary health campaign, reported that even among those motivated, the more educated knew more about diet and nutrition than the less educated.

Despite conflicting evidence on the role of motivational factors, it is clear that variables at both the individual level and the social structural level are important in explaining knowledge gaps; however, future studies need to do a better job of linking these different levels of analysis (Viswanath and Finnegan, 1995).

The importance of these subsequent studies is that they have given back to guided social change efforts some modifiable factors that if appropriately understood and addressed, can restore some of our optimism about the use of interventions to address public problems. However, unlike the unbounded optimism of the early days of public campaigns, the attitude of these studies is to urge us to be more sober and wiser in considering structural factors that pose barriers to public campaigns. Public health regards addressing problems of the whole population, information rich and information poor alike, as an ethical precept.

Agenda-Setting Hypothesis.
Mass communication research has long been concerned with the influence of mass media on public opinion, especially as these media affect politics and policy making. Early writers such as Walter Lippmann (1922) saw media behavior as a "restless searchlight" panning from one issue to

the next and seldom lingering long on any single issue. Later researchers such as Bernard Berelson (1948) noted that although the media influence public opinion, the reverse is also true: public opinion influences what the media report. Researchers Lazarsfeld, Berelson, and Gaudet (1948) also observed that media attention itself confers status on public issues and raises their importance. These insights coalesced in the 1970s to a focus on the mass media's role and influence in setting the public agenda of important issues and problems.

Agenda setting has received a great deal of scholarly attention, in part owing to the reemergence of media models that predict powerful media effects (McCombs and Shaw, 1972). An axiom underlying this approach is that mass media are not very successful in telling us *what* to think but they are surprisingly successful in telling us what to think *about*. The key idea here, quite simply, is that mass media are powerful in setting the public agenda of important issues and problems. To quote a related axiom, "If it doesn't appear in the media, it isn't news."

Studies have shown high correlations between media coverage of issues and the public's opinion of the importance and interest of issues. The agenda-setting hypothesis implies a strong if not direct link between the media's agenda of important issues (as reflected in news coverage) and the public's agenda of important issues (with the causal direction flowing from the media to the public). In essence, agenda setting attributes a kingmaking role to the media but also presents a number of opportunities for applications in public health interventions (Table 15.3). Researcher Jerry Kosicki (1993) has suggested that there are actually three types of agenda-setting research: (1) public agenda setting, which examines the link between media portrayal of issues and the impact on issue priorities assigned by the public; (2) policy agenda setting, which examines the connection between media coverage and the legislative agenda of policy-making bodies; and (3) media agenda setting, which focuses on factors that influence the media to cover certain issues.

Recent research has suggested refinements in agenda-setting theory (Kosicki, 1993). Initial somewhat crude studies have given way to more empirically sophisticated designs with clearer causal links (Iyengar and Kinder, 1987; Demers, Craff, Choi, and Pessin, 1989). In addition, the approach is being further refined through several changes in the agenda-setting perspective. One change has to do with the former idea that mass media do not tell us what to think. According to the newer view, the media not only tell us what is important in a general way, they also provide ways of thinking about specific issues by the signs, symbols, terms, and sources they use to define the issue in the first place. In this view, public problems are social constructions. That is, groups, institutions, and advocates compete to identify problems, to move them onto the public agenda, *and* to define the issues symbolically (Gamson and Modigliani; 1987; Hilgartner and Bosk, 1988; Entman,

TABLE 15.3. AGENDA-SETTING CONCEPTS, DEFINITIONS, AND APPLICATIONS.

Concept	Definition	Application
Media agenda setting	Institutional roles, factors, and processes that influence the definition, selection, and emphasis of issues in the media	Work with media professionals to understand their work needs and routines in gathering and reporting news.
Public agenda setting	The link between issues portrayed in the media and the public's issue priorities	Work with media professionals in advocacy or partnership contexts to build a public agenda for important health issues.
Policy agenda setting	The link between issues developed in policy-making institutions and issues portrayed by the media	Work with community leaders and policy makers to build importance of health issues on the media's and public's agendas.
Problem identification, definition	Factors and process leading to the identification of an issue as a "problem" by social institutions	Mobilize community leaders, advocacy groups, and organizations to define an issue and modes of solution or basis for action.
Framing	Organized public discourse about an issue leading to the selection and emphasis of some characteristics and dimensions and the exclusion of others	Public health advocacy groups "package" an important health issue for the media and the public (for example, secondhand smoke framed as the public's involuntary exposure to a toxic pollutant contrasted with the "smokers' rights" emphasis of tobacco advocates).

1993). This theoretical refinement is important because it suggests that the media's agenda-setting function is not completely independent but is built by various community groups, institutions, and advocates. It also has a basis in the sociology of knowledge, which emphasizes processes involved in the "social construction of reality" (Berger and Luckmann, 1966). This has obvious implications and applications for those in public health who seek to use the mass media to raise the salience and public awareness of specific problems.

Cultivation Studies. *Cultivation studies* are primarily concerned with the impact that mass media have on our perceptions of "reality." The pervasive presence of television underlies much of this approach. Simply stated, researchers propose that heavy exposure to television programs may lead individuals to accept the world portrayed by television as real (Gerbner, Gross, Morgan, and Signorelli,

1980). That is, the greater the exposure to television, the greater the congruence between viewers' perception of reality and the mythic reality portrayed on television (Gerbner, Gross, Morgan, and Signorelli, 1994). In essence, television *cultivates* within viewers a stilted view of the world.

Cultivation studies have involved two types of research. The first, *message system analysis*, seeks to examine the world that television constructs. For example, in a long series of studies, Gerbner, Gross, Morgan, and Signorelli (1980, 1994) have been tracking television's violent content. (They define violence as "overt expression of physical force" by characters to force victims to act against their will, and they measure the frequency of such violent acts.) In their 1980 report, they demonstrated that, on average, there were five acts of violence per hour of prime-time programming and twenty acts of violence on weekend daytime television. They also tracked and recorded the gender, age, ethnic, and occupational breakdown of characters who frequent TV dramas. For example, on television (unlike the real world), men outnumber women, young people and senior citizens are underrepresented, and professional and law enforcement personnel are overrepresented.

The second type of research is *cultivation analysis*. Gerbner, Gross, Morgan, and Signorelli (1994) have proposed that heavy exposure to television has a profound effect on viewers' perception of social reality. Their data show that heavy viewers are more likely than light viewers to give "television answers" to opinion and knowledge questions. Heavy viewers are more likely to perceive the world as violent and frightening out of proportion to reality, are less trusting of others, overestimate the number of people employed in law enforcement, and fear that they are more likely than is statistically true to become victims of crime. They also are likely to be more accepting of violence as a means of dealing with social problems. This cultivation of the television worldview is believed to occur through two distinct mechanisms: mainstreaming and resonance. *Mainstreaming* is the "sharing of commonality of outlooks." Interestingly, irrespective of their sociodemographic background, heavy viewers of television tend to share this worldview. As Gerbner, Gross, Morgan, and Signorelli (1980) assert, heavy viewing "may serve to cultivate beliefs of otherwise disparate and divergent groups toward a more homogeneous 'mainstream' view." *Resonance* is regarded as the more powerful mechanism. The reality of television programs for certain groups has resonance when it is in fact congruent with the reality of their lives. In such cases, they receive a double dose of the cultivation effect, and thus television has stronger effects for these groups.

Although other research has raised questions about the nature of the evidence supporting the cultivation hypothesis, most researchers agree that television affects our perception of reality depending on our level of exposure (Potter, 1994). Subsequent studies have added several contingent conditions that could affect cultivation. For example, Hughes (1980) suggested that television's powerful cultivation effects become weaker or disappear when controlled for other factors. The association between fear of crime and measures of social alienation on the one hand and heavy viewing of television on the other grows weaker after accounting for factors of age, gender, education, income, hours worked per week, social ties, and size of the city of residence. The fear of crime supposedly cultivated by heavy television viewing could be explained by the fact that heavy viewers often live in high crime areas (Doob and McDonald, 1979). That is, because of fear, they may stay home and watch more television. Some have also argued that the cultivation effect could be nonlinear. That is, television viewing may lead to a cultivation of a television worldview only up to a point (Potter, 1994).

Risk Communication. Communication about risk is a field of special concern in public health, one that bridges individual and community levels of analysis. At the individual level, researchers emphasize the cognitive mechanisms by which individuals are exposed to and attend to information about risk, how they interpret risk information in relation to themselves, and finally, whether and how they act upon risk information to alter their behavior (Slovic, Fischoff, and Lichtenstein, 1981; Weinstein, 1984; Glanz and Yang, 1996). This approach to the study of communication about risk owes much of its theoretical base to social psychological models of behavior (discussed in Part Two), including value expectancy theories such as the Health Belief Model and the Theory of Reasoned Action (for example, perception of personal risk susceptibility and severity), and also has a debt to self-regulatory models including Social Cognitive Theory (for example, self-efficacy beliefs that one can take effective action to reduce personal risk) (see Chapter Eight). This approach is also a staple of communication research at the individual level that examines media effects on knowledge, beliefs, and behavior.

At the community level, studies of communication about risk focus on the interaction of populations and social institutions (such as governmental agencies, advocacy groups, and the mass media) in the formation and management of public opinion and policy making about risk. Here, risk communication studies owe much of their theoretical basis to the agenda-setting and agenda-building perspectives and also to research into the definition and framing of public issues. Risk communication research in this vein has noted that risk is usually a *constructed* phenomenon arising from the communication activity of social institutions, advocates, and the public (Sandman, 1987; Griswold and Packer, 1991; Glanz and Yang, 1996). Public definitions of risk will usually include some form of scientifically assessed ("objective") risk information mediated by the political and social context of the risk (the outrage factor). Frequently, it is the later that prevails in the public definition of important risk issues. This can have both negative and positive consequences, depending on whether the low or high actual risk corresponds or contrasts with the low or high public "outrage." For example, a high level of outrage is a form of community conflict that can quickly propel important information throughout the population at all socioeconomic levels (this phenomenon relates to studies of the knowledge gap discussed earlier). In such a case, there will be little difference in the information held by all socioeconomic groups. Conversely, where outrage is low (or there is little publicity), we might expect to find socioeconomic group differences in knowledge about risk. Either situation, a well-informed or a ill-informed public, may have an impact on policy making about risk.

Media Studies Applications in Health

This section reviews examples of the usefulness of some previously discussed perspectives in understanding and evaluating health promotion and disease prevention efforts. Applying communication theories to health behavior in the media studies framework occurs mainly along the two dimensions described earlier: (1) effects of day-to-day interaction with media on health outcomes and (2) effects of the purposive use of media to achieve some health outcome, usually in the context of a planned campaign intervention.

Applications in the Day-to-Day Impact of Media on Health

The idea that there is a day-to-day impact of mass media on health has linked media studies and public health for much of this century, and this trend shows little sign of abating, to judge by the amount of research generated. Its major concern is the effect of media use itself on health behavior. As communication historians have noted, the emergence of each new media technology has carried with it a "legacy of fear" about its harmful effects on the social fabric, public health, and especially "vulnerable" groups such as children and adolescents (DeFleur and Dennis, 1985). Thus in the 1930s, the Payne Fund sponsored some of the first empirical studies examining the effects on youths of exposure to movies. The concern was whether movies engendered violent or other antisocial behavior, and these studies approached the question from a psychological or social-psychological perspective, but more recently, investigators have used the cultivation studies approach. The emphasis on vulnerable groups in such studies also stems from the fact that children and the elderly are the heaviest users of television.

Violence and Television. The concern with the impact of day-to-day media use has continued with the emergence of commercial television. Nearly twenty-five years ago, empirical studies examining the effects on children and youths of exposure to television violence in entertainment programming were conducted. They found disturbing connections between television use and aggressive behavior, a link amplified by thousands of subsequent studies (Comstock and others, 1987; Lande, 1993). Similar concerns have led to studies of the effects of exposure to violent pornography (Linz, Wilson, and Donnerstein, 1992). Many have noted the cumulative effect of such exposure, leading to desensitization toward violence in general or to important changes in perceptions about one's vulnerability to violence. This is of obvious concern at a societal level if widespread desensitization were to lead to public tolerance of violence or if public perceptions of violence that are out of proportion with reality were to lead to repressive policies.

Advertising and Entertainment. Advertising has raised additional public health issues, also with an emphasis on such vulnerable groups as children and adolescents. Both the social-psychological and cultivation approaches to communication effects have informed research in this area. Recent studies have suggested, for example, that cigarette advertising is extremely appealing to youths and plays a role in influencing their decisions to start smoking (Rombouts and Fauconnier, 1988; Pierce, Lee, and Gilpin, 1994). Studies of alcohol advertising and the depiction of drinking in entertainment programming suggest that their effect on youths is to alter perceptions in favor of the product's use by implying a false norm that everybody drinks and by suggesting the false notion that people cannot have a good time unless they drink alcohol (Iannotti and Bush, 1992; Grube and Wallack, 1994; Weintraub-Austin and Nach-Ferguson, 1995). Other studies have arisen from concerns that excessive television use influences children's adoption of sedentary lifestyles and may be partly responsible for increased rates of juvenile obesity, poor eating patterns, high cholesterol, and eating disorders and other mental health problems (Myers and Biocca, 1992; Wong and others, 1992; Lamontagne, 1993; Signorelli, 1993).

Although focusing on individual effects of media use, many of these studies also have public policy ramifications. For example, some public health advocates have proposed major restrictions on advertising or entertainment content or counteradvertising as solutions to the negative impact of media exposure on health (Mosher, 1991; Dorfman and Wallack, 1993; Sidney, and others, 1994).

Studies have also examined the positive effects on health of media use (Schilling and McAlister, 1990; Barker and others, 1993). These studies note that although media (especially television) may have negative impact, they can and should be used to create positive impact in public health. This view especially imbues the second application of media studies to health: effects of the purposive use of media in the context of planned interventions.

Applications in the Planned Use of Media:
Heart Disease Prevention and Media Communication

The planned use of media communication to accomplish some health outcome predates the founding of the United States and may have started as a uniquely American cultural phenomenon (Paisley, 1989). This American penchant for public campaigns continues unabated today but with a deeper understanding of the role of planning and a more systematic approach to it. Many of the media communication theories discussed earlier are relevant to public health community-based campaigns. In the development of campaign- and intervention-planning frameworks (discussed in Part Five), many media studies theories are useful in the formative analysis and strategy development stages and also in evaluating outcomes. The following section provides examples of such applications.

Beginning in the 1950s, epidemiological studies discovered that rates of heart disease varied greatly around the world. It became apparent that these differences were due largely to socially enculturated behavior patterns (Kromhout, Menotti, and Blackburn, 1994). To reduce mass levels of disease, investigators reasoned, would require multiple prevention strategies aimed at change in whole populations. The rationale underlying this approach was a chain of causal links hypothesizing that increasing exposure to such a campaign would increase people's participation and involvement in prevention, leading to behavioral change (Mittelmark and others, 1986). This in turn would result in increasing change in heart disease risk factors and eventually disease reduction.

In the United States, federally funded communitywide prevention campaigns were started by investigators in California, Minnesota, and Rhode Island. Multiple strategies were used in which media communication played an important role. The idea of using multiple strategies was also informed by the idea of synergy. That is, strategies used together can be more powerful in accomplishing behavioral change than if each were used alone (the effect of the whole being greater than the sum of the effects of the parts). The idea of synergy, in turn, is based on the idea that each individual strategy has strengths and weaknesses in the achievement of health behavior change. For example, group educational settings are strong in presenting an intensive, interactive experience, typically in the classroom, but weak in their capacity to reach a high proportion of the population. Conversely, mass media are strong in their capacity to reach large numbers of people but weaker in their capacity to provide an intense interactive experience. Campaign-planning frameworks seek to offset individual weaknesses through employing the strengths of diverse strategies.

Media were used initially in each of the state campaigns to increase public awareness of the problem of heart disease, its major risk factors and associated lifestyle change strategies, and the programs themselves. In this sense, media were used first to build a community agenda for heart disease prevention as a major concern worthy of public attention. A strength of mass media is their capacity to expose many persons simultaneously to the same information, and thus it is not surprising that public awareness of prevention messages and programs increased dramatically and rapidly (Viswanath and others, 1994).

But a key issue for these and all public health campaigns is the extent to which they attain exposure among all socioeconomic segments of the community. Exposure is regarded as a contingent condition for some kind of effect to occur (McGuire, 1989). Yet health campaign planners are confronted with a number of important factors that influence exposure leading to behavioral change. As knowledge gap theory suggests, the tendency is for higher socioeconomic status groups to acquire information faster than lower SES groups. In addition, people living in communities of varying size and complexity may be differentially exposed to campaigns because of differences in communication systems. These considerations require health campaign planners to ensure, in the development and evaluation of campaigns, that social structural factors are considered and do not pose serious barriers to the diffusion of exposure, other intermediate effects, and behavioral outcomes.

In the cardiovascular disease (CVD) prevention campaigns, a number of studies examined the question of exposure, intermediate effects such as the distribution of prevention information, and behavioral change itself.

Exposure and Prevention Information. As a measure of intermediate exposure to the campaign, the Minnesota program tracked changes in community awareness and the ability of the public to recall the program name. Of course, neither of these intermediate outcomes was necessary to achieve behavioral change, but they functioned importantly as a process measure of campaign delivery. That is, the question was whether people were aware of the CVD prevention activity due to the campaign and could they recall (unaided) the name of the specific institutional source of this activity? More importantly, did these effects vary by SES group?

During the five-year campaign, random population surveys were conducted in each of three communities about every six months to monitor such changes (Viswanath and others, 1994). Awareness in the smallest community (population 28,651) increased rapidly from 42 percent at six months to a peak of 91 percent at three years and 88 percent at five years. In the regional community (population 137,574), awareness increased from 30 percent at six months to a peak of about 86 percent at two years and 76 percent at five years. In the suburb (population 81,831), awareness increased from about 30 percent at six months to a peak of

84 percent at three years and 71 percent at five years. Recall of the program name grew at about the same rate but was lower in each community overall, due certainly to the more difficult task of recalling a name without prompting. The data were suggestive of the more difficult task posed when campaigns were conducted in the more complex communities. In the regional community and the suburb (part of a metropolitan area of 2 million), much more media communication was required to maintain levels of awareness and name recall, which in any case were somewhat lower than they were in the smallest community in the study. The level of media communication required was more intense due to the complexity of the larger communities: there were more available channels, more "noise" and distractions than in the smallest community. But what about effects by SES segment?

The study showed that as predicted by the knowledge gap studies, CVD awareness and program name recall were highest among high SES groups (measured by formal education) over the course of the five years. However, importantly, the less educated groups (those with some college, high school, or less education) showed net gains that were actually larger than the gains of the highest group (which started out higher at the beginning). So although gaps still existed, the campaign succeeded in narrowing them to a great extent as the result of targeted communication efforts. Moreover, it is important to recognize that changes among lower SES groups can and do occur but frequently lag behind changes for higher SES groups. In our view, the reason for this is primarily unequal access to channels of communication and education, a situation that even further raises the importance of channel influence analysis in campaign-planning stages—that is, asking what channels are used most and are most effective with which groups (Finnegan, Viswanath, Kahn, and Hannan, 1993).

Dietary Education. An early study of the Stanford Heart Disease Prevention Project (Fortmann and others, 1982) examined the problem of variable effects by SES, asking, "Does dietary health education reach only the privileged?" In this pioneering U.S. heart disease prevention campaign, investigators were concerned to learn whether dietary change efforts communicated through mass media and other education channels were reaching all SES segments equally, particularly Spanish-speaking people in the study's California communities. Investigators conducted three years of cross-sectional surveys—before, during, and after a campaign—in two communities and compared their results to one community that served as a reference. Surveys included questions about dietary patterns (saturated fat and dietary cholesterol intake) and blood cholesterol measures. The study found that all groups reported 20 percent to 40 percent reductions in dietary cholesterol and saturated fat. Importantly, these reductions were just as large in lower as in higher SES groups, with Spanish-speaking groups reporting greater decreases in saturated fat ($p = .02$). As would be expected from the difference in saturated fat intake, Spanish-speaking groups also demonstrated at least marginally lower blood cholesterol levels ($p = .06$).

This study is important in light of the structural barriers to change implied by knowledge gap theory. Such barriers need not be regarded as intractable. The Stanford investigators speculated that traditionally expected differences between SES groups did not materialize due in part to extensive analysis and planning in the early stages of the media and education campaign.

Applications in Media and Policy: Preventing Alcohol Use Among Adolescents

In the last five years, public health campaigns increasingly have emphasized policy strategies to influence populationwide behavioral change. Two Midwest campaigns using this approach seek to prevent and to delay alcohol use by adolescents (Perry and others, 1993; Wagenaar and others, 1994). The Project Northland campaign combines traditional school-based prevention programs aimed at children and their parents with a community coalition of leaders, volunteers, and young people. The goal is both to educate children and to affect the larger community environment, where norms of widespread and irresponsible use of alcohol are all too apparent. The second campaign, Communities Mobilizing for Change on Alcohol (CMCA), uses exclusively a community organization and citizen participation model whose goal is to politically empower young people and adults. An objective of both studies is to influence policy affecting youths' access to alcohol and use of alcohol.

Both studies include an important role for media communication that is related to the agenda-setting approach described earlier. Specifically, use of the mass media in these settings is designed to build the community agenda among leaders, volunteers, and the public for enforcement of existing alcohol policies and, where needed, to build public consensus and influence for passage of new policies. Effects of these activities will be evaluated for their impact on adolescent alcohol use and public opinion. Although at this writing final results are not yet available from either study, preliminary evidence is suggestive of improvements in policy enforcement. Some new policies have even been passed as a result of these programs. As of 1996, Project Northland reported that community task forces had advocated successfully for passage of five alcohol-related ordinances requiring responsible beverage server training, refinements in liquor license renewal, and requirements for liquor establishment closing hours. In addition, three resolutions were passed identifying underage drinking as an unacceptable behavior and supporting tighter enforcement of existing ordinances, establishing designated alcohol sales and consumption areas at outdoor public events, and blocking a proposal to extend Sunday liquor sales hours.

The key application of media communication in these studies is the use of advocacy groups to influence community media to increase their attention to and coverage of youth and alcohol issues. Although this application is related to the agenda-setting framework discussed earlier, it differs in some important ways. The agenda-setting framework emphasizes the media as key players in establishing important community issues. The approach applied here recognizes that media agendas are themselves heavily influenced by other community institutions, groups, and coalitions.

Successful use of this approach in public health settings means that advocacy groups must understand the dynamics of media news production and work requirements. For example, successful influencing of the media agenda requires that media gatekeepers (editors, reporters, producers) perceive the advocacy group as legitimate and mainstream rather than radical or peripheral to community interests (Donohue, Tichenor, and Olien, 1995). The media tend to shy away from coverage of groups they perceive as peripheral. Thus, formation of advocacy groups in public health settings frequently focuses on mobilizing community leaders, power centers, and volunteers on behalf of a public health issue.

A second factor in this approach is activity by the advocacy group that defines and identifies a problem for the media and is successful in framing discussion, debate, and potential conflict over the issue. Thus, in the youth and alcohol programs, advocates focus on protecting a vulnerable group such as adolescents by way of policies designed to control the supply and availability of alcohol (Wagenaar, 1994). Framing the issue in this way (and also as a grassroots movement of adult citizens and youth) is helpful in controlling and channeling potential conflict over the issue that could erupt between public health advocates and members of the alcohol and related industries, who usually have strong political influence and resources.

Applications in this framework have also been discussed recently as "media advocacy" approaches in public health (Wallack, Dorfman, Jernigan, and Themba, 1993).

Conclusion and Future Directions

There are several important issues in the application of media communication theory in health that will influence research into the next century. The first is continuing study of the media's influence on health as a function of day-to-day media use, particularly among vulnerable audiences such as children and adolescents. Although some in the baby-boom generation can recall a time without television, subsequent generations have been exposed to the medium unrelentingly almost from birth. The power of television and the mass media's socializing functions are not, of course, felt through single exposures to a medium but through cumulative effects. Mass media's purpose is not primarily to support the goals of public health improvement, especially in light of the mass media emphasis on advertising and entertainment, an emphasis that frequently collides with the goals of public health. Can the mass media, as message producers par excellence, be encouraged to do a better job—for example, to reduce content regarded as detrimental to public health goals?

The answer is an equivocal "maybe." There have been some successes, notably efforts by the Harvard University School of Public Health, to encourage television producers to include positive messages on designated drivers in their programs. Public health advocates have continued to criticize violence in film and on television. Further successes in encouraging the media to modify content at odds with the public health will depend in large measure on the effectiveness of public health advocates in building the national agenda for such changes.

A second issue that will continue to be debated into the next century is the purposive use of mass media to achieve health behavior change. Specifically, community health settings will continue to provide an ideal environment to examine communication effects across levels of analysis. Of particular interest is how communication at each level of analysis may influence or link to communication at other levels. There undoubtedly are both structural- and individual-level factors responsible. For example, social cognitive theorist Albert Bandura recently suggested that the "power" of any single channel of communication (mass media or interpersonal) may depend on the complexity of the behavioral change being sought. On the one hand, the less complex the change, the more the influence of a single channel leading to performance of the behavior (1994). On the other hand, the more complex the behavior, the greater the need for multiple exposure to multiple sources. In this setting, the influence of any single channel is relatively less.

A third issue continues to be the social structural influences on mass media use and its impact on health behavior change. Recent epidemiological studies suggest, for example, that the health gap between higher and lower SES groups in the United States is worsening rather than improving. Communication contributes to these circumstances, at least insofar as structural barriers of access and exposure continue to be too frequently ignored or overlooked.

Fourth, the emergence of new electronic communication technologies provides opportunities and challenges to health educators and researchers. The World Wide Web, newsgroups, and other Internet innovations offer information on an array of topics from diverse sources. Electronic technologies permit information to be available on demand to users, allowing users a great degree of control over the timing, pace, and topic of the information they seek. However, two potentially serious problems warrant closer examination. One potential difficulty has to do with access to new media technologies and to the skills to use them effectively. These technologies have the potential to widen the gap between those who can pay for access and have the skills, and those who cannot pay and have little opportunity to acquire the skills. If this gap does widen, a significant portion of the population, perhaps those most in need of prevention information, may be out of the communication loop for important health information. The second potential concern has to do with control of information. In traditional campaigns, campaign planners have a fair amount of control over the kind of information disseminated. On the Internet, users have much less control. On the positive side, this feature supports greater diversity and gives relative freedom and autonomy to audience subgroups to seek the information they require. On the negative side, health educators and health promotion advocates have less control over the accuracy and quality of health information. Despite these twin concerns, which are also twin challenges, the new media technologies will surely become a significant area of public health application and scholarly inquiry. They also offer the promise of linking interpersonal and mass media outcomes.

Finally, in light of the current preference in public health for community-based interventions, is there a place for national media campaigns in public health? Some suggest that national campaigns are a waste of time and that resources could be better spent mobilizing local communities for health behavior change. Our judgment at this writing is that national media campaigns are important because they help build a national prevention agenda on specific issues. The issues raised by national campaigns are usually of concern to every community big or small; thus, they create a foundation upon which local efforts can build. National campaigns can amplify local prevention efforts, which are typically more targeted and intense. But national media campaigns should not be regarded as a substitute for community prevention nor should they be expected to accomplish widespread behavioral change by themselves.

References

Bandura, A. "Social Cognitive Theory of Mass Communication." In J. Bryant and D. Zillmann (eds.), *Media Effects: Advances in Theory and Research*. Hillsdale, N.J.: Erlbaum, 1994.

Barker, C., and others. "You in Mind-A Preventive Mental-Health Television Series." *British Journal of Clinical Psychology*, 1993, *32*(3), 281–293.

Beniger, J. R., and Gusek, J. A. "The Cognitive Revolution in Public Opinion and Communication Research." In T. L. Glasser and C. T. Salmon (eds.), *Public Opinion and the Communication of Consent*. New York: Guilford Press, 1995.

Berelson, B. "Communications and Public Opinion." In W. Schramm (ed.), *Communications in Modern Society.* Urbana, Ill.: University of Illinois Press, 1948.

Berger, P. L., and Luckmann, T. *The Social Construction of Reality: A Treatise in the Sociology of Knowledge.* New York: Doubleday, 1966.

Blumler, J. G., and Katz, E. (eds.). *The Uses of Mass Communication: Current Perspectives on Gratifications Research.* Thousand Oaks, Calif.: Sage, 1974.

Bryant, J., and Zillman, D. (eds.). *Media Effects: Advances in Theory and Research.* Hillsdale, N.J.: Erlbaum, 1994.

Chaffee, S., and Roser, C. "Involvement and Consistency of Knowledge, Attitudes and Behaviors." *Communication Research,* 1986, *13*(3), 373–400.

Clarke, P., and Evans, S. "Field Definitions: Mass Communication." In *1984–85 U.S. Directory of Graduate Programs.* (9th ed.) Princeton, N.J.: Educational Testing Service, 1983.

Comstock, G. S., and others. *Television and Human Behavior.* New York: Columbia University Press, 1987.

DeFleur, M., and Dennis, E. *Understanding Mass Communication.* (2nd ed.) Boston: Houghton Mifflin, 1985.

Demers, D., Craff, D., Choi, Y. H., and Pessin, B. M. "Issues' Obtrusiveness and the Agenda Setting Effect of National Network News." *Communication Research,* 1989, *16,* 793–812.

Donohue, G. A., Tichenor, P. J., and Olien, C. N. "Mass Media and the Knowledge Gap: A Hypothesis Reconsidered." *Communication Research,* 1975, *2,* 3–23.

Donohue, G. A., Tichenor, P. J., and Olien, C. N. "A Guard Dog Perspective on the Role of Media." *Journal of Communication,* 1995, *45*(2), 115–132.

Doob, A. N., and McDonald, G. E. "Television Viewing and Fear of Victimization: Is the Relationship Causal?" *Journal of Personality and Social Psychology,* 1979, *37,* 170–179.

Dorfman, L., and Wallack, L. "Advertising Health—The Case for Counter-Ads." *Public Health Reports,* 1993, *108*(6), 716–726.

Entman, R. M. "Framing: Toward Clarification of a Fractured Paradigm." *Journal of Communication,* 1993, *43*(4), 51–58.

Ettema, J. S., Brown, J., and Luepker, R. V. "Knowledge Gap Effects in a Health Information Campaign." *Public Opinion Quarterly,* 1983, *47,* 516–527.

Ettema, J. S., and Kline, F. G. "Deficits, Differences and Ceilings: Contingent Conditions for Understanding the Knowledge Gap." *Communication Research,* 1977, *4,* 179–202.

Finnegan, J. R., and Viswanath, K. "Health and Communication: Medical and Public Health Influences on the Research Agenda." In E. Berlin-Ray and L. Donohew (eds.), *Communication and Health: Systems and Applications.* Hillsdale, N.J.: Erlbaum, 1989.

Finnegan, J. R., Viswanath, K., Kahn, E., and Hannan, P. "Exposure to Sources of Heart Disease Prevention Information: Community Type and Social Group Differences." *Journalism Quarterly,* 1993, *70,* 569–584.

Fortmann, S. P., and others. "Does Dietary Health Education Reach Only the Privileged? The Stanford Three Community Study." *Circulation,* 1982, *66*(1), 77–82.

Fredin, E., Monnett, T. H., and Kosicki, G. M. "Knowledge Gaps, Social Locators, and Media Schemata: Gaps, Reverse Gaps, and Gaps of Disaffection." *Journalism Quarterly,* 1994, *71,* 176–190.

Gamson, W., and Modigliani, A. "The Changing Culture of Affirmative Action." In R. G. Braungart and M. M. Braungart (eds.), *Research in Political Sociology.* Vol. 3. Greenwich, Conn.: JAI Press, 1987.

Gandy, O. H., Jr. *Beyond Agenda-Setting.* Norwood, N.J.: Ablex, 1982.

Gaziano, C. "Knowledge Gap: An Analytical Review of Media Effects." *Communication Research*, 1983, *10*, 447–486.

Gaziano, C. "Community Knowledge Gaps." *Critical Studies in Mass Communication*, 1988, *5*, 351–357.

Gerbner, G. "Field Definitions: Communication Theory." In *1984–85 U.S. Directory of Graduate Programs.* (9th ed.) Princeton, N.J.: Educational Testing Service, 1983.

Gerbner, G., Gross, L., Morgan, M., and Signorelli, N. "The 'Mainstreaming' of America: Violence Profile No. 11." *Journal of Communication*, 1980, *30*, 10–29.

Gerbner, G., Gross, L., Morgan, M., and Signorelli, N. "Growing Up with Television: The Cultivation Perspective." In J. Bryant and D. Zillmann (eds.) *Media Effects: Advances in Theory and Research*. Hillsdale, N.J.: Erlbaum, 1994.

Glanz, K., and Yang, H. "Communicating About Risk of Infectious Diseases." *Journal of the American Medical Association*, 1996, *275*(3), 253–256.

Griffin, R. "Energy in the Eighties: Education, Communication and the Knowledge Gap." *Journalism Quarterly*, 1990, *67*, 554–566.

Griswold, W., and Packer, C. "The Interplay of Journalistic and Scientific Conventions in Mass Communication About AIDS." *Mass Communication Review*, 1991, *18*(3), 9–20, 47.

Grube, J. W., and Wallack, L. "Television Beer Advertising and Drinking Knowledge, Beliefs, and Intentions Among Schoolchildren." *American Journal of Public Health*, 1994, *84*(2), 254–259.

Gunter, B. *Poor Reception: Misunderstanding and Forgetting Broadcast News*. Hillsdale, N.J.: Erlbaum, 1987.

Hawkins, R. P., Weimann, J. M., and Pingree, S. (eds.). *Advancing Communication Science: Merging Mass and Interpersonal Processes*. Thousand Oaks, Calif.: Sage, 1988.

Hilgartner, S., and Bosk, C. L. "The Rise and Fall of Social Problems: Public Arenas Model." *American Journal of Sociology*, 1988, *94*, 53–77.

Hovland, C. I., Janis, I. L., and Kelley, H. H. *Communication and Persuasion: Psychological Studies of Opinion Change*. Westport, Conn.: Greenwood Press, 1953.

Hughes, M. "The Fruits of Cultivation Analysis: A Reexamination of Some Effects of Television Watching." *Public Opinion Quarterly*, 1980, *44*, 287–302.

Hyman, H. H., and Sheatsley, P. B. "Some Reasons Why Information Campaigns Fail." *Public Opinion Quarterly*, 1947, *11*, 412–423.

Iannotti, R. J., and Bush, P. J. "Perceived vs. Actual Friends' Use of Alcohol, Cigarettes, Marijuana, and Cocaine—Which Has the Most Influence?" *Journal of Youth and Adolescence*, 1992, *21*(3), 375–389.

Iyengar, S., and Kinder, D. R. *News That Matters*. Chicago: University of Chicago Press, 1987.

Kosicki, G. M. "Problems and Opportunities in Agenda-Setting Research." *Journal of Communication*, 1993, *43*, 100–127.

Kromhout, D., Menotti, A., and Blackburn, H. B. *The Seven Countries Study: A Scientific Adventure in Cardiovascular Disease Epidemiology*. Utrecht, Netherlands: Brouwer, 1994.

Lamontagne, Y. "Influence of the Media on Mental Health." *Canadian Journal of Psychiatry—Revue Canadienne de Psychiatrie*, 1993, *38*(2), 117–121.

Lande, R. G. "The Video Violence Debate." *Hospital and Community Psychiatry*, 1993, *44*(4), 347–351.

Lasswell, H. D. "The Structure and Function of Communication in Society." In L. Bryson (ed.), *The Communication of Ideas*. New York: Institute for Religious and Social Studies, 1948.

Lazarsfeld, P., Berelson, B., and Gaudet, H. *The People's Choice.* New York: Columbia University Press, 1948.

Lee, C. C. *Media Imperialism Reconsidered.* Thousand Oaks, Calif.: Sage, 1980.

Linz, D., Wilson, B. J., and Donnerstein, E. "Sexual Violence in the Mass Media—Legal Solutions, Warnings, and Mitigation Through Education." *Journal of Social Issues,* 1992, *48*(1), 145–171.

Lippmann, W. *Public Opinion.* New York: Macmillan, 1922.

McCombs, M. E., and Shaw, D. "The Agenda-Setting Function of the Mass Media." *Public Opinion Quarterly,* 1972, *36,* 176–187.

McGuire, W. J. "Public Communication as a Strategy for Inducing Health Promoting Behavioral Change." *Preventive Medicine,* 1984, *13,* 299–313.

McGuire, W. J. "Attitudes and Attitude Change." In G. Lindzey and E. Aronson (eds.), *Handbook of Social Psychology.* (3rd ed.) Vol. 2. New York: Random House, 1985.

McGuire, W. J. "Theoretical Foundations of Campaigns." In R. E. Rice and C. K. Atkin (eds.), *Public Communication Campaigns.* (2nd ed.) Thousand Oaks, Calif.: Sage, 1989.

McLeod, J. M., Kosicki, G. M., and Pan, Z. "On Understanding and Misunderstanding Media Effects." In J. Curran and M. Gurevitch (eds.), *Mass Media and Society.* London: Edward Arnold, 1991.

McLeod, D. M., and Perse, E. M. "Direct and Indirect Effects of Socioeconomic Status on Public Affairs Knowledge." *Journalism Quarterly,* 1994, *71,* 433–442.

Mittelmark, M. B., and others. "Community-Wide Prevention of Cardiovascular Disease: Education Strategies of the Minnesota Heart Health Program." *Preventive Medicine,* 1986, *15*(1), 1–17.

Mosher, J. F. "The Need for a Responsible Advertising Policy." *American Journal of Public Health,* 1991, *81*(10), 1348.

Mosteller, F., and Moynihan, D. P. *On Equality of Educational Opportunity.* New York: Random House, 1972.

Myers, P. N., and Biocca, F. A. "The Elastic Body Image—The Effect of Television Advertising and Programming on Body Image Distortions in Young Women." *Journal of Communication,* 1992, *42*(3), 108–133.

Paisley, W. "Public Communication Campaigns: The American Experience." In R. E. Rice and C. K. Atkin (eds.), *Public Communication Campaigns.* (2nd ed.) Thousand Oaks, Calif.: Sage, 1989.

Perloff, R. M. *The Dynamics of Persuasion.* Hillsdale N.J.: Erlbaum, 1993.

Perry, C. L. and others. "Background, Conceptualization, and Design of a Community-Wide Research Program on Adolescent Alcohol Use: Project Northland." *Health Education Research,* 1993, *8*(1), 125–136.

Petty, R. E., and Cacioppo, J. T. *Attitudes and Persuasion: Classic and Contemporary Approaches.* Dubuque, Iowa: W.C. Brown, 1981.

Pierce, J. P., Lee L., and Gilpin, E. A. "Smoking Initiation by Adolescent Girls, 1944 Through 1988—An Association with Targeted Advertising." *Journal of the American Medical Association,* 1994, *271*(8), 608–611.

Potter, W. J. "Cultivation Theory and Research: A Methodological Critique." In *Journalism Monographs,* no. 147. Columbia, S.C.: Association for Education in Journalism and Mass Communication, 1994.

Ray, M., and others. "Marketing Communication and the Hierarchy of Effects." In P. Clarke (ed.), *New Models for Mass Communication Research.* Thousand Oaks, Calif.: Sage, 1973.

Rogers, E. M. *Diffusion of Innovations.* (4th ed.) New York: Free Press, 1995. (First edition published 1962.)

Rogers, E. M., and Storey, J. D. "Communication Campaigns." In C. R. Berger and S. H. Chaffee (eds.), *Handbook of Communication Science.* Thousand Oaks, Calif.: Sage, 1987.

Roloff, M. E., and Miller, G. R. (eds.). *Persuasion: New Directions in Theory and Research.* Thousand Oaks, Calif.: Sage, 1980.

Rombouts, K., and Fauconnier, G. "What Is Learnt Early Is Learnt Well? A Study of the Influence of Tobacco Advertising on Adolescents." *European Journal of Communication,* 1988, *3,* 303–322.

Roshco, B. *Newsmaking.* Chicago: University of Chicago Press, 1975.

Sandman, P. M. "Apathy Versus Hysteria: Public Perception of Risk." In L. R. Batra and W. Klassen (eds.), *Public Perception of Biotechnology.* Bethesda, Md.: Agricultural Research Institute, 1987.

Schilling, R. F., and McAlister, A. L. "Preventing Drug Use in Adolescents Through Media Interventions." *Journal of Consulting and Clinical Psychology,* 1990, *58*(4), 416–424.

Shinghi, P., and Mody, B. "The Communication Effects Gap: A Field Experiment on Television and Agricultural Ignorance in India." *Communication Research,* 1976, *3,* 171–190.

Shoemaker, P. J. *Gatekeeping.* Thousand Oaks, Calif.: Sage, 1991.

Sidney, S., and others. "Television Viewing and Cardiovascular Risk Factors in Young Adults—The Cardia Study." *Circulation,* 1994, *89*(2), 936–936.

Sigal, L. V. *Reporters and Officials: The Organization and Politics of Newsmaking.* Lexington, Mass.: Heath, 1973.

Sigal, L. V. "Sources Make the News." In K. Manoff and M. Schudson (eds.), *Reading the News.* New York: Pantheon Books, 1987.

Signorelli, N. *Mass Media Images and Impact on Health: A Sourcebook.* Westport, Conn.: Greenwood Press, 1993.

Slovic, P., Fischoff, B., and Lichtenstein, S. "Perceived Risk: Psychological Factors and Social Implications." In F. Warner and D. H. Slater (eds.), *The Assessment and Perception of Risk.* London: Royal Society, 1981.

Snyder, L. B. "Channel Effectiveness over Time and Knowledge and Behavior Gaps." *Journalism Quarterly,* 1990, *67,* 875–886.

Tichenor, P. J., Donohue, G. A., and Olien, C. N. "Mass Media Flow and Differential Growth in Knowledge." *Public Opinion Quarterly,* 1970, *34,* 159–170.

Tichenor, P. J., Donohue, G. A., and Olien, C. N. *Community Conflict and the Press.* Thousand Oaks, Calif.: Sage, 1980.

Tuchman, G. *Making News: A Study in the Construction of Reality.* New York: Free Press, 1978.

Turow, J. *Media Systems in Society: Understanding Industries, Strategies, and Power.* New York: Longman, 1992.

Viswanath, K. "Knowledge Gap Effects in a Cardiovascular Disease Prevention Campaign: A Longitudinal Study of Two Community Pairs." Unpublished doctoral dissertation, University of Minnesota, 1990.

Viswanath, K., and Finnegan, J. R. "The Knowledge Gap Hypothesis: Twenty-Five Years Later." In B. Burleson (ed.), *Communication Yearbook.* Vol. 19. Thousand Oaks, Calif.: Sage, 1995.

Viswanath, K., Finnegan, J. R., Hannan, P. J., and Luepker, R. V. "Health and Knowledge Gaps: Some Lessons from the Minnesota Heart Health Program." *American Behavioral Scientist,* 1991, *34,* 712–726.

Viswanath, K., and others. "Motivation and the 'Knowledge Gap': Effects of a Campaign to Reduce Diet-Related Cancer Risk." *Communication Research*, 1993, *20*, 546–563.

Viswanath, K., and others. "Community Type and the Diffusion of Campaign Information." *Gazette*, 1994, *54*, 39–59.

Wagenaar, A. C., and others. "Communities Mobilizing for Change on Alcohol: Design of a Randomized Community Trial." *Journal of Community Psychology*, 1994 (CSAP special issue), 79–101.

Wallack, L., Dorfman, L., Jernigan, D., and Themba, M. *Media Advocacy and Public Health: Power for Prevention*. Thousand Oaks, Calif.: Sage, 1993.

Weinstein, N. D. "'Why It Won't Happen to Me': Perceptions of Risk Factors and Susceptibility." *Health Psychology*, 1984, *3*, 431–457.

Weintraub-Austin, E., and Nach-Ferguson, B. "Sources and Influences of Young School-Age Children's General and Brand-Specific Knowledge About Alcohol." *Health Communication*, 1995, *7*(1).

Wong, N. D., and others. "Television Viewing and Pediatric Hypercholesterolemia." *Pediatrics*, 1992, *90*(1), 75–79.

Yows, S., Salmon, C. T., Hawkins, R., and Love, R. "Motivational and Structural Factors in Predicting Different Kinds of Cancer Knowledge." *American Behavioral Scientist*, 1991, *34*, 727–741.

Zandpour, F., and Fellow, A. R. "Knowledge Gap Effects: Audience and Media Factors in Alcohol-Related Health Communication." *Mass Communication Review*, 1992, *19*(3), 34–41.

CHAPTER SIXTEEN

PERSPECTIVES ON GROUP, ORGANIZATION, AND COMMUNITY INTERVENTIONS

Karen Glanz

The chapters in Part Four present four models for health behavior change in groups, organizations, and communities. The aim of these chapters is to demonstrate the utility and promise of each theory or framework in health promotion and health education.

The central theme of Part Four is that we need to understand, predict, and know how to work with people through the social structures that are the context for their health behavior. We also need to be able to foster change and to assist populations in their efforts to create healthier institutions and communities. The concepts of social networks, change within and among systems, organizational processes, and communication channels are apparent across each of the chapters.

New Concepts and Strategies for Macro-Level Change

The chapters in this section bring together long-standing ideas and new concepts and strategies for understanding behavior and facilitating change. In Chapter Twelve, Minkler and Wallerstein add the concept of community building for health to their discussion of the now familiar principles and methods of community organization. Important aspects of community building as an orientation derive from a feminist perspective, emphasizing *power to* and *power with* in contrast to *power over* communities and their members. Organizing is seen as a holistic endeavor, dealing with both rational and nonrational elements of the human experience. Chapter Twelve also discusses new developments in measurement and evaluation of community organization strategies and community activation. Emerging methodologies and cross-cutting research issues will be discussed later in this chapter.

Chapter Thirteen, by Oldenburg, Hardcastle, and Kok, analyzes diffusion theory, its main concepts, and its applications in health care and school settings. The chapter is particularly noteworthy because its authors are from Australia and the Netherlands and demonstrate that some organizational issues cross geographical boundaries and that many health promotion challenges are shared internationally. The authors also examine diffusion as it applies to both change strategies and adoption of health promotion programs.

Goodman, Steckler, and Kegler analyze three theories of organizational change in Chapter Fourteen: stage theory, organizational development theory, and interorganizational relations theory. The latter theory is new in the second edition of this book, and its considerable overlap with community organization and community building reveals how these models are complementary. Chapter Fourteen raises intriguing questions about the uncontrollability of many aspects of community health practice and about the types of outcomes health promotion experts need to examine.

In Chapter Fifteen, Finnegan and Viswanath tackle the enormous literature on communication theories, focusing on theories and hypotheses with special relevance to public health and health behavior change. They emphasize a media studies framework, as distinct from interpersonal communication (covered in Part Three). Four media effects perspectives are introduced: the knowledge gap hypothesis, agenda setting, cultivation studies, and risk communication. These models cut across a range of considerations about mass media: their differential impact on high and low socioeconomic status populations; their application in social action and advocacy; their impact on people's worldviews, and their communications regarding health risks, especially those risks with broad public health implications.

These four chapters offer new concepts and strategies as well as expanded and updated coverage of all the issues at hand. The constraints of the present perspectives chapter preclude coverage of all the issues at hand. Instead, this chapter highlights the new concepts and strategies included in Part Four of this second edition of *Health Behavior and Health Education*, discusses similarities among the models, draws common themes, and critiques their usefulness for research and practice in health promotion.

Multiple Levels of Influence and Action

A central premise of this book is that improvements in health require both an understanding of the multilevel determinants of health behavior and a range of change strategies at the individual, interpersonal, and community or larger levels. Critiques of the tendency for health promotion programs to focus excessively on individuals abound in the literature (McKinlay, 1993; Winett, 1995). Indeed, there is substantial overlap between public health and health promotion approaches and disease prevention and control strategies in clinical settings (Rimer, Glanz, and Lerman, 1991). Nevertheless, the view that societal changes and supportive environments are necessary to address major health problems successfully *and* to maintain individual behavioral changes is promulgated widely (Schmid, Pratt, and Howze, 1995; Rimer, Glanz, and Lerman, 1991) and seems generally accepted. The chapters in this section clearly exemplify a multilevel perspective, which builds on both intrapersonal and interpersonal theories to explain or affect community change.

Minkler and Wallerstein describe the Adolescent Social Action Program (ASAP) as drawing on protection-motivation theory, an individual-level model, along with empowerment education and community-building approaches. Oldenburg, Hardcastle, and Kok remind us that Social Cognitive Theory (SCT) and the Theory of Reasoned Action (TRA) are very helpful for understanding diffusion at the organizational level, and they describe a risk-reduction intervention in health care settings based on SCT and the stages of change construct. Goodman, Steckler, and Kegler begin with the premise that organizations have multiple levels or layers, and these authors carry through with the theme of the ecology of organizations. Finally, Finnegan and Viswanath organize their review of communication studies according to multiple levels, from intrapersonal processes (for example, information processing) and interpersonal interactions (for example, patient-provider communication) to the level of community and macro social structure. They advance the central thesis that various levels of analysis are appropriate to considering various types of effects and aims of interventions.

An important message at the heart of these chapters is that the broader community- or organization-level models and concepts are not intended to stand alone at the expense of neglecting the individuals who constitute groups, organizations, and communities. Nor should the charge of excessive focus on individuals cause us to turn away from well-established theories and strategies. It is collectives of *individuals* who create organizational structures, provide leadership in communities, choose to participate—or not participate—in coalitions, and make decisions about local, state, and federal policies and priorities. Also, it would be a mistake to assume that the answers to all health promotion challenges lie in policy development, social action, and environmental change. For example, a recent evaluation of thirty-seven community AIDS prevention projects found that the health promotion strategies rated most effective were small-group discussions, outreach workers, trained peers and volunteers, and the provision of safer-sex kits. These small-group and individually oriented strategies were more likely to be implemented, in contrast with protest marches and strategies to educate policy makers, approaches that were either seldom done or were rated ineffective (Janz and others, 1996). Thus, the most suitable approaches, not necessarily the most far-reaching methods, should be adopted for health promotion initiatives.

Models for Change

The chapters in Part Four examine models for community activation, planned change, and collaboration.

Community Activation and Planned Change

Two general domains define the scope of the models included in Part Four: social activation and processes for changing attitudes, behaviors, and policies. The former is usually characterized by internal or *intra*group stimuli for change, whereas the latter are more likely to inform external change agents about how to facilitate changes identified as needed or desirable. (None of the models is purely of one domain or the other, but all break down roughly into these categories.) These generalized approaches reflect implicit assumptions about power and social control versus empowerment and self-control.

Social activation is central to community organization, organizational development, interorganizational relations, and media advocacy. As Minkler and Wallerstein note in Chapter Twelve, several of the key principles of community organizing relate directly to creating the conditions for change: empowerment, community competence, and the principles of participation and relevance. Two of the three models of community organization proposed by Rothman and Tropman (1987)—locality (community) development and social action, as well as community building—stress consensus, cooperation, group identity, and mutual problem solving.

Organizational development (OD) theory aims to improve organizational performance and the quality of work life. Its roots are in human relations and humanist psychology. It is concerned with members of organizations, and organizational problems are diagnosed by gathering information directly from the members or workers through formal surveys, interviews, and other methods. OD interventions include such strategies as team building, group development, and T-groups to promote interpersonal exchanges. As Goodman, Steckler, and Kegler point out in Chapter Fourteen, face-to-face contact and group interaction are integral to this approach.

Agenda-setting approaches to media communication suggest that media tell people *what to think about*. Media advocacy strategies are an extension of this view: advocacy groups in the community define, identify, and frame a problem and stimulate media coverage of it as a public health issue (Wallack, 1990). Media advocacy activates forces in a social system (that is, media coverage) to stimulate public concern and action.

Processes for facilitating large-scale *changes in attitudes and behaviors* are the province of diffusion of innovations theory, stage theory of organizational change, and the branch of communication studies that emphasizes changes in cognitions, beliefs, and behavior. Each of these frameworks offers guideposts for professionals wishing to promote specific changes in individuals in a larger society and within organizations. The term *diffusion of innovations* describes the spread of ideas, products, and behaviors within a society or from one society or social system to another. Stage theory is closely allied to diffusion of innovations because it focuses on understanding and matching the organizational stages of change with efforts to introduce or encourage organizational change. The communication studies areas of message production and media effects are rooted in theory and research on communication and persuasion dating back to the work of Lasswell (1948) and Hovland, Janis, and Kelley (1953) more than forty years ago.

These contrasting orientations to change—social activation and planned change—raise issues about who has power and control, who defines needs and problems, and the extent to which existing institutions (including the mass media) act as instruments of social control, issues that will be discussed further in a later section of this chapter. As Kipnis (1994) noted, there has been a recent surge in behavioral techniques based on reducing restraints against change (for example, social support, empowerment, personal growth) rather than on pushing people to change. But even when these methods are used to promote social justice, there remains an exercise of power that may be disquieting to target audiences (Kipnis, 1994). Of particular interest is the paradox that Minkler and Wallerstein suggest: that community needs and wants should be superseded by social justice concerns in cases where communities are mobilizing to restrict civil rights (through such devices as anti–gay rights legislation). This paradox underscores the dilemma of professionals whose personal values are not consistent with those of a given community.

Collaboration

Collaboration, through partnerships among health promotion experts and other providers (educators, medical personnel, and media producers, for example) or through coalitions with interorganizational representation emerges as a strategy for change across the chapters of Part Four. The relevance of social support and social networks concepts underpins these strategies. It is logical to expect that there is strength in numbers and that partnerships and coalitions can mobilize material and human resources and be more effective at achieving desired goals than individuals working alone. Collaborations have enormous potential for community and systems change, too: they can achieve valued public health outcomes while also transforming power relations and revitalizing a sense of shared power and shared responsibility (Himmelman, 1992). Yet collaborative efforts are complex, successful coalitions are not easy to develop, and the processes and outcomes of collaboration may be imperfectly correlated. There is a small but growing literature that may reveal the best practices for developing partnerships and helping them to succeed in achieving desirable changes.

Interorganizational relations theory, discussed in Chapter Fourteen, articulates several stages for developing and sustaining community coalitions. The extent of the external control and the coalition structure affects task orientation, extent of conflict, and effectiveness of coalitions. Butterfoss, Goodman, and Wandersman (1996) studied the determinants of participation and satisfaction in coalitions for alcohol, tobacco, and other drug abuse prevention and these determinants' association with the quality of resultant plans. Community leadership, shared decision making, linkages with other organizations, and a positive organizational climate were correlated with participation and satisfaction among coalition members. However, neither these factors nor reports of satisfaction were related to the quality of coalition plans. Butterfoss and others suggest that their measure of "plan quality" was preliminary and that this might explain the negative findings. Nevertheless, these results remind us that a satisfied, active coalition does not guarantee effective products or results anymore than worker happiness guarantees greater productivity.

Collaborations take many forms and proceed in many different ways. For a coalition in Virginia that was advocating for public health efforts to reduce premature and preventable death and disability, diffusion of innovations theory was a valuable practical tool. It helped coalition members shape a work plan, guide their work with opinion leaders, tailor the innovation to achieve its objectives, and create information exchange relationships (Howze and Redman, 1992). Mobilization of a coalition in an African American community around tobacco control was achieved through heavy reliance on community-organizing and community-building strategies (Ellis, Reed, and Scheider, 1995).

Approaches to Defining Needs, Problems, and Aims

The roots of change efforts for health enhancement lie in the early phases of needs assessment or problem definition. Several philosophical and methodological questions for developing and implementing health promotion strategies are either explicitly decided or implicitly addressed when researchers and practitioners define needs, problems, and program aims or objectives. *Who* will decide what is a problem? What is the balance between professional (outsider or change agent) definition of needs and the lay or community (insider or target audience) expression of needs? The concepts of felt ownership, participation, and relevance are shared by community organization, organizational change, diffusion of innovations, and media communication studies, but their applications vary significantly.

Once needs or problems are defined (by whomever, by whatever methods), strategies are identified to achieve certain aims and objectives—usually to improve the situation or to prevent, reduce, or eliminate the problem(s). The questions that parallel these issues involve defining the appropriate or desirable outcome(s). Is a smoothly functioning participatory process sufficient in itself? Is awareness of a health issue or program a meaningful endpoint? Must we aim for improvements in specific health behaviors, health risks, or health status outcomes, or are these impacts compromised due to their narrow definition of physical health? Pressures for accountability for health improvement and even for cost savings are growing at the same time that some health promoters contend that these expectations are inappropriately narrow and limiting.

Indeed, a fundamental ideological conflict about the goal of health promotion has arisen: should health promotion improve health status or serve as an instrument of social change in general and social justice in particular (Robertson and Minkler, 1994)? Labonte (1994) comments that health promotion, while not a social movement per se, is a professional response to the challenges of social movements. He suggests that it is both empowering and disempowering, but critiques the narrow view that focuses on physical and categorical health outcomes as disempowering *unless* it is combined with a view of clients in terms of their family, community, and economic lives as well. The Healthy Cities movement, with its focus on citizen participation, community, information, problem solving, and shared power (Flynn, Ray, and Rider, 1994), embodies a view of health promotion as part of a large movement to improve the quality of life. Thus, some Healthy Cities projects focus on housing and unemployment and others focus on transportation, crime, drugs, pollution, or health education (Duhl, 1996).

It is unclear whether the health promotion efforts of Healthy Cities and related initiatives represent a broadening of the mission of health promotion, or merely a renaming of a collection of activities that include health promotion *as well as* health services, social welfare, human services, criminal justice, and urban planning. While professional training in health education and promotion usually includes community organization techniques, it may not equip graduates to be any more than consultants in these diverse areas. Robertson and Minkler (1994) suggest that what appears as an ideological conflict may be best understood as boundary issues and that health promotion benefits from using multiple frameworks. They stress the importance of evaluating and demonstrating the benefits (or lack thereof) of whichever methods are chosen, a point I will return to later.

Similarities Between Models

Each community and group intervention theory and model in Part Four of this second edition of *Health Behavior and Health Education* is distinctive in its perspective, emphasis, and research base. At the same time, there are many similarities among these models and also similarities between these models and the intrapersonal and interpersonal models of health behavior presented in Part Two and Part Three. This section highlights some of those similarities and the related differences in the models. It compares and contrasts (1) community organization and organizational change, (2) diffusion of innovations and organizational change, (3) diffusion of innovations and Social Cognitive Theory, and (4) diffusion of innovations and communication-persuasion models of attitude change. The question of stages, steps, and phases across models is also addressed. This chapter does not offer in-depth analyses of these related models because each comparison would require a chapter in itself (and these tasks have been accomplished in other books).

Community Organization and Organizational Change

Chapter Twelve presents key principles and models of community organization and community building along with the theoretical foundations that form a base for these activities. There is no single theory of community organization that applies adequately to health promotion work (Bracht, 1990). Rather, we must borrow from other theories (some of which are integral to the organizational change frameworks discussed in Chapter Fourteen). Social support theory, community development concepts, and network analysis are most pertinent to OD theory as a component of organizational change. Interorganizational relations theory is consonant with coalition building as it is used in community organizing. Another important consideration relates to the final stage of stage theory that Goodman, Steckler, and Kegler present. That phase, institutionalization, is the adoption of an innovation (a new idea or practice) as an ongoing part of an organization's structure and activities. The relationship to community organization lies in the virtual necessity to consider community organization principles (such as participation, relevance, and community competence) if institutionalization is to occur.

Diffusion of Innovations and Organizational Change

Chapters Thirteen and Fourteen put forth concepts from diffusion theory and organizational change that bear remarkable resemblance to one another. A reason for this similarity is that Oldenburg, Hardcastle, and Kok emphasize diffusion of health promotion innovations through organizational structures, notably health care settings and schools. Both chapters include multistage models (adoption, implementation, maintenance, and so on). Also, both describe trials of interventions to promote adoption, implementation, and institutionalization of health promotion strategies of demonstrated efficacy, with diffusion or organizational change occurring with varying degrees of success. A recent analysis of the diffusion of school-based drug abuse prevention programs by Rohrbach, D'Onofrio, Backer, and Montgomery (forthcoming) reflects a combined application of diffusion and organizational change theories, noting the need for different strategies at different stages of the diffusion process, system barriers to diffusion, and innovation barriers to diffusion.

Diffusion of Innovations and Social Cognitive Theory

Albert Bandura's 1986 volume on Social Cognitive Theory includes a chapter on social diffusion and innovation. In it, Bandura notes that "understanding how new ideas and social practices spread . . . has important bearing on personal and social change." Thus, even before the relatively recent attention to diffusion, the linkages between social learning (or cognition) and diffusion were set in place. The most apparent recent difference, reflected in the structure of this book, is that diffusion concepts and research emphasize social change (a macro function), whereas social learning emphasizes intrapersonal and interpersonal change (a micro function). Winett (1986) succinctly outlined some of the similarities and differences between social cognition and diffusion. Similarities include the focus on behavioral change, the importance of interpersonal networks for behavioral change, the essential role of information exchange, and the movement toward two-way influence processes. SCT and diffusion differ in their research traditions, as reflected in the dominant measurement methods and research designs; but they may be coming closer together, as seen in the two health care case studies in Chapter Thirteen. Historically, diffusion research has primarily involved naturalistic field surveys, whereas SCT research designs have been primarily experimental and often conducted in the laboratory. The difference mirrors the distinct conceptual perspectives of these two theories and exemplifies the way that macro models of behavioral change depart from intrapersonal and interpersonal approaches.

Diffusion of Innovations and Communication Persuasion

Diffusion frameworks are useful for understanding how the mass media contribute to the spread of innovations in populations. The phases of diffusion can also be examined as phases of psychological change in individuals. The correspondence suggests parallels between models of communication and persuasion on the one hand and information processing at the individual level and the community framework of adoption and diffusion on the other. Communications can be designed to promote effects on individuals at each stage of the individual models and disseminated to promote optimal diffusion in social systems (Rogers, 1983).

Stages, Steps, and Phases

The chapters on organizational change and diffusion of innovations (Chapter Twelve and Thirteen) include explicit discussions of staged models of organizational and social change. The innovation in the cardiovascular risk reduction case study in Chapter Thirteen also used a staged approach to health counseling by physicians. Chapter Fifteen, on communication theory, describes multistage processes as they apply to some of the communication models with relevance to public health. The influence of Lewin's work ([1942] 1951), in particular his stage model of unfreezing, moving, and refreezing, is basic to concepts of group and organizational change. The exact number of stages varies across the models. Goodman, Steckler, and Kegler propose the need for greater consensus on, or better specification of, the number of stages. While such consensus might add precision and clarity to a given model, it may also be arbitrary. The editors of this book believe that a pragmatic approach serves well at this stage of the field: the number of stages (steps, or phases) should fit the situation and behavior, while striving for as much parsimony as possible without losing meaning.

Research Issues

Each of the theories and action models presented in Part Four is complex and multimodal and aims to influence not only large groups of individuals but organizational structures as well. An assessment of the impact of interventions based on these frameworks typically requires more complex and less-controlled evaluation designs than the designs used at the intrapersonal or interpersonal level. Evaluations may also require surveying unusually large numbers of people in order to allow detection of statistically significant differences, especially if organizations or communities are used as the unit of randomization and analysis. Further, access to information at the organizational level may be difficult to obtain and even more difficult to validate, given the divergent perspectives of organizations' managers and workers or members and constituents (or clients).

Action research has been proposed as an integral approach to intervention and evaluation when community or organizational change is attempted. The participatory research methods often used in action research include active roles for clients or consumers in defining their own health needs, setting priorities, and evaluating health improvement efforts (Green and others, 1995). These methods are consistent with community participation, shared decision making, and facilitating ownership of change strategies, but they also pose great challenges in establishing valid and unbiased results from evaluations. Community intervention research and evaluation require a balance of scientific rigor and community dynamics with ethical concerns (Glanz, Rimer, and Lerman, 1996). Partnership research models are not all-or-nothing phenomena; they are continua with varying degrees of community and scientist participation and control (Glanz, Rimer, and Lerman, 1996).

The use of both quantitative hypothesis-testing research methods and qualitative methods is illustrated in each chapter in Part Four. These methods complement each other (Janz and others, 1996; McKinlay, 1993), and both lend strength to an understanding of the processes and impacts of health promotion efforts. New developments in measurement are increasing our toolbox of community-level indicators (Cheadle and others, 1992), thus enabling better assessments of whether environments have changed and closer examination of the associations between individual- and community-level effects.

Additional research challenges involve the study of community change and societal change as two-way processes, the need to attend to personal influence as well as the content of interventions, and the need to ensure that evaluation occurs prospectively, thus minimizing bias and ensuring that valuable information is not lost. We have an obligation to use our professional skills and resources for high-quality evaluation, even in the most process-driven change efforts. Models that work warrant wide dissemination, and models and strategies that are ineffective need to be improved or discarded. It is a disservice to health promotion's constituents to promulgate models based on ideology alone if they are not useful in achieving worthwhile aims.

Conclusion

Societal, community, and institutional factors are critical to promoting health because certain of them can provide a fertile environment for health enhancement and directly shape individuals' health behavior. The power of policy is evident in health education settings such as workplaces and schools. Both broad social changes and specific organizational and governmental policies have been linked to individual behavior and perceptions. The impact of social historical events on individuals is complex: such events appear to interact with individual receptivity to change as reflected in life stages and other key developmental markers. Their impacts can be seen, for example, in changes in women's work, family roles, and health behavior as certain social historical events differentially influence each generation of women (Stewart and Healy, 1989).

Macro-level approaches of health education and health promotion can complement intrapersonal and interpersonal approaches. Blended models suggest integrated strategies for reaching various units of practice in communitywide programs. Some health issues—for example, environmental protection through control of hazardous waste and infectious diseases—cannot be influenced through individual efforts alone. However, they may be affected positively through methods based on individual behavior analysis frameworks combined with two-way communication with public health leaders and media efforts to promote wide awareness and prompt community action (Glanz and Yang, 1996; Weinstein and Sandman, 1993).

The integration of group, organizational, and community intervention frameworks with individual and interpersonal models of health behavior has potential for real-world impact that will exceed the use of any one approach. Our most challenging public health problems require increased attention to organizational and environmental factors. Because behavior is highly influenced by settings, rules, organizational policy, community norms, and opportunities for action, changes in these factors are promising targets for change. Individual change will follow successful organizational and environmental changes (Winett, 1995).

Ideally, comprehensive health promotion efforts build on strategies that have been tried and found effective for reaching health and health behavior goals. However, although particular strategies have been shown effective in many behavioral arenas (the marketing and political arenas, for example), there are currently few health issues for which a variety of demonstrably effective strategies are known. Smoking prevention and control is one of the few areas for which effective interventions have been developed and evaluated at each level of change (Advocacy

Institute, 1989). It is to be hoped that the armamentarium of effective strategies for other health behaviors will grow to the same level.

The theories and methods of community organization and community building, diffusion of innovations, organizational change, and media communication provide a strong foundation for understanding and positively influencing health behavior. Advances in research will clarify the operational mechanisms of these theories and models and refine our understanding of how best to use them. Health education and health promotion strategies will achieve greater success through informed application of these frameworks for social activation and community attitude and behavior change.

References

Advocacy Institute. *Action Handbook for Tobacco Control.* Washington, D.C.: Advocacy Institute, 1989.

Bandura, A. *Social Foundations of Thought and Action: A Social Cognitive Theory.* Englewood Cliffs, N.J.: Prentice Hall, 1986.

Bracht, N. (ed.). *Health Promotion at the Community Level.* Thousand Oaks, Calif.: Sage, 1990.

Butterfoss, F. D., Goodman, R. M., and Wandersman, A. "Community Coalitions for Prevention and Health Promotion: Factors Predicting Satisfaction, Participation, and Planning." *Health Education Quarterly,* 1996, *23*(1), 65–79.

Cheadle, A., and others. "Environmental Indicators: A Tool for Evaluating Community-Based Health-Promotion Programs." *American Journal of Preventive Medicine,* 1992, *8*(6), 345–350.

Duhl, L. "An Ecohistory of Health: The Role of 'Healthy Cities.'" *American Journal of Health Promotion,* 1996, *10*(4), 258–261.

Ellis, G., Reed, D., and Scheider, H. "Mobilizing a Low-Income African American Community Around Tobacco Control: A Force Field Analysis." *Health Education Quarterly,* 1995, *22*(4), 443–457.

Flynn, B., Ray, D., and Rider, M. "Empowering Communities: Action Research Through Healthy Cities." *Health Education Quarterly,* 1994, *21*(3), 395–405.

Glanz, K., Rimer, B. K., and Lerman, C. "Ethical Issues in the Design and Conduct of Community-Based Intervention Studies." In S. Coughlin and T. Beauchamp (eds.), *Ethics in Epidemiology.* New York: Oxford University Press, 1996.

Glanz, K., and Yang, H. "Communicating About Risk of Infectious Diseases." *Journal of the American Medical Association,* 1996, *275*(3), 253–256.

Green, L. W., and others. *Study of Participatory Research in Health Promotion: Review and Recommendations for the Development of Participatory Research in Health Promotion in Canada.* Vancouver: University of British Columbia, 1995.

Himmelman, A. T. "On the Theory and Practice of Transformational Collaboration: Collaboration as a Bridge from Social Service to Social Justice." *Communities Working Collaboratively for Change.* Minneapolis, Minn.: Himmelman Consulting Group, 1992.

Hovland, C. I., Janis, I. L., and Kelley, H. H. *Communication and Persuasion: Psychological Studies of Opinion Change.* Westport, Conn.: Greenwood Press, 1953.

Howze, E. H., and Redman, L. J. "The Uses of Theory in Health Advocacy: Policies and Programs." *Health Education Quarterly,* 1992, *19*(3; special issue: *Roles and Uses of Theory in Health Education Practice*), 369–383.

Janz, N. K., and others. "Evaluation of 37 AIDS Prevention Projects: Successful Approaches and Barriers to Program Effectiveness." *Health Education Quarterly,* 1996, *23*(1), 80–97.

Kipnis, D. "Accounting for the Use of Behavior Technologies in Social Psychology." *American Psychologist,* 1994, *49*(3), 165–172.

Labonte, R. "Health Promotion and Empowerment: Reflections on Professional Practice." *Health Education Quarterly,* 1994, *21*(2), 253–268.

Lasswell, H. D. "The Structure and Function of Communication in Society." In L. Bryson (ed.), *The Communication of Ideas.* New York: Institute for Religious and Social Studies, 1948.

Lewin, K. "Field Theory and Learning." In K. Lewin, *Field Theory in Social Science: Select Theoretical Papers* (D. Cartwright, ed.). New York: HarperCollins, 1951. (Originally published 1942.)

McKinlay, J. B. "The Promotion of Health Through Planned Sociopolitical Change: Challenges for Research and Policy." *Social Science and Medicine,* 1993, *36*(2), 109–117.

Rimer, B. K., Glanz, K., and Lerman, C. "Contributions of Public Health to Patient Compliance." *Journal of Community Health,* 1991, *16*(4), 225–240.

Robertson, A., and Minkler, M. "New Health Promotion Movement: A Critical Examination." *Health Education Quarterly,* 1994, *21*(3), 295–312.

Rogers, E. M. *Diffusion of Innovations.* (3rd ed.) New York: Free Press, 1983.

Rohrbach, L. A., D'Onofrio, C., Backer, T., and Montgomery, S. "Diffusion of School-Based Substance Abuse Prevention Programs." *American Behavioral Scientist,* forthcoming.

Rothman, J., and Tropman, J. E. "Models of Community Organization and Macro Practice: Their Mixing and Phasing." In F. M. Cox, J. L. Erlich, J. Rothman, and J. E. Tropman (eds.), *Strategies of Community Organization.* (4th ed.) Itasca, Ill.: Peacock, 1987.

Schmid, T. L., Pratt, M., and Howze, E. H. "Policy as Intervention: Environmental and Policy Approaches to the Prevention of Cardiovascular Disease." *American Journal of Public Health,* 1995, *85*(9), 1207–1211.

Stewart, A., and Healy, J. "Linking Individual Development and Social Changes." *American Psychologist,* 1989, *44*, 30–42.

Wallack, L. "Media Advocacy: Promoting Health Through Mass Communication." In K. Glanz, F. M. Lewis, and B. K. Rimer (eds.), *Health Behavior and Health Education: Theory, Research, and Practice.* San Francisco: Jossey-Bass, 1990.

Weinstein, N. D., and Sandman, P. M. "Some Criteria for Evaluating Risk Messages." *Risk Analysis,* 1993, *13*(1), 103–114.

Winett, R. A. *Information and Behavior: Systems of Influence.* Hillsdale, N.J.: Erlbaum, 1986.

Winett, R. A. "A Framework for Health Promotion and Disease Prevention Programs." *American Psychologist,* 1995, *50*(5), 341–350.

PART FIVE

USING THEORY IN RESEARCH AND PRACTICE

Karen Glanz

One of the greatest challenges for public health professionals is to learn to analyze the "fit" of a theory or model for issues and populations with which they are working. A working knowledge of a handful of theories and how they have been applied is the first step. Mastering the challenges of using theories appropriately and effectively is the logical next step. Effective practice depends on marshaling the most appropriate theory or theories and practice strategies for a given situation. Theory-based research and evaluation further require appropriate designs, measures, and procedures for the health problem, organization, and unique population at hand.

No one theory or model will be right in all cases. Depending on the unit of practice and type of health behavior or issue, different theoretical frameworks will have a good fit and be practical and useful. Often, more than one theory is needed to adequately address an issue. For comprehensive health promotion programs, this is almost always true. It is also evident in the use and description of applied theories in the professional literature.

The preceding sections of this book make clear that theories often overlap and that some actually fit easily within broader models. Theories are often most effective if they are integrated within a comprehensive planning framework. Such a system assigns a central role to research, as input to determine the situation and needs of the population to be served, the resources available, and the progress and effectiveness of the program at various stages. Planning is a continual process, in which new information is constantly being gathered to build or improve the program.

Part Five gives specific examples of combining theories for greater impact. Two well-developed planning models that can be used to integrate and apply diverse theoretical frameworks are discussed in this section. In Chapter Seventeen, Gielen and McDonald describe the PRECEDE-PROCEED planning model for health promotion planning and present a case study of theory-driven program planning that used this model for a comprehensive injury prevention program at a well-child clinic. In Chapter Eighteen, Lefebvre and Rochlin describe the key components and methods of social marketing. They illustrate its application in a federal breast cancer education program and a program for the social marketing of Vitamin A–rich foods in Thailand.

Chapter Nineteen, by Sallis and Owen, describes the current status of ecological models for health promotion and proposes principles that should be followed if these models are to contribute substantially to health promotion research and practice. This chapter clarifies the various ecological models that have been advanced and their historical development and implications. Because ecological models are emerging comprehensive frameworks for health promotion, the authors focus on needs for greater clarity, precision, and understanding about how these models operate.

In Chapter Twenty, Pasick addresses moderating factors in developing, selecting, and applying health behavior theory in practice and research—namely, cultural and socioeconomic factors. She challenges all health professionals to become aware of the importance of these characteristics of individuals and communities and elucidates how theories can and should assist practitioners and researchers in developing programs responsive to and appropriate for diverse populations. She provides applied examples that deal with cancer control for Asian, Pacific Islander, and Latina populations living in California.

Chapter Twenty-One summarizes key issues from each of the four preceding chapters, comments on the state of the art, and discusses emerging developments and challenges.

Using theory thoughtfully and appropriately is not simple but it can be most rewarding. Our aim in Part Five is to bring together many constructs and models and equip readers to work effectively with them in their own practice settings.

CHAPTER SEVENTEEN

THE PRECEDE-PROCEED
PLANNING MODEL

Andrea Carlson Gielen
Eileen M. McDonald

Individual theories, interpersonal theories, community change theories, pamphlets, videotapes, counseling, support groups, public service announcements, grassroots organizing—these represent but a few of the tools available to health professionals for designing, implementing, and evaluating health behavior change programs. The appropriate selection and application of these tools can mean the difference between program success and failure. Typically, a problem and target audience have been identified and the health professional wants to *do something* to fix the problem. Examples of problems include inappropriate use of urgent care facilities for nonurgent problems by health maintenance organization enrollees, low birth weight babies born to mothers in a specific urban area, and high rates of smoking among the pregnant women seen in a prenatal clinic. The health professional's ability to apply theories of health behavior is one of the most critical skills needed in designing programs to address such problems.

A planning model like PRECEDE-PROCEED can guide this process (Green, Kreuter, Deeds, and Partridge, 1980; Green and Kreuter, 1991). Unlike the theories

The SAFE Home Project of the Johns Hopkins University School of Public Health and the Johns Hopkins Children's Center is an intervention trial funded by the Maternal and Child Health Bureau of the U.S. Department of Health and Human Services, with additional support provided by the Johns Hopkins Center for Injury Research and Policy. The original needs assessment work was supported by the faculty development fund of the Johns Hopkins University.

described in previous chapters, PRECEDE-PROCEED is not a theory per se. It does not attempt to *predict or explain* the relationship among factors thought to be associated with an outcome of interest. Rather, it provides a structure for *applying theories*, so that the most appropriate intervention strategies can be identified and implemented. PRECEDE-PROCEED can be thought of as a *road map* and theories as the specific *routes* to a destination. The road map presents all the possible avenues, and the theory suggests certain avenues to follow. Even though the emphasis in PRECEDE-PROCEED is typically on service programs delivered in practice settings, the framework may be equally useful to researchers conducting health behavior change trials.

This chapter begins with an overview of PRECEDE-PROCEED that describes each step in the process and presents examples from the literature about the process as applied to health promotion programs. In the second section of the chapter, we present a case study of theory-driven program planning that employed the PRECEDE-PROCEED planning model to develop a comprehensive injury prevention program for a well-child clinic. The objectives of the chapter are to enable readers to use PRECEDE-PROCEED to choose and apply relevant behavioral change theories in their work, and to incorporate into a PRECEDE-PROCEED planning process the constructs from individual-, interpersonal-, and community-level theories and models presented in previous chapters.

Overview of PRECEDE-PROCEED

The PRECEDE-PROCEED framework originated in the 1970s and was developed to enhance the quality of health education interventions by offering practitioners a systematic planning process. The acronym stands for Predisposing, Reinforcing, and Enabling Constructs in Educational Diagnosis and Evaluation, and the model is based on the premise that just as medical diagnosis precedes a treatment plan, so should educational diagnosis precede an intervention plan (Green, Kreuter, Deeds, and Partridge, 1980). In 1991, PROCEED (Policy, Regulatory, and Organizational Constructs in Educational and Environmental Development) was added to the framework, in recognition of the emergence of and need for health promotion interventions that go beyond traditional educational approaches to changing unhealthy behaviors (Green and Kreuter, 1991) (Figure 17.1).

The PRECEDE-PROCEED model is a nine-phase process that begins with the proposition that health behaviors are complex, multidimensional, and influenced by a variety of factors. While PRECEDE-PROCEED is not considered a behavioral theory per se, it is a conceptual framework for practice, or a planning model (see

FIGURE 17.1. PRECEDE-PROCEED PLANNING MODEL.

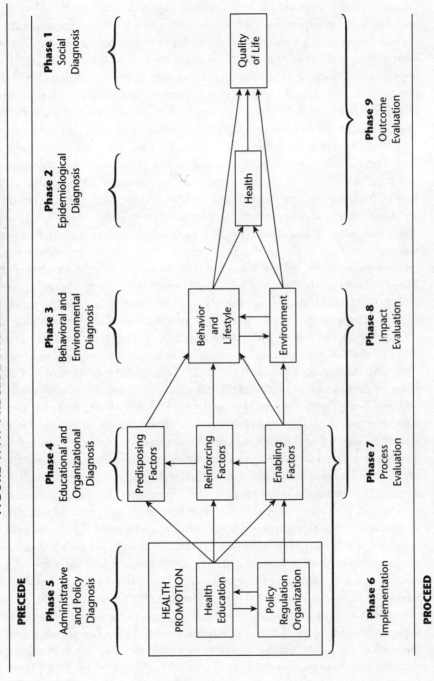

Source: Green and Kreuter, 1991, p. 24.

Chapter Two). Its systematic approach offers specific guidelines for priority setting, and with its aid, intervention resources can be more efficiently and effectively used. For example, a well-constructed public service announcement might help inform the public about the health consequences of a high-fat diet yet be an inappropriate strategy for teaching low-fat cooking skills. A planning model can indicate this kind of appropriateness or inappropriateness. Without a careful analysis of the extent to which a target population lacks knowledge or skills, program resources can be misdirected and the impact of the program compromised.

The planning process outlined in PRECEDE-PROCEED also rests on a practice fundamental, the principle of participation. The principle of participation states that success in achieving change is enhanced by the active participation of members of the target audience in defining their own high-priority problems and goals and in developing and implementing solutions (Green and Kreuter, 1991; Minkler, 1990; Freudenberg and others, 1995). This principle derives from the community development roots of the profession as well as the empowerment education models exemplified by Freire's early work and by the more recent work of Wallerstein, Minkler, Israel, and others (see Chapter Twelve). Accordingly, at each phase in a PRECEDE-PROCEED diagnosis, efforts should be made to include the target audience in all aspects of program planning, implementation, and evaluation.

PROCEED, the recent addition to PRECEDE, highlights another overarching tenet of the diagnostic process—that is, the important role of environmental factors as determinants of health and health behaviors. Over the past two decades, it has become clear that individual lifestyles contribute significantly to public health and well-being (McGinnis and Foege, 1993). Patterns of diet and exercise, use of cigarettes and alcohol, sexual practices, and stress all have been linked to greater or lesser longevity and quality of life. While these are considered individual behaviors, it is also true that they are not wholly volitional behaviors. Rather, they are in many ways influenced by powerful forces outside of the individual, such as industry, the media, politics, and social inequities. Recognition and understanding of this larger context that constrains or facilitates individual behavior is a hallmark of health promotion programming and a central focus of ecological approaches to health promotion (see Chapter Nineteen). Through a series of diagnostic steps, the PRECEDE-PROCEED planning model facilitates consideration of both individual and environmental factors that influence health and health behaviors. The model begins at the end, focusing on the outcome of interest, and works backward to determine how best to achieve that outcome. Descriptions of the components of PRECEDE-PROCEED presented here are summarized from the work of the model's creators, and readers are referred to their books for more detailed information (Green, Kreuter, Deeds, and Partridge, 1980; Green and Kreuter, 1991).

Phase 1: Social Diagnosis

The purpose of a social diagnosis is to determine people's perceptions of their own needs and quality of life. At this stage, the planners expand their understanding of the community in which they are working by conducting multiple data collection activities such as interviews with key opinion leaders, focus groups with members of the community, observations, and surveys. The term *community* is typically used to mean a geographical area with defined boundaries. However, it may also be used in a more general sense to describe a group with shared characteristics, interests, values, and norms (see Chapter Twelve).

There are many reasons why a social diagnosis is important. First, the relationship between health and quality of life is reciprocal, with each affecting the other. For example, living in poverty is associated with poor health and being unhealthy makes it more difficult to escape impoverished living conditions. Related to this is the notion that health is an instrumental value rather than a terminal value. That is, people value their health because being healthy enables them to achieve other goals, such as enjoying work and recreation. Finally, by understanding the target population's concerns, practitioners design a program that is relevant to the intended audience, thus increasing the chances that the program will be well received and effective.

At this phase of the program-planning process, community organization theories and principles are relevant (Table 17.1). Community organization "emphasizes the active participation and the development of communities that can better evaluate and solve health and social problems" (Glanz and Rimer, 1995). Minkler's work (1985) in the Tenderloin Project with low-income elderly and Eng and Blanchard's work (1991) conducting a community action diagnosis in a rural county are good examples of the importance of social diagnosis and its use of community-organizing strategies.

Phase 2: Epidemiological Diagnosis

An epidemiological diagnosis helps planners determine which health problems are most important for which target groups in a community. Using a *reductionist* approach, the planner takes information on the most important quality-of-life concerns that emerged from the social diagnosis and identifies the contributing health problems. Using an *expansionist* approach, the planner begins with an important health problem that is then linked to a quality-of-life concern. The latter approach has been more commonly used, primarily because funding is typically available for specific health problems and target populations.

Even when starting with an epidemiological diagnosis, it is important to identify the related quality-of-life concerns because that helps ensure that limited resources

TABLE 17.1. PRECEDE-PROCEED AS AN ORGANIZING FRAMEWORK FOR APPLICATION OF THEORY AND PRINCIPLES.

Change Theories and Principles by Level of Change	*PRECEDE-PROCEED Planning Phases*				
	Phase 1 Social Diagnosis	Phase 2 Epidemiological Diagnosis	Phase 3 Behavioral and Environmental Diagnosis	Phase 4 Educational and Organizational Diagnosis	Phase 5 Administrative and Policy Diagnosis
Community level					
Participation and relevance	X	X	X	X	X
Community organization	X		X		
Organizational change				X	X
Diffusion of innovations				X	X
Interpersonal level					
Social Cognitive Theory			X	X	
Adult learning				X	
Interpersonal communication				X	
Individual level					
Health Belief Model				X	
Stages of change			X	X	
Theory of Reasoned Action				X	
Theory of Planned Behavior			X	X	
Information processing				X	

Source: Adapted from Glanz and Rimer, 1995.

are being used to address health problems that contribute significantly to larger societal priorities. Epidemiological diagnosis typically does not draw on specific theories (Table 17.1), although to the extent that the community is involved in the process of choosing the health problems to be addressed, community-level theories do apply.

In an epidemiological diagnosis, it is often useful to conduct secondary data analysis, using existing data sources (vital statistics, state and national health surveys, medical and administrative records, and the like). These data provide indicators of morbidity and mortality in a population and can specify subgroups at particularly high risk. Characteristics of these subgroups can include age, gender, ethnicity, occupation, education, income, family structure, geographical location, and so on. Sometimes it is inappropriate to extrapolate from national data to a smaller region, and original data collection will be necessary. For example, household surveys in a nationally representative sample may have inadequate numbers of respondents from a single state to provide reliable state data. Data collection and analysis for an epidemiological diagnosis should yield reliable and valid indicators for setting measurable objectives for the program.

With data on the community's health problems in hand, the planner is ready to begin setting priorities and writing program goals. Decisions should be guided by the desires of the community members themselves, with consideration given to health problems with the greatest impact, those that have been previously underserved, and those for which solutions are realistically available. The program goal will be a statement of the program's ultimate benefit (for example, "Improve infant health by reducing infant mortality"), whereas program objectives should answer specific questions. The question, "What health improvements will be achieved, in whom, by when?" for example, might be answered by this objective: "Infant mortality will be reduced by 25 percent in County X by the year 2000." Measurable program objectives are essential to guide the allocation of resources and to evaluate the program's success. (Note, however, that sometimes specific program objectives cannot be established until after phase 3 or phase 4.) The availability of national and regional policy documents should be investigated for the guidance these documents offer in setting reasonable targets for change. For example, in the United States, the Public Health Service's year 2000 health objectives for the nation provide data and objectives for the major health problems across the United States (U.S. Department of Health and Human Services, 1991).

Phase 3: Behavioral and Environmental Diagnosis

The purpose of phase 3 is to identify the behavioral and environmental determinants of (or risk factors for) the health problem selected in phase 2. Behavioral factors are those behaviors or lifestyles of the individuals at risk that contribute to the occurrence and severity of the health problem. The environmental factors are those social and physical factors that are external to the individual, often beyond his or her personal control, that can be modified to support the behavior or influence the health outcome. For example, elevated serum cholesterol is a function of a high-fat diet (behavioral factor) that in turn is affected by the lack of available low-fat food choices (environmental factor). While biological and genetic factors certainly contribute to health problems, these are not changeable through a health promotion program. Such factors are carefully considered, however, in determining target groups that can benefit most from interventions (for example, a breast cancer screening program might focus on reaching women at high risk due to family history of the disease).

Using theory, literature, and the wisdom of the planning group, an inventory should be made of influential behavioral and environmental factors. Interpersonal theories of behavior change can be useful at this stage of applying the PRECEDE-PROCEED framework because of the emphasis on the interaction between individuals and their environments. For example, Social Cognitive Theory posits that behavior, cognition, other personal factors, and environment have reciprocal relationships, influencing one another continually (Bandura, 1986). In addition, individual behavior is thought to be influenced by learning that takes place from observing others and by receiving reinforcement for behavioral change. Both of these influences speak to the importance of the individual's social environment. Thus, at this stage of the diagnosis, the planner should consider ways in which these constructs help specify behavioral and environmental factors that contribute to the health problem of interest. For example, in planning a program to reduce low birth weight, it should be considered whether there are women in the community who model appropriate use of prenatal care and whether community leaders and health professionals reinforce that model.

Each of the enumerated factors is rated in terms of its importance to the health problem. The most important factors are those that are highly prevalent or strongly associated with the health problem. Principles derived from community organization theory (for example, participation and relevance) apply here to assure that selected factors are indeed important to the target population.

Each factor is then rated in terms of changeability. Theories of organizational change, community organization, and diffusion of innovations are helpful for estimating changeability of environmental influences. Organizational change theories are relevant if the policies of formal organizations have been identified as an environmental factor (Ross and Mico, 1980): for example, in a worksite, organizational policies restricting smoking may need to be made more restrictive or be better enforced. In this situation, planners need to understand the process of changing organizational policy if they are to make a reasonable estimate of the changeability of tobacco control policies. Community organization may be used to effect change in environmental conditions that directly influence individuals' health or their health behaviors. Similarly, diffusion of innovations theory describes and predicts the process by which new ideas are adopted. If, for example, the diagnosis at this point suggests that a potential behavioral factor is bicycle helmet use, then an evaluation of its changeability (according to diffusion theory) should consider such features as the relative advantage, compatibility with existing norms, and observability of helmet use.

Intervention targets are chosen by combining importance and changeability ratings. Directing program resources toward those factors that are most important and most changeable helps to ensure program efficiency and effectiveness. Finally, measurable objectives are written to specify the desired behavioral impact (How much of what will be changed by when?) or environmental change (Who will do how much of what by when?).

Phase 4: Educational and Organizational Diagnosis

After planners select the appropriate behavioral and environmental factors for intervention, phase 4 identifies those antecedent and reinforcing factors that initiate and sustain the change process. Green and Kreuter (1991) classify these factors as predisposing, reinforcing, and enabling and note that collectively, they increase the likelihood that behavioral and environmental change will occur. *Predisposing factors* are the antecedents that provide the rationale or motivation for a behavior. They include individuals' knowledge, attitudes, beliefs, personal preferences, existing skills, and self-efficacy beliefs. *Reinforcing factors* are those elements that appear subsequent to the behavior and that provide continuing reward or incentive for the behavior to become persistent. Examples of such factors are social support, peer influence, significant others, and vicarious reinforcement. *Enabling factors* are antecedents that enable (allow) motivation to be realized; they can affect behavior directly or indirectly through an environmental factor. They include the programs, services, and resources necessary for behavioral and environmental outcomes to be realized and, in some cases, the new skills needed to enable behavior change. As in the previous diagnostic step, these factors are enumerated, rated in terms of importance and changeability, and priority targets for intervention are selected. Finally, measurable objectives are written: How many will know, believe, or be able to do what by when? How much of what resource will be available to whom by when? This process, as in all the previous diagnostic steps, should be driven by a thorough knowledge of the relevant empirical literature, an understanding of theory, and input from the specific target population.

All three levels of health behavior theories—community, interpersonal, individual—can be useful at this stage of the diagnostic process. For example, planners of a program to promote maternal and infant health through family planning may identify negative attitudes toward contraception as a predisposing factor to be changed. However, these negative attitudes may in fact be the result of deeply held religious beliefs in the community, making them inappropriate targets for change. Without adherence to the principles of participation and relevance included in community-organizing theory, planners could easily misdirect program resources and alienate the community.

By contrast, in a community with high teen pregnancy and sexually transmitted disease (STD) rates, community norms may support contraception, but teens may lack access to confidential, sensitive health services. In this case, organizational change theories will provide more effective guidance than will individually oriented theories. Individually oriented theories would suggest ways to change predisposing beliefs, when these are already favorable. Alternatively, organizational change theories would suggest ways to enable the delivery of services to the target population. Enhancing the delivery of services, whether through organizations such as on-site school-based clinics or other structures in the community, would require a thorough understanding of the selected organization's policies, procedures, and ability to change.

In another example, planners of a program to promote bicycle helmet use might learn from their community and the literature that children find helmets uncomfortable, fear "looking nerdy," and believe that they will not get hurt on their bikes. This would suggest, from a diffusion theory perspective, that the relative advantage, compatibility, and observability attributes of the helmet need to be addressed, in efforts to shape more favorable predisposing factors within the community. Drawing also on Social Cognitive Theory, these findings suggest that social influence plays an important role in both predisposing and reinforcing helmet use. The personal belief that bike riding poses no risks suggests that an individual-level theory such as the Health Belief Model (Janz and Becker, 1984) will help bike riders understand the factors associated with helmet use. The Health Belief Model includes the construct of perceived susceptibility, which in this case appears to be an important predisposing factor for helmet use.

The reason for making determinations about the relative importance of predisposing, reinforcing, and enabling factors and for incorporating different theoretical orientations is to choose appropriate points of intervention and appropriate strategies. In general, individual-level theories are most appropriate for addressing predisposing factors, and they help the planner identify communication messages for media and face-to-face encounters. Interpersonal-level theories are most appropriate for reinforcing factors, and they suggest communication channels (for example, significant others and social networks) and methods (for example, incentives and social support). Community-level theories are most appropriate for enabling factors, and they suggest environmental changes (for example, organization and delivery of services; availability of products; and policies, laws, and regulations that govern products and behaviors) and strategies such as advocacy and redesign of products or hazards. Due to the complexity of lifestyle-related health problems typically addressed by health promotion programs, multiple levels of factors and strategies are generally needed. Combining ideas from various theoretical orientations into a comprehensive program is a hallmark of most effective health promotion interventions.

Phase 5: Administrative and Policy Diagnosis

Delineating the intervention strategies and final planning for their implementation occurs in the phase known as administrative and policy diagnosis. Its purpose is to identify the policies, resources, and circumstances prevailing in a program's organizational context that could facilitate or hinder program implementation. Green and Kreuter (1991) define the PRO in PROCEED as follows: *policy* is the set of objectives and rules guiding the activities of an organization or administration; *regulation* is the act of implementing policies and enforcing rules or laws; and *organization* is the bringing together and the coordination of resources necessary to implement a program.

At this stage, the intervention strategies are enumerated based on the previous diagnostic steps, and the planner must now assess the availability of necessary resources (time, people, funding, and so on). Barriers to implementation such as staff commitment or lack of space should be assessed, and plans to address them put in place. Also, any organizational policies or regulations that could affect program implementation should be considered and planned for accordingly. Administrative and policy diagnosis is specific to the context of the program and the sponsoring organization(s) and requires political savvy as much as theoretical or empirical knowledge.

Administrative and policy diagnoses can be informed by theories, particularly community-level theories. Community organization theories encourage health planners to involve key community members. The definition and identification of those key members will differ for every community and health issue. Organizational change theory informs public health practitioners about the processes and strategies for creating and sustaining changes in health policies and procedures that influence the success of health promotion programs.

Phases 6 to 9: Implementation and Evaluation

At this point, the health promotion program is ready for implementation (phase 6). Data collection plans should be in place for evaluating the process, impact, and outcome of the program, the final three steps in the PRECEDE-PROCEED planning model (phases 7, 8, and 9). Typically, process evaluation determines the extent to which the program was implemented according to protocol. Impact evaluation assesses change in predisposing, reinforcing, and enabling factors, as well as in the behavioral and environmental factors. Finally, outcome evaluation determines the effect of the program on health and quality of life indicators. Generally, the measurable objectives that are written at each step of the PRECEDE-PROCEED planning model serve as milestones against which accomplishments are evaluated. Because the emphasis in this chapter is on the application of theory to program planning, the details of these steps will not be reviewed. Rather, their application will be described in a case study.

Summary of PRECEDE-PROCEED

PRECEDE-PROCEED is a widely used planning model that has guided the design of programs for numerous health problems (Morisky and others, 1983; Worden and others, 1990; Bertera, 1990, 1993; Windsor, 1986; Windsor and others, 1993; Eriksen and Gielen, 1983; Rimer, 1995; Gielen, 1992; Green, 1994). It has also been incorporated into national policy documents for community health (Centers for Disease Control, 1992) and injury control (National Committee for Injury Prevention and Control, 1989). Programs that have used this model and demonstrated significant improvements in health indicators include interventions for high blood pressure control (Morisky and others, 1983), breast cancer screening (Rimer, 1995), breast self-examination (Worden and others, 1990), smoking cessation (Windsor and others, 1993), worksite health promotion (Bertera, 1993), and correct use of car safety seats (Gielen, Bernstein-Cohen, and Radius, 1985).

Evaluation and Critique

Because PRECEDE-PROCEED is an integrative planning model that includes constructs from numerous other theories, it has not been systematically evaluated in comparison with other theoretical models of health behavior, with one exception, a study conducted by Mullen, Hersey, and Iverson (1987). In a longitudinal study of 326 adults who were interviewed twice over an eight-month interval, Mullen, Hersey, and Iverson compared PRECEDE, the Health Belief Model, and the Theory of Reasoned Action in terms of their predictive power, parsimony, acceptability to respondents, and specificity for program planning. The outcomes were self-reported changes in smoking, exercise, and consumption of sweet and fried foods. The results demonstrated that PRECEDE explained more of the variance in all outcomes (except attempts to quit smoking), and it was the most inclusive of the models, although it required a considerably larger number of variables than the Health Belief Model. The study concluded that PRECEDE "can sensitize the planner to draw on certain categories of variables, particularly the enabling and reinforcing. It does not, however, specify relationships. . . . In particular, the predisposing category is too broad to provide a basis for judging which types of variables ought to be emphasized." Despite its considerable success, potential users of PRECEDE-PROCEED should be aware of some of the challenges in applying it. The model is heavily data driven, and its application may require more substantial financial and human resources than are available in some situations. For example, Bertera's (1990) experience using the model for a worksite health promotion program in the DuPont company led him to conclude that smaller companies might have difficulty implementing the model because of the need for record keeping, survey capabilities, and skilled health education staff. An evaluation of four PATCH programs (which incorporate much of the PRECEDE-PROCEED model) found that the process of planning was slow and that those responsible needed substantial training or technical assistance to carry it out (Orenstein and others, 1992).

Case Study: The SAFE Home Project

This case study illustrates how the PRECEDE-PROCEED framework and social science theories were helpful in the development of the SAFE Home Project, an intervention trial aimed at reducing in-home childhood injuries among low-income inner-city families. This example highlights how the framework was used not only in program planning but also in applying and integrating social science theories within real-world constraints.

In practice, a new program must fit into an existing context. This program's context was the Johns Hopkins University School of Public Health and the Johns Hopkins Children's Center. Specifically, several faculty had a long-standing interest in the prevention of childhood injury and had collaborated on projects in the past. They supported and influenced the development of this program through their disciplinary expertise and professional roles, responsibilities, and access to resources. One such resource that was critical to this program was access to the pediatric primary care clinic that was to serve as the program's focal point. This outpatient continuity clinic provides medical care to children living in the East Baltimore community, one of the most impoverished areas of the city. The clinic also serves as a pediatric residency training site. Although the program was designed to serve this particular clinic's population, an overarching goal was that the intervention strategies developed would be generalizable to a variety of other pediatric care settings.

Social and Epidemiological Diagnosis (Phases 1 and 2)

The health problem (pediatric injuries) and its associated impact on quality of life were defined at the outset based on clinical observation, potential for change, professional interests, and funding priorities (Figure 17.2). Of particular interest were in-home injuries, because they are numerous, costly, and often preventable and because relatively simple prevention measures are available for parents.

The first two phases of PRECEDE-PROCEED—the social and epidemiological diagnoses—relied heavily on a review of the literature and the data on injuries among our target audience. Below is a sample of the data we found:

> Injury is the leading cause of death for children in the United States and children from birth to four years old are particularly vulnerable to injuries (Baker, O'Neill, Ginsburg, and Li, 1992).

> In 1985, there were over four million medically attended injuries (Rice and MacKenzie, 1989) and numerous nonmedically attended injuries among the preschool age population.

> Motor vehicle crashes are the leading cause of fatal injuries for preschoolers; falls, poisonings, and burns are the leading cause of their nonfatal injuries, and the majority of these latter injuries happen in and around home (Baker, O'Neill, Ginsburg, and Li, 1992; Rice and MacKenzie, 1989).

> The American Academy of Pediatrics recommends that pediatricians promote specific injury prevention practices to parents (American Academy of Pediatrics, 1994).

> The extent to which pediatricians provide injury prevention counseling is not known, although there are recent studies indicating that when provided, it can be effective (Bass and others, 1993; Miller and Galbraith, 1995).

We also assessed the prevalence of injuries in patients seen at either the pediatric clinic or at a pediatric emergency department for the year 1993. Both locations were selected because they are two of the clinical training sites for pediatric residents. More than six thousand injury diagnoses were made during this one-year period alone.

FIGURE 17.2. APPLICATION OF PRECEDE-PROCEED TO INJURY PREVENTION.

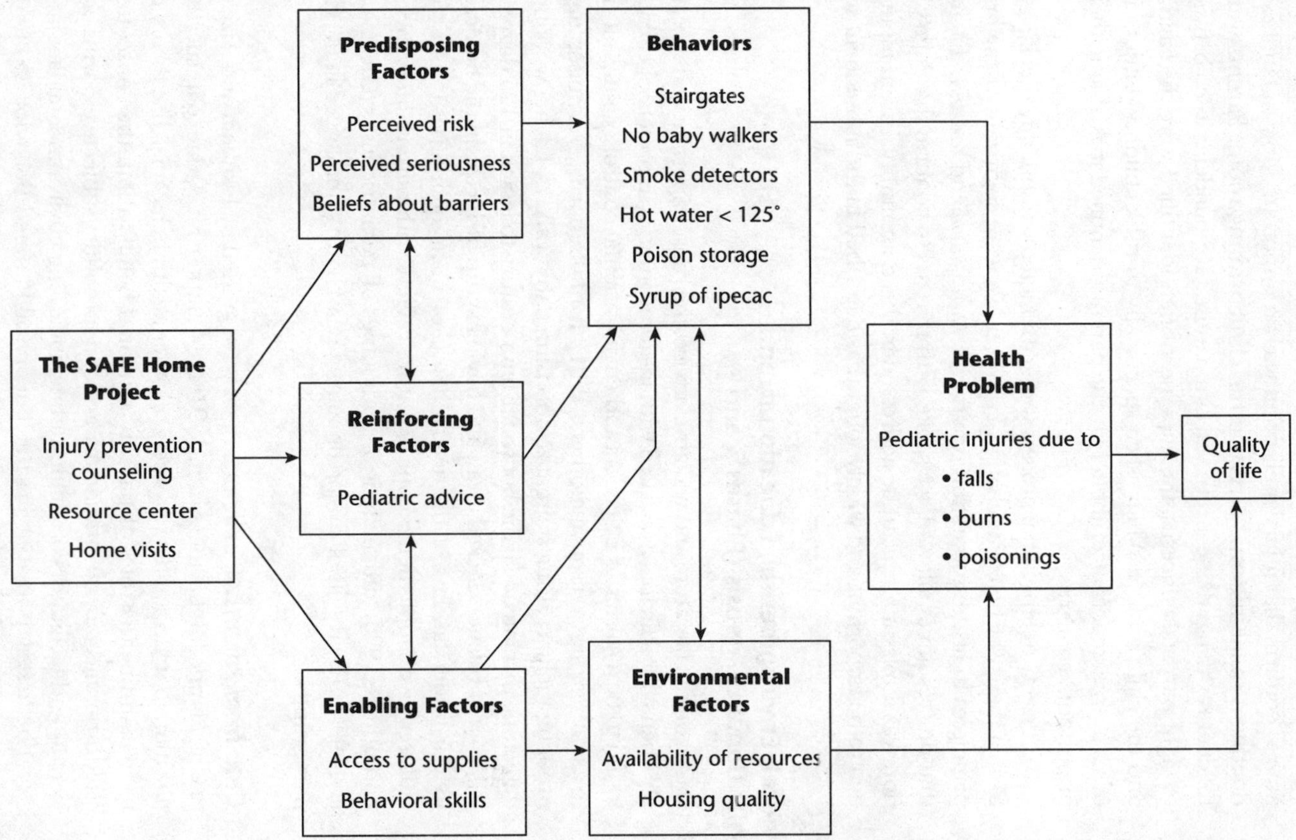

The SAFE Home Project

Injury prevention counseling

Resource center

Home visits

Predisposing Factors

Perceived risk

Perceived seriousness

Beliefs about barriers

Reinforcing Factors

Pediatric advice

Enabling Factors

Access to supplies

Behavioral skills

Behaviors

Stairgates

No baby walkers

Smoke detectors

Hot water < 125°

Poison storage

Syrup of ipecac

Environmental Factors

Availability of resources

Housing quality

Health Problem

Pediatric injuries due to
- falls
- burns
- poisonings

Quality of life

In preparing data collection instruments for the intervention trial, we were able to confirm that injury prevention was an important topic to families by conducting a small informal survey in the clinic waiting room. Parents were asked to identify "things that concern you as a parent." Respondents listed between three to eight parental concerns; the ones most often identified were the child's health and the child's safety. When asked specifically to rank childhood injury in terms of its overall importance, about half the parents identified it as among their "most important" concerns.

These two steps in the process were conducted without any specific guidance from a theory of behavior change. However, we were cognizant of the important principles in health promotion practice of *participation* and *relevance*. To the extent that our resources allowed, we spoke with parents to confirm that injury prevention was a relevant topic to be addressed in this community. Parent input continued to be important and widely sought, as described in the subsequent steps.

Behavioral, Environmental, Educational, and Organizational Diagnosis (Phases 3 and 4)

Based on the literature and pediatric advice, the most important and most changeable behavioral factors associated with in-home injuries in preschool children were found to be a cluster of behaviors and environmental controls, commonly referred to as *childproofing* (Wilson and others, 1991). For falls, burns, and poisonings, childproofing includes using stairgates, not using baby walkers, having working smoke detectors, turning down the hot water temperature to less than 125 degrees, keeping toxic substances locked away, and having syrup of ipecac in the home. To clarify our understanding of the determinants of in-home injuries to preschool age children, we supplemented our literature review with parent interviews (Gielen and others, 1995) and analysis of audiotapes of pediatric visits (Gielen and others, 1996). The results of this preliminary research are summarized in the following paragraphs.

Data from Parents. Parent interviews were guided by Fishbein and Ajzen's Theory of Planned Behavior (Ajzen, 1991; see Chapter Five), due to its successful application to understanding a variety of other health behaviors. The theory directed us to examine the roles of parents' personal beliefs about the consequences of childproofing, general attitude toward childproofing, subjective norms, and barriers to and facilitators of childproofing, including environmental factors.

The first step in applying the Theory of Planned Behavior was to conduct elicitation interviews with a sample that represented the target population. The elicitation interview used semistructured items to elicit parents' perceptions of childproofing—what the term meant to them, what its advantages and disadvantages and barriers and facilitators were, and whose opinions about childproofing were important to them. Responses to these elicitation interviews confirmed that parents understood the concept of childproofing and many of its specific behavioral components. Advantages included peace of mind and enhanced safety; few disadvantages were identified. Parents generated an extensive list of barriers and facilitators, most of which centered on the environmental factors associated with successful childproofing (for example, moving less often and knowing where to get supplies and materials). Parents commonly identified pediatricians (as well as family members) as people whose opinions about child safety mattered to them.

The results of these informal interviews were used to develop a structured interview that was administered to a convenience sample of 150 parents in the clinic (Gielen and others, 1995) to provide quantifiable data on parents' injury prevention practices (behavioral factors) and associated environmental factors, as well as predisposing, reinforcing, and enabling determinants.

We found that 88 percent of parents did not have syrup of ipecac, 63 percent did not know if their hot water temperature was at a safe setting, 59 percent did not use a stairgate, 27 percent did not have a smoke detector, and 11 percent did not store poisonous substances safely. Moreover, only 5 percent of respondents reported doing all five of the childproofing practices. Despite these low rates of safety practices, virtually all respondents expressed favorable personal beliefs and attitudes about childproofing and the majority reported positive subjective norms favoring childproofing. In terms of environmental factors, housing quality, income, and barriers to childproofing—such as having help from others and moving less often—were significantly associated with the number of childproofing practices reported.

Constructs from the Theory of Planned Behavior were helpful in demonstrating to us the importance of barriers in parental practices but did not help us identify key beliefs that distinguished parents who adopted the recommended childproofing from those who did not. We concluded that a risk-based theoretical orientation might be useful in this endeavor. The Health Belief Model (Chapter Three) and Weinstein's Precaution Adoption Model (1988; also see Chapter Seven) suggest that parents' perceptions of the *risk of injury* and the *salience of this threat* might better explain their adoption of safety practices.

From our data, we concluded that disadvantaged living conditions, including a lack of resources and skills, interfere with parents' ability to implement safety practices. Also, uniformly favorable attitudes and norms suggest that a risk-oriented theory may be more useful for understanding the individual-level factors associated with parents' safety practices.

Data from Pediatricians. One of the social environmental factors suggested by the parent interviews was that parents believed their pediatricians thought child-proofing was extremely important. Discussions among the project team, however, revealed that pediatricians did not receive much education in effective counseling about injury prevention during their residency training, and there was some question as to the extent to which pediatricians were actively encouraging parents. From a pragmatic standpoint, the role of the pediatrician was critical because the intervention being planned was going to be delivered in the clinic. From a theoretical standpoint, the role of the pediatrician was critical because there is strong empirical evidence that the communication style of physicians has an impact on patient outcomes and that adherence to principles of adult learning increases the likelihood of behavioral change (see Chapter Ten; Roter, 1989; U.S. Preventive Services Task Force, 1989; Green and Kreuter, 1991). Thus, we needed a better understanding of pediatricians' current injury prevention counseling skills and efforts.

In a prior study (of mental health issues), a member of the project team had audiotaped all pediatric medical visits to the clinic over a one-year period (Wissow, Roter, and Wilson, 1994). From these tapes, we selected all well-child visits for children under the age of five ($n = 214$) and developed a coding protocol to document the types of injury topics discussed and the communication skills used (Gielen and others, 1996). The majority (61 percent) of visits did not include any discussion of injury prevention. Among the remaining 83 visits in which families did receive some counseling, the average length of time spent on injury topics was 1.08 minutes per child. The most common communication pattern used by physicians was information giving, with little involvement of parents in any discussion.

From our analysis of these tapes, we concluded that injury prevention counseling was not a routine component of pediatric well-child care, potentially effective behavioral change counseling skills were not widely evident, and prioritizing injury topics and enhancing communication skills should help pediatricians use limited time more effectively and efficiently.

At this point in the PRECEDE-PROCEED process, data collection and planning had incorporated numerous theoretical constructs and principles of practice. Involvement of the target population included both the primary audience, parents, and an equally important secondary target audience, pediatricians. Both individual-level theories (the Theory of Planned Behavior, Health Belief Model, and Precaution Adoption Model) and principles derived from interpersonal-level theories (adult learning and interpersonal communication) were incorporated into the data collection and analysis strategies. A considerable amount of data had been generated: data about injury prevalence; data about parents' and medical residents' childproofing knowledge, attitudes, and practices; and data about residents' clinical skills related to injury prevention counseling. The PRECEDE-PROCEED model prompted us to organize the data into predisposing, enabling, and reinforcing factors. It was through this mechanism that we could explore possible interventions to influence health behavior that contributes to the selected health problem.

In the case of predisposing factors, we found both parents and pediatricians to have extremely favorable attitudes toward childproofing; however, little was known about our parents' perceptions of their child's risk to injury and their perceptions of the potential seriousness of injuries to their child's health. Moreover, our needs assessment data pointed to beliefs about barriers as an important predisposing factor impeding parents from adopting recommended safety practices. With regard to reinforcing factors, our needs assessment suggested that some reinforcements were in place. For instance, mothers reported that their social support networks felt childproofing the home was important. Professional associations endorsed injury prevention counseling by pediatricians during well-child visits. One potentially important reinforcing factor was clearly missing: effective pediatric advice regarding childproofing. Finally, in terms of enabling factors, access to safety supplies and the help or skills to use them effectively were identified as important. Translating these findings into effective intervention strategies was the next step in the process.

Administrative and Policy Diagnosis and Implementation (Phases 5 and 6)

An administrative and policy diagnosis identified the resources needed (as well as the barriers and supports present within the organization) to positively influence mothers' childproofing practices. This diagnosis identified the need for three distinct yet related interventions: enhancing pediatricians' injury prevention counseling, developing a clinic-based safety resource center, and conducting home visits. Planning for each of these interventions again incorporated several theories and principles of practice.

Enhanced Pediatric Counseling. The enhanced pediatric counseling was designed primarily to address predisposing and reinforcing factors that influence parents' childproofing practices. Pediatric residents participated in special training sessions that covered injury prevention content areas (falls, burns, and poisonings) and specific communication skills for behavioral change counseling. Instituting the training program within the organizational constraints of the clinic schedule and the residency training program required the support of the pediatric faculty, who (fortunately) were committed to making it possible for the residents to attend. In fact, three pediatric faculty served as trainers, which provided effective role modeling, reinforcement, and high credibility.

A number of theories were useful in the development and implementation of the enhanced pediatric counseling component. The primary objective was to enable pediatricians to heighten parents' perceptions about the risk and seriousness of childhood injuries and to help them overcome specific barriers to injury prevention that are associated with living conditions in the inner city. In addition to drawing on the constructs identified in the parent interview, we also drew on the stages of change construct and theories of information processing in the training. We educated pediatricians about the notion that behavioral change is a process and that individuals are at different levels of readiness to change (Prochaska, DiClemente, and Norcross, 1992). The training also focused on information-processing capacity: pediatricians received instruction about the need to select the most important injury prevention advice to communicate, because people are limited in the amount of information they can use and remember (Rudd and Glanz, 1990).

Principles of adult learning and Social Cognitive Theory were keys to successfully implementing the enhanced pediatric counseling training. First, because residents brought to the training a considerable amount of experience communicating with parents, we drew on these experiences in discussions during the training. We also used a number of experiential teaching techniques, such as *skills stations* for hands-on practice with safety supplies (for example, smoke detectors, stairgates), shopping trips (for example, to purchase syrup of ipecac), and demonstrations (for example, falling downstairs in a walker). Perhaps most important, we provided opportunities through role-playing for residents both to observe and to model effective communication and counseling skills.

On-Site Safety Resource Center. The safety resource center is aimed primarily at reducing barriers of access to and costs of safety supplies, those enabling factors identified in earlier diagnostic steps. However, because education is provided by a trained health educator at the center, predisposing factors are also being addressed. The objective of the center is to improve parents' access to needed safety supplies and to provide supplies at reduced cost. Numerous administrative and organizational constraints surfaced in our planning for this intervention component—finding space in the clinic for the center, paying the renovation costs for the space, staffing, selecting and stocking supplies and educational materials, and arranging access to the center for families other than those receiving care in the clinic. At least a year of planning will have been devoted to these issues by the time the center becomes operational in July 1996.

The principles of participation and relevance continue to be high priorities for development of the safety resource center. Focus groups with parents are being conducted to obtain their ideas about the center's role, the supplies the center should carry, and its operating policies and procedures. The notion of *empower-*

ment from community organization theories is also relevant to this component of the project. The clinic has a parent advisory board that is being consulted about plans for the center (and for the home visit component described later). An additional goal for the project is to work with this advisory board to identify local retailers and foundations who would be willing to become partners with the project and provide additional resources. Because pediatric residents will be making referrals to the center, informal interviews with them will be conducted to allow them opportunities to shape center policies and procedures.

Home Visiting. The third intervention, home visits, will address another identified enabling factor, skills to adopt childproofing practices. Home visits will be conducted by a community health worker trained in injury prevention counseling and the reduction of household hazards. Through the community health worker, parents will receive the technical assistance they need to use or install safety supplies in their homes. Home visits will address primarily enabling factors but also predisposing and reinforcing factors. Predisposing factors, such as perceptions of injury risk and seriousness, will be addressed through the education that the community health worker will provide. Social networking, using a health worker from the same community to make the visits, will reinforce the outreach and education.

The administrative and organizational aspects of implementing this intervention are significant. In addition to having funding available for this component of the project, there are numerous other resource issues. Training, supervising, and providing for the safety of community health workers making home visits require attention from the project administrators. Safety protocols for the health workers and lists of community referrals for a wide array of needs that may arise need to be developed before home visits begin. Of particular importance in this project is the need for a mechanism to make referrals for housing code violations, because poor housing quality was identified by parents as a barrier to implementing safety practices.

The application of both community-organizing and interpersonal theories was useful in development and implementation of the home-visiting intervention. The principle of participation is acknowledged through the use of focus groups and collaboration with the clinic's Parent Advisory Board, which will allow us to incorporate parents' ideas about the home-visiting intervention into our protocol. Community empowerment and capacity building are evidenced by employing health workers who are from the same community as the families being served. Moreover, the tasks of the community health workers are informed by the Social Cognitive Theory constructs of role-modeling and self-efficacy. Health workers will first model the appropriate injury prevention behaviors (changing a smoke detector battery or testing the hot water temperature, for example), then allow mothers the opportunity to practice and master the necessary skills.

Process, Impact, and Outcome Evaluation (Phases 7, 8, and 9)

As mentioned earlier, the final three steps in the PRECEDE-PROCEED planning model deal with evaluation of the intervention in terms of its process, impact, and outcome. The SAFE Home Project is a randomized control trial involving two cohorts of pediatricians and their patients' parents, who are enrolled during visits to the pediatric primary care clinic when their infants are between zero and six months of age. Our first cohort of pediatricians was randomized to either the standard or enhanced injury prevention counseling group. Both groups received a one-hour seminar on pediatric injuries provided by the director of general pediatrics. Pediatricians in the enhanced counseling group also received the special training in injury prevention counseling described earlier. The goal of the enhanced counseling is that pediatricians will heighten parents' perceptions about the risk and seriousness of injury and will help them overcome specific barriers to childproofing associated with inner-city living conditions.

When twelve-month follow-up with this group is completed, the on-site safety resource center will be opened, and a second cohort of pediatricians and their patients' families will be recruited. All pediatricians in this second cohort will receive the special training in enhanced injury prevention counseling, and the parents will have access to the safety resource center. The on-site resource center will improve access to needed safety supplies at reduced cost. Educational materials and a health educator will also be available in the center. One-half of this second cohort of pediatricians will be randomly assigned to the home visit intervention, and their patients' families will be visited by specially trained community outreach workers who will provide technical assistance in using or installing safety supplies.

To assist with process, impact, and outcome evaluation, measurable objectives were written for each step in PRECEDE-PROCEED. However, due to our research context, our measurable objectives were written in the form of specific hypotheses predicting differences between control and intervention groups. At the level of impact evaluation, we will use baseline and follow-up parent interviews to assess changes in knowledge, attitudes, beliefs, skills, and social influences (predisposing, enabling, and reinforcing factors) and home observations to determine changes in safety practices and household hazards (behavioral and environmental factors). Because injuries are rare events and current funding limitations prohibit following families beyond one year, outcome evaluation of the differences in injury experiences between intervention and control groups is not possible.

Process evaluation is critical in an intervention trial because it enables researchers and practitioners to interpret the impact evaluation results more completely. We are audiotaping all pediatric visits with families enrolled in the project and asking both the parent and the physician to complete a visit checklist describing their reactions to the visit and the counseling provided. These activities will be used to document the extent to which enhanced injury prevention counseling actually took place. Use of the safety resource center and acceptance of the home visits will also be monitored to document implementation of these intervention components. Parent satisfaction with each of the intervention components will also be measured.

Conclusion

For the public health professional in practice, the usefulness of theory lies in its application to solving real-world problems. In this chapter, we outlined a model for planning interventions that incorporates multiple theories of how individuals and communities change. The PRECEDE-PROCEED planning model is an approach to health promotion program planning that is at once structured and flexible. Its systematic diagnostic approach forces the planner to think critically about where and how to intervene. The categories of behavioral determinants are sufficiently broad to incorporate the most relevant theoretical constructs for the problem under study and also help to ensure a comprehensive approach to problem solving. By incorporating different levels of analysis of the problem (individual, behavioral, and social environmental) and by linking determinants to intervention strategies, the process broadens the approach to health promotion planning beyond that typically included in a single theory or framework. PRECEDE-PROCEED should not be confused with a predictive theory but rather should be considered an integrative planning model that can be used to assist in the rigorous application of theory to practice.

References

Ajzen, I. "The Theory of Planned Behavior." *Organizational Behavior and Human Decision Processes*, 1991, *50*, 179–211.

American Academy of Pediatrics. *TIPP: The Injury Prevention Program: A Guide to Safety Counseling in Office Practice.* Chicago: American Academy of Pediatrics, 1994.

Baker, S. P., O'Neill, B., Ginsburg, M. J., and Li, G. *The Injury Fact Book.* (2nd ed.) New York: Oxford University Press, 1992.

Bandura, A. *Social Foundations of Thought and Action: A Social Cognitive Theory.* Englewood Cliffs, N.J.: Prentice Hall, 1986.

Bass, J. L., and others. "Childhood Injury Prevention Counseling in Primary Care Settings: A Critical Review of the Literature." *Pediatrics,* 1993, *92*(4), 544–550.

Bertera, R. L. "Planning and Implementing Health Promotion in the Workplace: A Case Study of the DuPont Company Experience." *Health Education Quarterly,* 1990, *17*(3), 307–327.

Bertera, R. L. "Behavioral Risk Factor and Illness Day Changes with Workplace Health Promotion: Two-Year Results." *American Journal of Health Promotion,* 1993, *7*(5), 365–373.

Centers for Disease Control, National Center for Chronic Disease Prevention and Health Promotion. "PATCH: Planned Approach to Community Health." *Journal of Health Education,* 1992, *23*(3), 129–192.

Eng, E., and Blanchard, L. "Action-Oriented Community Diagnosis: A Health Education Tool." *International Quarterly of Community Health Education,* 1991, *11*(2), 93–110.

Eriksen, M. P., and Gielen, A. C. "The Application of Health Education Principles to Automobile Child Restraint Programs." *Health Education Quarterly,* 1983, *10*(1), 30–55.

Freudenberg, N., and others. "Strengthening Individual and Community Capacity to Prevent Disease and Promote Health: In Search of Relevant Theories and Principles." *Health Education Quarterly,* 1995, *22*(3), 290–306.

Gielen, A. C. "Health Education and Injury Control: Integrating Approaches." *Health Education Quarterly,* 1992, *19*(2), 203–218.

Gielen, A. C., Bernstein-Cohen, L., and Radius, S. "Case Study of Program Evaluation Activities for Child Passenger Safety Programs in Local Health Department Settings." Paper presented at the 113th annual meeting of the American Public Health Association, Washington, D.C., Nov. 1985.

Gielen, A. C., and others. "In-Home Injury Prevention Practices for Infants and Toddlers: The Role of Parental Beliefs, Barriers, and Housing Quality." *Health Education Quarterly,* 1996, *22*(1), 85–95.

Gielen, A. C., and others. "Injury Prevention Counseling in an Urban Pediatric Clinic: Analysis of Audiotaped Visits." Unpublished manuscript, 1996.

Glanz, K., and Rimer, B. K. *Theory at a Glance: A Guide for Health Promotion Practice.* NIH publication no. 95–3896. Bethesda, Md.: National Institutes of Health, National Cancer Institute, 1995.

Green, L. W. "Published Applications of the PRECEDE Model, Sept. 18, 1994." Unpublished manuscript, University of British Columbia, Vancouver, 1994.

Green, L. W., and Kreuter, M. W. *Health Promotion Planning: An Educational and Environmental Approach.* (2nd ed.) Mountain View, Calif.: Mayfield, 1991.

Green, L. W., Kreuter, M. W., Deeds, S. G., and Partridge, K. B. *Health Education Planning: A Diagnostic Approach.* Mountain View, Calif.: Mayfield, 1980.

Janz, N. K., and Becker, M. H. "The Health Belief Model: A Decade Later." *Health Education Quarterly,* 1984, *11,* 1–47.

McGinnis, J. M., and Foege, W. H. "Actual Causes of Death in the United States." *Journal of the American Medical Association,* 1993, *270*(18), 2207–2212.

Miller, T. R., and Galbraith, M. "Injury Prevention Counseling by Pediatricians: A Benefit-Cost Comparison." *Pediatrics,* 1995, *96*(1), 1–4.

Minkler, M. "Building Supportive Ties and Sense of Community Among the Inner-City Elderly: The Tenderloin Senior Outreach Project." *Health Education Quarterly,* 1985, *12*(4), 303–314.

Minkler, M. "Improving Health Through Community Organization." In K. Glanz, F. M. Lewis, and B. K. Rimer (eds.), *Health Behavior and Health Education: Theory, Research, and Practice*. San Francisco: Jossey-Bass, 1990.

Morisky, D. E., and others. "Five-Year Blood Pressure Control and Mortality Following Health Education for Hypertensive Patients." *American Journal of Public Health*, 1983, *73*(2), 153–162.

Mullen, P. D., Hersey, J. C., and Iverson, D. C. "Health Behavior Models Compared." *Social Science and Medicine*, 1987, *24*(11), 973–981.

National Committee for Injury Prevention and Control. *Injury Prevention: Meeting the Challenge*. New York: Oxford University Press, 1989.

Orenstein, D., and others. "Synthesis of the Four PATCH Evaluations." *Journal of Health Education*, 1992, *23*(3), 187–193.

Prochaska, J. O., DiClemente, C. C., and Norcross, J. C. "In Search of How People Change: Applications to the Addictive Behaviors." *American Psychologist*, 1992, *47*(9), 1102–1114.

Rice, D. P., and MacKenzie, E. J. "Cost of Injury in the United States: A Report to Congress." San Francisco: Institute for Health and Aging, University of California, and Injury Prevention Center, Johns Hopkins University, 1989.

Rimer, B. K. "Audiences and Messages for Breast and Cervical Cancer Screening." *Wellness Perspectives: Research, Theory and Practice*, 1995, *11*(2), 13–39.

Ross, H. S., and Mico, P. R. *Theory and Practice in Health Education*. Mountain View, Calif.: Mayfield, 1980.

Roter, D. L. "Which Facets of Communication Have Strong Effects on Outcome—A Meta-Analysis." In M. Stewart and D. L. Roter (eds.), *Communicating with Medical Patients*. Thousand Oaks, Calif.: Sage, 1989.

Rudd, J., and Glanz, K. "How Individuals Use Information for Health Action: Consumer Information Processing." In K. Glanz, F. M. Lewis, and B. K. Rimer (eds.), *Health Behavior and Health Education: Theory, Research, and Practice*. San Francisco: Jossey-Bass, 1990.

U.S. Department of Health and Human Services. *Healthy People 2000: National Health Promotion and Disease Prevention Objectives*. DHHS publication no. PHS 91–50213. Washington D.C.: U.S. Government Printing Office, 1991.

U.S. Preventive Services Task Force. *Guide to Clinical Preventive Services: An Assessment of the Effectiveness of 169 Interventions*. Baltimore, Md.: Williams & Wilkins, 1989.

Weinstein, N. D. "The Precaution Adoption Process." *Health Psychology*, 1988, *7*(4), 355–386.

Wilson, M.E.H., and others. *Saving Children: A Guide to Injury Prevention*. New York: Oxford University Press, 1991.

Windsor, R. A. "An Application of the PRECEDE Model for Planning and Evaluating Education Methods for Pregnant Smokers." *International Journal of Health Education*, 1986, *5*, 38–43.

Windsor, R. A., and others. "Health Education for Pregnant Smokers: Its Behavioral Impact and Cost Benefit." *American Journal of Public Health*, 1993, *83*(2), 201–206.

Wissow, L. S., Roter, D. L., and Wilson, M.E.H. "Physician Interview Style and Mothers' Disclosure of Psychosocial Issues Important to Child Development." *Pediatrics*, 1994, *93*, 289–295.

Worden, J. K., and others. "A Community-Wide Program in Breast Self-Examination Training and Maintenance." *Preventive Medicine*, 1990, *19*, 254–269.

CHAPTER EIGHTEEN

SOCIAL MARKETING

R. Craig Lefebvre
Lisa Rochlin

Since the first edition of *Health Behavior and Health Education,* social marketing has come of age, especially in the field of public health. This maturity is reflected in increased numbers of publications and professional activity in the area. Since 1990, there have been two reviews of the field (Ling, Franklin, Lindsteadt, and Gearon, 1992; Walsh, Rudd, Moeykens, and Maloney, 1993), a new textbook on the subject (Andreasen, 1995), the establishment of two annual conferences devoted exclusively to social marketing, and the appearance of a peer-reviewed journal, *Social Marketing Quarterly.* In the last six years, the practice of social marketing has expanded from a few federal, state, and private-sector agencies to virtually all federal agencies with a charge to conduct public health education efforts (for example, the Centers for Disease Control and Prevention, the National Eye Institute, and the Environmental Protection Agency), voluntary health organizations, and numerous private-sector agencies. However, this explosion of interest in social marketing by public health professionals has also been met with concern about whether social marketing is an appropriate (or even necessary) model to use in public health education (Buchanan, Reddy, and Hossain, 1994; Tones, 1994; Vanden Heede and Pelican, 1995). And some social marketers have voiced concern about the ways certain social marketing advocates and practitioners think about and practice the activity (Lefebvre, 1992).

Rather than begin with an historical narrative of social marketing (a task ably performed by others, see, for example, Elliot, 1991; Ling, Franklin, Lindsteadt, and Gearon, 1992; Walsh, Rudd, Moeykens, and Maloney, 1993), we review several models of social marketing with the goal of describing core features of the social marketing approach. We then examine the research support for social marketing approaches to health behavior change. Finally, two case studies illustrate how social marketers apply the key principles and concepts.

What Is Social Marketing?

Before we discuss models of social marketing, it will be useful to define it. Lefebvre and Flora (1988) note that definitions of *social marketing* have included such descriptions as a process for increasing the acceptability of ideas or practices in a target group, a process for problem solving, a process to introduce and disseminate ideas and issues, and a strategy to develop effective communication messages. More recently, opinion has converged, defining social marketing at its most basic as a strategy for changing behavior on a populationwide basis (Andreasen, 1995; Kotler and Roberto, 1989; Lefebvre and others, 1995a). A definition put forth by Andreasen (1995) is, "Social marketing is the application of commercial marketing technologies to the analysis, planning, execution, and evaluation of programs designed to influence the voluntary behavior of target audiences in order to improve their personal welfare and that of their society." This definition encompasses several key aspects of the social marketing approach: it is seen as (1) a key benefit to individuals and society, not focused on profit and organizational benefits as commercial marketing practices are; (2) a focus on behavior, not awareness or attitude change; and (3) an approach centered on the target audience's having a primary role in the process.

A second definition issue is determining what constitutes social marketing practice. The term social marketing has often been inappropriately used to describe an agency's activities. For example, the development and implementation of a public service announcement campaign, a nutrition education program for cardiac patients, a condom marketing program, and the marketing of prenatal services and of alcohol treatment programs have all been labeled social marketing. More appropriate labels for these activities would be, respectively, social advertising, nutrition education, product marketing, and services marketing. The practice of social marketing lies in developing and implementing integrated elements that have the shared purpose of leading to a specific change in behavior. This shared purpose is referred to as the program objective. One or more strategies are then developed to guide program planners in developing specific tactics to meet this objective. These strategies dictate which tactics are appropriate and which inappropriate to pursue. Tactics might range from the development and distribution of print or audiovisual self-help materials to increase levels of physical activity, to worksite programs designed to develop peer support systems for regular physical activity, to the development of community coalitions to advocate for safe areas where individuals can exercise. Each of these elements may lead to behavioral change, but it is the strategic combination and integration of these tactics that constitutes a social marketing program.

Social marketing has also been conceived of as a theoretical approach to behavior change (Tones, 1994). However, social marketing in and of itself is not a theory. Most classical notions of social marketing note that its theoretical base lies in the world of economics where *exchange theory* is used to describe, predict, and design marketing programs that address consumer behavior (Kotler, 1975; Lefebvre and Flora, 1988). Exchange theory has also been extended, in what is known as *social exchange theory*, to examine and explain relations between individuals and their environments. Here, research has focused on such issues as equity, distributive justice, power, and exploitation (Emerson, 1987). A critical review of exchange theory by Elliot (1991) concludes that although it may be central to marketing, it is not necessary for, or even relevant to, social marketing. Likewise, Novelli (1990) notes that social marketing is theory based. But he continues, "[Social marketing] is predicated on theories of consumer behavior, which in turn draw upon the social and behavioral sciences." This position allows a social marketer to employ any number of theories of behavior to guide research, development, implementation, and evaluation of a program.

Finally, and most importantly, all social marketing efforts are characterized by their dedication to being consumer driven. While many approaches to individual and social change have likewise proclaimed an emphasis on starting with the patient, client, individual, or community, the emergence of social marketing has brought new life to that old but important concept. As Ling, Franklin, Lindsteadt, and Gearon (1992) have noted: "Social marketing has had a beneficial impact on how the public health sector educates the public and persuades communities and individuals to adopt healthy practices. With its emphasis on clients, social marketing has sharpened the focus on the public. It has brought more precision to audience analysis and segmentation. . . . These data provide critical information for the formulation of better targeted and more effective messages, thus leading to more appropriate message design, more effective delivery, and, above all, better reception by the public."

We turn next to reviewing a component model of social marketing (what are its essential ingredients?), a process model (how is it done?), and finally a strategic model for execution or implementation (how is strategy developed?). The models are followed by a summary of research on the effectiveness of social marketing, and two case studies that exemplify social marketing approaches to public health problems.

Program Component Model

Lefebvre and Flora (1988) contributed one of the first articles about a program component model. It began with the conclusion, based on their respective experiences at the Pawtucket Heart Health Program and the Stanford Five City Project, that "social marketing is an invaluable referent from which to design, implement, evaluate, and manage large-scale, broad-based, behavior-change focused programs." Their eight-component model included the following elements (see Table 18.1 for definitions of the five key components):

1. A consumer orientation that recognizes that consumer needs should drive health initiatives, as opposed to expert-driven or top-down approaches that have little consumer input and little regard for consumer satisfaction.
2. An emphasis on voluntary exchanges of goods and services between providers and consumers. This needs to be explicitly understood in the development of programs. Exchanges should be win-win: consumers should exchange their resources for those expended by the agency that provide the desired messages, products, or services.
3. Research in audience analysis and segmentation strategies to group the population into meaningful target audiences and characterize these audiences in ways that are meaningful. Variables include people's current participation in health promotion behaviors, their future likelihood to engage in such behaviors, their communication networks, and their motivations related to the desired behaviors.
4. The use of formative research in concept testing and product or message design, and the pretesting of materials with target audience representatives to determine relevance, comprehensibility, motivational characteristics, and impact.
5. An analysis of distribution or communication channels to determine those times, places, and situations where the target audience is likely to be most attentive and responsive to the message, product, or service offering.
6. Use of the marketing mix to maximize the use and blending of message, product, and service offerings and to establish their price, place, and promotion characteristics in intervention planning and implementation.
7. A process-tracking system with both integrative and control functions that help the marketing manager monitor and adjust the marketing program.
8. A management process that involves problem analysis, planning, implementation, and feedback functions to ensure that the program meets timelines, reaches appropriate audiences, and meets behavioral objectives.

TABLE 18.1. SOCIAL MARKETING CONCEPTS.

Concept	Definition	Application
Consumer orientation	Focus of research, planning, implementation, and evaluation is consumer driven.	Use research methods to understand consumer reality; pretest materials with members of target group; use citizen advisory panels.
Audience segmentation	Differentiation of large groups of people into smaller, more homogeneous subgroups.	Determine behavior, motivational, cultural, and other variables that may affect the communication strategy, and create specific target groups who share the same qualities and are distinct from other subgroups who share other attributes.
Channel analysis	Determination of the appropriate methods to reach target audience members where and when they are most likely to attend to and respond to the message.	Determine those places, times, and states of mind when the target audience may have the predisposition to be thinking about the subject area.
Strategy	Overarching concept(s) that focus program planning on achieving the stated objectives.	After determining the objective(s), create broad areas of program impact that can be refined by selecting related tactics.
Process tracking	Mechanisms established to monitor program implementation.	Determine if program is implemented as planned; feedback results to redirect, refine, or revise implementation.

In noting the limitations of the social marketing approach, Lefebvre and Flora reiterated the problems and challenges facing social marketing. These had been highlighted earlier by Bloom and Novelli (1981), and little progress had been achieved in the intervening years. Lefebvre and Flora also noted that the often-professed view that social marketing was another form of placing "blame" on individuals for unhealthy behaviors was a narrow conceptualization of social marketing, and that, in fact, many social marketers understood and addressed the antithetical consumer-marketing practices of the private sector, lack of supportive public policies, and a lack of consensus and coordination among health authorities and agencies (see also Manoff, 1985). In a brief review of ethical issues faced by social marketers, Lefebvre and Flora noted that while social marketers must address issues related to the techniques used to market certain behaviors to particular target audiences, they must also be concerned about people who use social marketing practices but with limited knowledge and skills. Finally, Lefebvre and Flora also called for controlled studies of social marketing's effectiveness (an issue we will return to in the next section).

In concluding an article that also codified the components of social marketing, Walsh, Rudd, Moeykens, and Maloney (1993) recognized several limitations of social marketing, particularly the lack of a consistent theoretical base on which social marketers could develop their programs, few empirical studies of social marketing effectiveness, and the potential for social marketing programs, like their commercial marketing counterparts, to "skim the cream off the top" of difficult public health problems and not address the needs of disadvantaged population groups (a point, Walsh, Rudd, Moeykens, and Maloney note, that many social marketers do not agree with). Yet Walsh, Rudd, Moeykens, and Maloney point to social marketing as providing public health practitioners with "sense-making techniques to convert communication from a process of transmission to a process of dialogue, something health educators are increasingly eager to do."

Marketing Process Model

Many public health professionals' first exposure to a social marketing model has likely been through a marketing process *wheel*, or iterative cycle. This process model was introduced to social marketing by Novelli (1984) and popularized by its centrality in the publication *Making Health Communications Work* (U.S. Department of Health and Human Services, 1989). The marketing process model poses six sequential stages, designed to take into account audience wants, needs, expectations, and satisfactions or dissatisfactions; to formulate program objectives; to employ an integrated marketing approach and mix; and to continually track consumer and market response to the program. The six stages are defined as follows.

Market analysis (planning and strategy). This stage includes consideration of the overall organization's mandates and goals, an economic analysis of the context of the behavior that is the issue, the geographical scope of the market, the distribution outlets, the market trends and projections (that is, is the behavior increasing or decreasing), and the resources available for conducting the marketing program. Market analysis also examines the target consumer. Here, research with the target audience should include but not be limited to such variables as demographic, geographical, and psychographic attributes of the audience, including benefits sought by audience members and these members' media usage patterns. A third level of market analysis is institutional analysis—the review of financial, management, and staff resources available (or not) to mount a successful program. Practitioners should also look at other organizations active in the same marketplace (competitor analysis). Both friendly and unfriendly competitors need to be understood so that the program will be correctly positioned to consumers and take advantage of opportunities to leverage other resources.

Planning (selecting channels and materials). The planning phase is the time when the program's structure and organization are established; program objectives are specified; the target market is segmented; strategy for entry into the marketplace is selected; the marketing mix strategy (the mix of behavior or product, price, place, and promotion) that is the essence of the marketing program is developed; and the action plan, including all tactics, schedules, milestones, process and outcome measures, and budgets, is created.

Developing, testing, and refining plan elements. This stage is the first step in executing the action plan. It is here that each element of the marketing mix is developed and tested with the target audience, and the program is refined as needed. This pretesting phase is a hallmark of the social marketing approach. It might involve any of a variety of qualitative research methods to pretest specific tactics or program elements. It might also involve pilot testing of the entire program prior to the larger rollout. Often, it also involves working with intermediary organizations that are part of the implementation or distribution plan, to provide them with the materials and training necessary for the program's success.

Implementation. At this stage, the program is fully implemented. The details of the plan, the schedules, milestones, and budgets need to be carefully reviewed and managed if the program is to be implemented as planned. The process evaluation should be carefully monitoring key implementation variables to assure managers that the program is proceeding on course.

Assessing effectiveness. This stage involves the systematic assessment of whether, and how, the program is meeting its objectives. When integrated with the ongoing process evaluation, the data gathered in this assessment should constitute an effective management information system. This system, in turn, can provide information to program managers about any necessary midcourse corrections in the implementation; the need to act on new or unanticipated opportunities; and the need to begin planning for the next cycle of the marketing process.

Feedback to stage 1 (feedback to refine program). As an iterative process, this model takes into account marketplace changes over time, target audience responses to program shifts, organizational mandates and objectives change, and budgets that expand and contract. At this stage, all these changes, along with the evaluation data, should be carefully reviewed to uncover problems with the implementation, identify deficiencies to be addressed, highlight program strengths to be capitalized on, and review opportunities to be exploited in the next cycle.

While effective as a process, the marketing process model provides little strate-gic guidance to the practitioner who is thinking through the key issues of *how* to systematically go about the process of changing behavior among a large group of people. This process model has been refined and incorporated as a framework for health communication programs at the Centers for Disease Control and Preven-tion. The wheel is shown in Figure 18.1.

Consumer-Based Health Communications: A Strategic Model for Implementation

This section presents a recent contribution to researchers' and practitioners' think-ing. It translates strategy development as practiced in the advertising world to social marketing practice. Sutton, Balch, and Lefebvre (1995) have developed the Consumer-based Health Communications (CHC) Model for translating marketing concepts and techniques into messages designed to improve the health behavior of

FIGURE 18.1. SOCIAL MARKETING WHEEL.

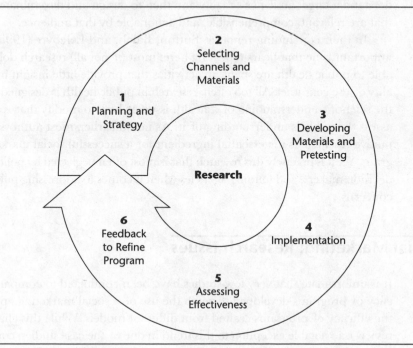

Source: Glanz and Rimer, 1995.

the target audience. The CHC Model is an adaptation of the ROI (relevance, originality, impact) process developed by Bill Wells for the advertising agency DDB Needham Worldwide (Wells, 1989). The CHC process transforms scientific recommendations for health promotion and disease prevention and treatment into message strategies that are relevant to the target audience. The model's premise is that, just as great care and rigor are used to establish the empirical base for these recommendations, equal care and weight should be given to the consumer research that illuminates the reality of consumers. "Scientific reality" is blended with "consumer reality" as planners develop a message strategy document that addresses six strategic questions: Who will be the target audience, and what are they like? Exactly what action do we want our target to take as a direct result of experiencing the communication? What reward should our message promise the consumer? How will we support our promise to make it credible? What communication openings and vehicles should be used? What image should distinguish the action?

In a paper and in a subsequent chapter that provides more detail, Lefebvre and others (1995b) illustrate how the 5 A Day for Better Health Program brings these questions and their answers to life. Using a variety of formative research techniques including focus groups, intercept interviews, and commercial databases, the authors demonstrate the process a practitioner can undertake to understand a target audience's reality and then to design and disseminate messages that are relevant, comprehensible, and actionable by that audience.

In their concluding remarks, Sutton, Balch, and Lefebvre (1995) raise an important issue that bears repeating here: most (if not all) research dollars available to public health are spent on activities that provide little insight into the reality of the consumer. All too often, research in public health is designed to further the scientific understanding of a health issue or how to modify that issue, not to assess the public's understanding of it. As noted earlier, most authors view formative research as the essential ingredient for a successful social marketing program. Yet it is precisely this research that is most often neglected by policy makers, decision makers, and funding agencies when it comes to addressing public health concerns.

Social Marketing: Research Issues

It is unfortunate that very few studies have been conducted to compare the efficacy of programs developed through the use of a social marketing approach to the efficacy of programs crafted from different models. While this chapter does review one notable exception to this trend in one of the case studies, comparative data are lacking. This point recently was underscored by the Board on Health Promotion and Disease Prevention of the Institute of Medicine (Leviton, Mrazek, and Stoto, 1996). Upon review of the extant literature, the board posed a number of questions for further research, including (1) How much research do social marketing approaches actually put into formative research? (2) Is consumer input achievable, especially with minority and adolescent populations? (3) Does this approach enhance the likelihood of achieving the desired behavioral outcome? (4) Does a social marketing approach favor a focus on influencing individual change as opposed to influencing the social context of the behavior? (5) Are there other appropriate theoretical frameworks for social marketing to use? (6) Can social marketing approaches be used equally effectively by public health departments, community organizations, and commercial firms?

The board concluded that answers to these questions and similar ones will help establish a scientific basis for social marketing that practitioners can draw upon for future efforts in the development of effective health promotion and disease prevention programs. The challenge for the field is to provide the answers to these and other questions.

Applications

This section describes two applications of social marketing: a national breast cancer education program and a program to improve nutrition in Thailand.

Case Study: The Breast Cancer Education Program of the Office of Cancer Communication

The National Cancer Institute's Office of Cancer Communications (NCI/OCC) is charged with communicating research findings and relaying messages on prevention, early detection, and state-of-the art treatment to the public through the development and dissemination of cancer education programs and information. The following selective review of activities that OCC developed for the Breast Cancer Education Program (BCEP) is organized around the process model of social marketing program development and covers approximately a five-year span of the program.*

*OCC's Breast Cancer Education Program is the result of many people's efforts and expertise. The authors want to especially acknowledge the contributions of Sharyn Sutton, Ruth Mattingly, Nelvis Castro Morales, Peter Garrett, and Becky Thorpe.

Review Background Information. An extensive array of background information exists on breast cancer and mammography. For the purposes of this discussion, only a sample of the available data will be highlighted to show how it was used to develop the framework for a communications strategy for the BCEP. In 1987, the National Health Interview Survey found that only one-third of white women aged fifty years and older reported ever having been screened. Compared to these women, approximately one-third fewer African American and Hispanic women had ever been screened. Roughly half of the women who were ever screened had obtained a mammogram within the past year.

Set Communication Objectives. With the background data pointing to the underutilization of mammography (especially among minorities) and to the benefits of screening, the communications objectives for the BCEP could be established. They included (1) increasing awareness of the importance of regular screening for breast cancer and (2) increasing appropriate mammography use.

Analyze and Segment Target Audiences. The initial target audience for OCC's efforts was women aged forty and older. In 1989, eleven medical organizations, including NCI, supported mammography screening guidelines for women aged forty to forty-nine. These guidelines suggested that a woman should get a screening mammogram every one to two years and a clinical breast exam annually. OCC placed particular emphasis on reaching African American and Hispanic women.

In 1994, NCI evaluated new clinical trials evidence on the value of screening mammography and found that no statistically significant reduction in mortality could be shown for women aged forty to forty-nine. In turn, there was no scientific agreement on the benefit of screening mammography for women aged forty to forty-nine. Therefore, NCI refocused its communications efforts on women aged fifty and older, where there was general scientific agreement and demonstration that breast cancer mortality could be reduced by one-third.

Later, OCC further segmented its target audience to women aged sixty-five and older. Data pointed to the fact that women sixty-five and older were two times as likely to develop breast cancer and two times as likely to die from it compared to younger women (aged forty to sixty-four) and were also least likely to get mammograms.

Identify Message Concepts. With a clear evolution in the target audience over the years, the messages designed to reach these women evolved as well. A sample of the messages that were designed follow. Developed to emphasize the importance of annual screening, the initial message for women forty to forty-nine was "Once a Year . . . For a Lifetime." Understanding the importance of creating culturally appropriate and relevant messages for different minority groups, OCC developed distinct messages for Hispanic and African American women. Focus groups emphasized the importance in Hispanic culture of family in making major decisions, including health decisions. Applying this information led to the message *"Hagalo hoy. . . . Por su salud y su familia"* ("Do It Today . . . For Your Health and Your Family") for Hispanic women.

Select Communication Channels. OCC's Breast Cancer Education Program used a variety of channels to reach diverse target audiences over the span of the program. These channels included print and broadcast media (both mainstream and minority); intermediary groups including state health departments and community, health professional, religious, voluntary health, and service organizations; and NCI's outreach network: the Cancer Information Service, the National Black Leadership Initiative, the National Hispanic Leadership Initiative, and the National Appalachian Leadership Initiative.

Create Materials and Pretest. A range of educational materials was developed for the BCEP, and choice of materials depended on the target audience and the selected channel. Educational materials included brochures and videos; media materials such as print and broadcast public service announcements, press kits, satellite media tours, and videotaped news releases; community intervention guidebooks; intermediary program activity kits; speaker kits; and giveaways such as bookmarks, pins, and mirrors. Pretesting was a component of the materials development process, addressing elements such as message comprehension, cultural appropriateness, reading level, and user friendliness.

Develop Promotional Plans. Throughout the BCEP, the Office of Cancer Communications used several consistent approaches when developing promotion plans. Each product or activity had its own promotional plan. An integrated approach using a combination of distribution channels was chosen to realize maximum reach. In addition, OCC often took advantage of national events such as National Breast Cancer Awareness Month or National Minority Cancer Awareness Week to release new materials, highlight a new activity, or reemphasize a message.

Implement Communication Strategies. OCC developed several effective and unique broadcast vehicles to reach women, particularly African American and Hispanic women. To reach African American and white women, OCC developed a twenty-six-minute educational film entitled *Once a Year . . . For a Lifetime* that told the stories of five women whose lives were forever changed by breast cancer. With celebrity hosts Phylicia Rashad and Jane Pauley, the film was broadcast by NBC stations in several major cities and was distributed via satellite to 950 members of the National Association of Broadcasters.

An outgrowth of *Once a Year* was the first Spanish-language film targeted to Hispanic women and their families. Introduced during National Minority Cancer Awareness Week in 1992, *Una vez* featured Latino celebrities, was accompanied by educational outreach and two press conferences, and was distributed via partnership with Univision, the largest Spanish-language network. In addition, *Una vez* was made available to community organizations targeting Hispanic audiences. A seven-minute version was created to facilitate the use of the program in educational settings. The film has also been distributed to other organizations including hospitals, clinics, churches, and community libraries.

OCC also helped launch an innovative program to bring together public and private national and community groups to provide underserved women with breast cancer education, mammography, clinical breast exams, and follow-up medical care. Project Awareness originally occurred as a pilot effort in four cities and then was employed again in eight cities. Each city was funded to recruit one hundred eligible low-income women, aged forty and older, with an emphasis on women over fifty. A guidebook instructed community groups how to develop and implement the three-tiered program that included educating women on the importance of early detection of breast cancer and instructing them on breast self-examination, providing free screening mammograms and clinical breast exams to participants, and providing follow-up medical care (when needed).

Assess the Effects. Whenever possible, the BCEP had built-in process and outcome evaluation measures. Process and outcome evaluation methods for all the program components described cannot be explained here. Instead, the focus is on the methods used to assess the outcome of one activity, *Una vez*.

Una vez premiered on Univision on April 12, 1992, and has been rebroadcast several times throughout Univision's more than 600 affiliates. Since the Spanish-language network did not have a system to measure viewing audiences at the time, OCC conducted a telephone survey among four hundred Hispanic women in nineteen selected markets two weeks after the film aired to determine its estimated reach. Thirty-nine percent of the women forty and older who were interviewed reported seeing the program. Extrapolating the data nationally, it was projected that approximately 1.7 million targeted women saw the initial airing of the program. International reactions were also positive with more than 2,500 requests for the tape in the United States and abroad.

Obtain Feedback. Feedback received on many BCEP components resulted in program refinement in a number of ways. For example, the *Project Awareness User's Guide* was revised based on input from the community groups that used it in the pilot phase of the program. Information exchange also resulted in product spin-offs such as the Spanish-language film *Una vez* in response to the success of *Once a Year*. The feedback OCC received also helped it refine the technical assistance that its field offices provided to intermediary groups interested in developing breast cancer education programs.

OCC's BCEP was one of many breast cancer education efforts occurring at the time, so its singular contribution to mammography education efforts and reductions in breast cancer–related morbidity and mortality rates cannot be isolated. Other federal, state, and local agencies, nonprofit groups, and voluntary health organizations dedicated extensive resources to reaching women with mammography messages. Whether taking a leadership role or supporting the efforts of other organizations, the positive effects of these overall national breast cancer education efforts were clear. Data from the 1992 National Health Interview Survey showed that the number of women who had ever had screening had nearly doubled for all populations and those screened within the past year had more than doubled. In addition, the gap in mammography use between minority women and white women was closed.

Case Study: The Social Marketing of Vitamin A–Rich Foods

Smitasiri (1994) presented an extensive description of the application of social marketing to address a specific nutritional deficiency. Her description is organized around the social marketing component model and illustrates how strategic insights about target audiences can be used to guide tactical choices in program development. This case study covers a three-year period (from 1988 to 1991).

In Thailand, an epidemiological study found that 80 percent of preschool children, 75 percent of pregnant women, and 82 percent of lactating mothers had Vitamin A intakes below the recommended daily allowance (RDA). This result was startling to the investigators as foods high in Vitamin A were readily available and affordable in local markets throughout the year. In response, the Social Marketing of Vitamin A Rich Foods (SM/VAF) project was developed with four objectives: increase dietary intake of Vitamin A–rich foods among the target audiences; improve knowledge, attitudes, and practices regarding Vitamin A–rich foods among these audiences; raise the status of Vitamin A among the target groups; and develop a model for improving individuals' Vitamin A status through nutrition.

The SM/VAF project employed a quasi-experimental research design using two comparable districts of Kanthararom (population 122,000) and Trakan Phutphon (population 105,000), both in Thailand. Kanthararom was selected as the intervention site because the only AM/FM radio station did not reach the reference area. Although the two sites are only 100 kilometers apart, there are no direct rail or road links between them and no shared commercial activities. Thus, possible contamination of the reference area by intervention activities was minimal. A carefully developed program was created based on several theoretical frameworks including systems theory, community organization frameworks, Social Cognitive Theory, social campaign theories, and social marketing. Seven steps were involved in the program's development and intervention:

Formative Research. This research involved in-depth interviews with 165 people in the intervention region, including mothers with children aged zero to seventy-two months, headmasters of schools, village heads, volunteer community health workers, traditional midwives, and monks.

Audience Segmentation. Based on the formative research, the primary target audience was identified as pregnant and lactating mothers and mothers of preschoolers. Schoolchildren were later added to this group because of their role in caring for younger siblings. The second target group consisted of all women of reproductive age and also elderly women, traditional midwives, fathers, and community health workers because of their influence on the primary target audience. Tertiary groups included monks, community leaders, headmasters, district and provincial officers, and local politicians and business leaders.

Intervention Development. Three major intervention strategies were initially developed. First, create a nutrition information environment in the intervention region so that its members would be more aware of the importance of a good diet and nutrition and their impact on a family's well-being. Second, change negative attitudes toward Vitamin A–rich dark green vegetables and increase the availability of these sources in the area. Third, provide training for traditional midwives and community health volunteers in remote areas to ensure that mothers' insecurity about difficult deliveries and illnesses after giving birth would be reduced. After discussions of these intervention strategies with both practitioners and academic experts, a fourth and a fifth strategy were added to the intervention. Fourth, develop a collaborative system between academicians and practitioners to enable them to work together to improve the nutritional status of the intervention area. Fifth, disseminate general Vitamin A information in all nutrition information activities.

To test these strategies, seventy representative mothers were randomly selected from seven villages in the intervention area. Using twenty-four-hour recall methods, the researchers took baseline data for both these mothers' and their children's dietary intake. The mothers were then encouraged to increase consumption of several types of dark green vegetables for both themselves and their children. A week later, the team returned and repeated the dietary recall and interviewed the mothers. The researchers found that more than half of the mothers could feed themselves and their children more Vitamin A–rich foods. With greater effort, almost 70 percent of them could attain the desired level of consumption of these foods. Based on the interviews, intervention strategies were modified to focus on home gardening of Vitamin A–rich foods to increase their availability in the area; an emotional appeal based on "a mother's love" was added to the nutrition information pieces; and special attention was given to the poor mothers in the area.

With this information, an implementation plan was developed with the following tactics: (1) a school vegetable gardening program conducted under the auspices of the district office of education; (2) an ivy gourd home and school gardening program integrated into the ongoing services of the district's agriculture office; (3) a comprehensive agricultural promotion program to increase vegetable production for family consumption, run by the project team in consultation with the provincial and district agricultural offices; (4) training sessions for midwives and health volunteers so they could ensure safe deliveries and offer appropriate information about maternal and child nutrition and child-rearing practices to mothers; (5) a mass educational and communication program to educate the area's residents in general nutrition knowledge and to provide information about Vitamin A through local radio stations and village public address systems and billboards; (6) an educational and communication program aimed at pregnant and lactating mothers and delivered through print materials available at local health offices, at a local hospital, and through traditional midwives, and local health officers also received a manual to assist their interpersonal communications with mothers, and posters were provided; (7) an educational and communication program designed to change elderly women's traditional beliefs about foods to be eaten during pregnancy and lactation, aimed at both grandmothers and traditional midwives—monks were provided with basic nutrition information that they could impart to elderly women during their religious visits to temples; (8) an educational and communication program that trained community leaders and health volunteers to incorporate nutrition messages into their ongoing programs; (9) an educational and communication program for schoolchildren that included a children's drama group, teacher workshops, a school lunch cookbook, and posters and exhibitions to promote better nutrition, along with activities designed to transfer nutrition information from the school environment to the family; (10) the SM/VAF project promotion program, which positioned the project as belonging to the community and concerned with family well-being; and (11) a program that established support networks to facilitate improved Vitamin A consumption among the disadvantaged.

Creative Strategies Development. To facilitate increased consumption of Vitamin A–rich foods, the decision was made to focus on one specific vegetable rather than talking generally about "green leafy vegetables." Ivy gourd (*tum leung*) was selected as that specific vegetable as it has the highest level of Vitamin A among green leafy vegetables. The promotion campaign had three phases with three key messages—phase 1: "Let's eat *tum leung* for our health"; phase 2: "Let's grow *tum leung*"; and phase 3: "Let's eat a *tum leung* soup," "Let's eat a *tum leung* omelet," "How to cook *tum leung* dishes," and "How to take good care of *tum leung.*"

Posters, pamphlets, radio broadcasts, public address systems, and visits by famous radio personalities were the primary channels employed to reach the general audience. Direct mail and manuals were used to reach mothers; prerecorded messages were played in the temples to reach grandmothers; and direct mail pieces and manuals were produced for community leaders and monks.

Implementation. Implementation occurred in three phases. During phase 1, the public relations element (SM/VAF program) was deployed in which the project was promoted to key governmental officers and local leaders. After this process was begun, general nutrition information communications began, with the purpose of mobilizing the community to become involved in the effort. Phase 2 marked the introduction and acceleration of other educational and communication activities and the introduction of a *tum leung* growing competition to increase lagging food production. Phase 3 addressed horticultural problems with *tum leung* that had not been previously identified (it was not as insect resistant as believed).

Monitoring. Throughout the implementation phases, monitoring was accomplished through meetings with local governmental officers, random visits by the field coordinator and other members of the project team, and participant observations by trained research assistants. As noted above, this monitoring process resulted in two additions to the implementation plan: the *tum leung* competition (as people were not acting on the phase 2 "grow" message), and the development of messages about controlling of insects for those who were growing *tum leung.*

Final Evaluation. A two-stage sampling technique was used to gather representative samples of twelve and sixteen villages from the intervention and reference areas, respectively, and pregnant and lactating mothers in each village. Knowledge, attitude, and behavior surveys and dietary assessments were conducted with respondents.

The results of *t* tests for K-A-P (knowledge-attitudes-practice) changes in the intervention and reference areas showed greater increases in the intervention area. More importantly, the analysis of data from pre- and postintervention dietary assessments for Vitamin A consumption found significant differences among both pregnant and lactating women in intervention areas as compared with those residing in the reference areas. Dietary data were not statistically different among preschoolers residing in one of the two conditions.

The results of several types of qualitative assessments found that these changes in the intervention area were primarily due to (1) use of a comprehensive educational and communication approach, (2) the decision to focus on *tum leung* in message development and delivery, (3) success in attaining cooperation and community involvement, and (4) effective management.

These results led Smitasiri to conclude that the SM/VAF project is one of only a few comprehensive community-based projects in health and nutrition "that includes education/communication components and attention to the necessary and feasible environmental changes in order to facilitate required behavior changes. . . . [A] well-planned and managed education/communication program which utilizes a solid theoretical framework and applies the social marketing approach can be effective in changing health and nutrition behaviors" (Smitasiri, 1994).

Conclusion

Social marketing provides a framework within which program planners, developers, implementers, and evaluators can apply knowledge, theories, and techniques to effecting population-based changes in health behavior. The utility and effectiveness of social marketing as a behavioral change technology depends heavily on how well the target audience is understood and listened to, how well barriers and benefits to new behaviors are strategically and tactically addressed, and how well program components are integrated and managed. It is not a panacea for people unwilling to exercise the time, thought, and energy needed to contribute to improving public well-being. However, it often provides a structured method for applying health behavior theories for health improvement.

References

Andreasen, A. R. *Marketing Social Change: Changing Behavior to Promote Health, Social Development, and the Environment*. San Francisco: Jossey-Bass, 1995.

Bloom, P. N., and Novelli, W. D., "Problems and Challenges of Social Marketing." *Journal of Marketing*, 1981, *45*, 79–99.

Buchanan, D. R., Reddy, S., and Hossain, Z. "Social Marketing: A Critical Appraisal." *Health Promotion International*, 1994, *9*, 49–57.

Elliot, B. J. "A Re-Examination of the Social Marketing Concept." Unpublished master's thesis, Sydney, University of New South Wales, 1991.

Emerson, R. M. "Toward a Theory of Value in Social Exchange." In K. Cook (ed.), *Social Exchange Theory.* Thousand Oaks, Calif.: Sage, 1987.

Glanz, K., and Rimer, B. K. *Theory at a Glance: A Guide for Health Promotion Practice.* NIH publication no. 95–3896. Bethesda, Md.: National Institutes of Health, National Cancer Institute, 1995.

Kotler, P. *Marketing for Nonprofit Organizations.* Englewood Cliffs, N.J.: Prentice Hall, 1975.

Kotler, P., and Roberto, E. L. *Social Marketing: Strategies for Changing Public Behavior.* New York: Free Press, 1989.

Lefebvre, R. C. "The Social Marketing Imbroglio in Health Promotion." *Health Promotion International,* 1992, *7,* 61–64.

Lefebvre R. C., and Flora, J. A. "Social Marketing and Public Health Interventions." *Health Education Quarterly,* 1988, *15*(3), 299–315.

Lefebvre, R. C., and others. "Social Marketing and Nutrition Education: Inappropriate or Misunderstood." *Journal of Nutrition Education,* 1995a, *27*(3), 146–150.

Lefebvre, R. C., and others. "Use of Database Marketing and Consumer-Based Health Communication in Message Design: An Example from the Office of Cancer Communications' '5 A Day for Better Health' Program." In E. Maibach and R. Parrott (eds.), *Designing Health Messages: Approaches from Communication Theory and Public Health Practice.* Thousand Oaks, Calif.: Sage, 1995b.

Leviton, L., Mrazek, P., and Stoto, M. "Social Marketing to Adolescents and Minority Populations." *Social Marketing Quarterly,* 1996, *3,* 6–23.

Ling, J. C., Franklin, B. A., Lindsteadt, J. F., and Gearon, A. N. "Social Marketing: Its Place in Public Health." *Annual Review of Public Health,* 1992, *13,* 341–362.

Manoff, R. K. *Social Marketing: New Imperative for Public Health.* New York: Praeger, 1985.

Novelli, W. D. "Developing Marketing Programs." In L. W. Frederiksen, L. Solomon, and K. Brehony (eds.), *Marketing Health Behavior.* New York: Plenum, 1984.

Novelli, W. D. "Applying Social Marketing to Health Promotion and Disease Prevention." In K. Glanz, F. M. Lewis, and B. K. Rimer (eds.), *Health Behavior and Health Education: Theory, Research, and Practice.* San Francisco: Jossey-Bass, 1990.

Smitasiri, S. *Nutri-Action Analysis: Going Beyond Good People and Adequate Resources.* Bangkok, Thailand: Amarin, 1994.

Sutton, S. M., Balch, G. I., and Lefebvre, R. C. "Strategic Questions for Consumer-Based Health Communication." *Public Health Reports,* 1995, *110,* 725–733.

Tones, K. "Marketing and the Mass Media: Theory and Myth: Reflections on Social Marketing." *Health Education Research,* 1994, *9,* 165–169.

U.S. Department of Health and Human Services. *Making Health Communications Work.* NIH publication no. 89–1493. Washington, D.C.: National Institutes of Health, National Cancer Institute, Office of Cancer Communications, 1989.

Vanden Heede, F. A., and Pelican, S. "Reflections on Social Marketing as an Inappropriate Model for Nutrition Education." *Journal of Nutrition Education,* 1995, *27,* 141–145.

Walsh, D. C., Rudd, R. E., Moeykens, B. A., and Maloney, T. W. "Social Marketing for Public Health." *Health Affairs,* 1993, *12,* 104–119.

Wells, W. D. *Planning for R.O.I.: Effective Advertising Strategy.* Englewood Cliffs, N.J.: Prentice Hall, 1989.

CHAPTER NINETEEN

ECOLOGICAL MODELS

James F. Sallis
Neville Owen

This chapter describes the current status of ecological models of health behavior and health promotion and proposes principles of ecological models that should be followed if these models are to contribute substantially to health promotion research and practice. Because ecological models and their terminology are not widely understood, we first describe the general usage of key terms and provide some working definitions.

What Are Ecological Models and Environmental Variables?

As described by Stokols (1992), the term *ecology* is derived from biological science and refers to the interrelations between organisms and their environments. The ecological perspective, as it has evolved in sociology, psychology, economics, and public health, focuses on the nature of people's transactions with their physical and sociocultural surroundings. Thus, *ecological* refers to models, frameworks, or perspectives rather than specific variables.

Because ecological models consider the connections between people and their environments, it is important to clarify the term environment. Although it is reasonable to conceive of *psychological environments* existing within individuals, in ecological models of behavior *environment* typically means the space outside the individual. Many models of behavioral change acknowledge the importance of the intrapsychic and social environments, but few explicitly specify the role of the physical environment. For purposes of this chapter, we consider the explicit treatment of relations between the individual and the physical environment to be a hallmark or defining feature of ecological models.

Behavior setting is another term that we believe to be very helpful in understanding the effects of the environment on behaviors. *Behavior settings* are those social and physical situations in which behaviors take place (Barker, 1968).

The ecological models we review in this chapter attempt to explain how environments affect behavior and how environments and behavior affect each other. The following statement captures the flavor of our chapter, the explicit environmentalist stand that we have taken, and the focus that we have chosen to use in presenting the ecological approach: "people are but one component of the larger behavior-setting system, which restricts the range of their behavior by promoting and sometimes demanding certain actions and by discouraging or prohibiting others" (Wicker, 1979). For example, bans on cigarette smoking in the workplace restrict the range of smokers' behaviors, significantly changing the temporal distribution of smoking behavior over a working day, the behavior settings in which smoking takes place, and how other people are affected by the smoke. The availability of a variety of low-fat foods in a school or workplace cafeteria can facilitate more healthful food choices. Bicycle racks and easily accessible stairs in public places can promote choices by individuals to be more physically active as part of their daily routines.

Although there are several ecological models, and the field is developing rapidly, we propose a working definition. *Ecological models of health behavior* posit that behaviors are influenced by intrapersonal, social and cultural, and physical environment variables; posit that these variables are likely to interact; and describe multiple levels of social and cultural and physical environment variables as relevant for understanding and changing health behaviors.

Applications Outpace Research

We believe there is some urgency in stimulating increased research based on ecological models because an examination of contemporary health promotion practice makes it clear that these models have already been adopted. The influence of ecological perspectives on the planning of national and international health agencies is particularly clear (and is illustrated in Table 19.1). The selection of objectives and strategies related to environmental changes indicates the types of environmental variables believed to control health behaviors.

Changing the environmental context of health behaviors in whole populations is a central element in the health promotion strategies of industrialized countries (see, for example, U.S. Department of Health and Human Services, 1991;

Commonwealth Department of Human Services and Health, 1994). Along with behavioral change targets, these national objectives specify environmental and regulatory changes to support healthful behaviors. The changes include such items as eliminating tobacco product advertising, increasing the miles of walking or cycling paths available in communities, and increasing the number of low-fat food items available in the mass food supply. Table 19.1 includes examples from the *Healthy People 2000* objectives and from the strategies of the Australian National Health goals and targets that demonstrate the extent to which implicit ecological models are being used as a basis for national health promotion policies.

TABLE 19.1. U.S. AND AUSTRALIAN YEAR 2000 HEALTH PROMOTION OBJECTIVES THAT EXEMPLIFY IMPLICIT ECOLOGICAL MODELS.

United States

Increase to at least 75 percent the proportion of worksites with a formal smoking policy that prohibits or severely restricts smoking at the workplace.

Increase community availability and accessibility of physical activity and fitness facilities (includes hiking, biking, and fitness trail rides, public swimming pools, acres of park and recreation open space).

Achieve useful and informative nutrition labeling for virtually all processed foods and at least 40 percent of fresh meats, poultry, fish, fruits, vegetables, baked goods, and ready-to-eat carry-away foods.

Extend adoption of alcohol and drug policies for the work environment to at least 60 percent of worksites with fifty or more employees.

Increase to at least thirty the number of states that have design standards for signs, signals, markings, lighting, and other characteristics of the roadway environment to improve visual stimuli and protect the safety of older drivers and pedestrians.

Australia

At the state and local government level, investigate structural changes that encourage people to walk or cycle instead of using motor transport wherever possible; possibilities are car-free areas in cities (except for the disabled and elderly) and strategies to encourage cycling instead of driving.

At the state and territory level, restrict the places where tobacco vending machines are available to supervised areas or to areas where young people under eighteen are unlikely to be found unsupervised.

Encourage public- and private-sector food services, food manufacturing companies, and all levels of government to adopt nutrition policies.

Encourage education departments, local governments, sporting bodies, and other groups controlling outdoor areas regularly used by the public to increase the amount of natural and structural shade available (for sun protection); this encouragement can come from commonwealth and state and territory governments and Australian Cancer Society members.

Expedite the introduction and adoption of a new Australian standard for playground safety that covers the design, manufacture, installation, maintenance, undersurfacing, and use of playground equipment (for prevention of falls among children).

Source: Data from U.S. Department of Health and Human Services, 1991; Commonwealth Department of Human Services and Health, 1994.

These national objectives are influencing the priorities, funding opportunities, and actions of health promotion researchers and practitioners, and they define key aspects of health promotion and disease prevention initiatives that will be pursued beyond the year 2000. Those of us with an interest in the potential of ecological models to lead to improved health promotion efforts are pleased by the interest of practitioners and policy makers, but we are concerned by the lack of scientific foundation for many environmental interventions. Environmental variables are targeted for change in some cases in the absence of data linking these variables with specific behavioral and health outcomes. Environmental interventions are starting to be implemented widely in the absence of data on their intended and unintended outcomes. Large-scale changes in poorly understood environmental variables may or may not be cost-effective uses of scarce resources, and they may or may not produce beneficial results. In general, we advocate applying ecological models to the design of health promotion programs, but we are concerned that premature or uninformed applications that lead to disappointing results could cause a complete rejection of environmental change approaches before these approaches are adequately tested. Thus, it is important to explicitly identify, develop, and test the ecologically based hypotheses that now play a key role in guiding local health promotion practice and national and international health promotion policies.

Background

The current interest in ecological approaches to health promotion has developed out of several historical trends, which have been reviewed previously (McLeroy, Bibeau, Steckler, and Glanz, 1988; Moos, 1980; Stokols, 1992). The most relevant conceptual traditions are drawn from public health and psychology. In the field of public health, environmental influences on disease have been recognized in some Western cultures for centuries. As early as the mid-1800s, systematic study of such ecological factors as poverty and social class was beginning. For example, a typhus epidemic was attributed by Rodolf Virchow to social, economic, and political factors as strongly as to biological factors (Moos, 1980). The host-agent-environment model is basic to public health analyses of infectious diseases, but it can also be applied to chronic diseases (McLeroy, Bibeau, Steckler, and Glanz, 1988).

There are multiple traditions of ecological analyses of behavior within the field of psychology. In contrast to earlier theories that posited an intrapsychic determination of behavior, Skinner's position (1953) was that antecedent and consequent events in the observable environment controlled behavior, and this view can be considered an early and influential forerunner of some current ecological models. The Skinnerian approach certainly focused investigators on physical environment factors outside of the person.

Early psychological theorizing about the role of broadly defined environmental influences is strongly evident in the work of Kurt Lewin, who coined the term *ecological psychology* to describe the study of the influence of the outside environment on the person (Lewin, 1936). Lewin's concept of the *life space,* the psychological representation of the environment, stimulated research in many fields. In this approach, the role of the environment is limited in that only *perceptions* of the external environment are deemed to be important.

The ecological approach was further developed in Roger Barker's long-term observational studies (1968) of children in their everyday environments. Barker developed the concept of the *behavior setting,* which referred to the social and physical aspects of environments, and he concluded that the characteristics of behavior settings were strongly associated with a wide range of psychological states and behaviors. Whereas Lewin hypothesized that environments influenced behavior indirectly, through effects on psychological variables, Barker developed the more radical view that environments directly affect behavior. He came to believe that "behaviors of children could be predicted more accurately from knowing the situations the children were in than from knowing individual characteristics of the children" (Wicker, 1979). Barker's broad hypothesis was not adequately investigated by his studies, and questions still remain about the relative strengths of intrapersonal and environmental influences on health behaviors.

The work of Urie Bronfenbrenner (1979) is also relevant to the development of ecological models as applied to health promotion (McLeroy, Bibeau, Steckler, and Glanz, 1988). Bronfenbrenner described three levels of environmental factors that reciprocally interact with individual variables. The *microsystem* consists of interpersonal interactions in specific settings, with family members, social acquaintances, and work groups, for example. The *mesosystem* refers to the interactions among settings, among family, school, and work, for example. The *exosystem* is the larger social system, which can affect individuals and settings through economic forces, cultural beliefs and values, and political actions. This model demonstrates the principle that environments can be conceptualized at various levels of integration. Among the many research challenges that face ecological theorists, the identification and categorization of environmental factors remains important.

Bandura's Social Cognitive Theory (1986) has been at least as influential as any other theory in health behavior research (see Chapter Eight), and it shares some features with ecological models. The structure of the theory is simple in that it specifies that behavior can be influenced by personal and environmental factors.

In the environmental realm, social factors have been most thoroughly studied. These studies include Bandura's own well-known work (1986) on modeling and vicarious learning. Although Bandura's works rarely explicate the role of physical environments, some models of health behavior based on Social Cognitive Theory have posited multiple influences of the physical environment (for example, Sallis and Hovell, 1990; Winett, King, and Altman, 1989).

Ecological Models and Health

Since the 1970s, Rudolph Moos has produced a great deal of theoretical and empirical work in the area of social ecology, focusing on the social context including institutional and cultural variables and describing how the social ecology model can be applied to the understanding of health issues. Moos (1980) specifies four sets of environmental factors relevant to health studies.

The first set is *physical settings*, which can include features of the natural environment such as geography and weather as well as features of the constructed environment such as architectural and urban designs. Moos argues that physical environments can be directly associated with health problems such as arthritis symptoms, allergy episodes, and heart attacks. The second set of environmental factors is *organizational;* the size and functions of organizations affect a wide range of behaviors. The third set is the *human aggregate*. These factors can be thought of as the sociodemographic or sociocultural characteristics of the people inhabiting a given environment. Social, economic, educational, ethnic, and cultural backgrounds of groups are known to influence a wide range of health behaviors (see Chapter Twenty). The fourth set of environmental factors is *social climate*, the perceived aspects of the social environment that relate to such variables as the supportiveness of a particular social setting and the clarity of expectations. Moos (1976) developed scales to measure social climates within several types of organizations, and these have been found to be associated with health status indicators.

Ecological Models and Health Promotion

The genesis of health promotion as a distinct field is often traced to a document commonly known as the Lalonde Report (Lalonde, 1974). This Canadian document presented a comprehensive approach to controlling chronic diseases that is consistent with the use of ecological models. The Lalonde Report proposed that health is influenced by four major elements: human biology, environment, lifestyle, and health care organizations. It was highly successful in presenting the case that specific health promotion initiatives are needed because health care alone is not effective for improving public health.

The Lalonde Report was later criticized for an overemphasis on the health effects of individual lifestyle, so the *Ottawa Charter for Health Promotion* (1986) made the case even more strongly for the need to consider sociocultural and physical environment influences on health. This report from an international conference convened by the World Health Organization and Canadian agencies has been very influential. The *Ottawa Charter* explicitly calls for an approach to health promotion that gives equal status to the creation of supportive environments alongside the development of personal skills and a reorientation of health services. Thus, the environmental goals in Table 19.1 are a logical outgrowth of the approach prescribed in the *Ottawa Charter.*

Stokols (1992) offers a detailed exposition of the need for a social ecological approach to health promotion. Four assumptions underlie the application of social ecology to the goal of improving the effectiveness of health promotion programs. The first assumption, reminiscent of Bandura (1986) and Moos (1980), is that health is likely to be influenced by multiple facets of the physical and social environments but that the role of personal attributes is also acknowledged. The second assumption is that environments are complex, and efforts to understand environmental effects on health must take into consideration environments' multiple dimensions. Environments can be described as social or physical and as actual or perceived. Environments can also be described as discrete attributes (such as temperatures or spatial arrangements) or as constructs (such as behavior settings or social climates). The third assumption recognizes that participants in environments can be described at varying levels of aggregation: individuals, families, organizations, communities, and populations. The understanding of environment-behavior relations may be enhanced by studying multiple levels of aggregation with diverse methodologies. Similarly, health promotion may be more effective when coordinated efforts operate across levels of aggregation: when family members work together to change behavior, for example, or corporate decision makers shape health-promoting policies or public health officials provide consistent health services and media messages. The fourth assumption is that there are multiple levels of feedback across different levels of environments and aggregates of persons. People-environment transactions occur in cycles: people influence their settings, and these settings then exert some influence over people's health behavior. Models that describe such cyclical and reciprocal processes have been proposed for workplace health promotion by Abrams and others (1986) and for health behavior more generally by Ewart (1990).

The *health-promotive environment* is an important concept in Stokols' model (1992), and his description of it is an extension of some of the concepts found in the *Ottawa Charter*. Stokols argues that health promotion interventions must address the environmental resources that may either facilitate or hinder the targeted health behavior changes. In addition to having indirect environmental effects on health through influencing health behavior, sociophysical environments can have more direct effects through the kind of emotional health and social cohesion they encourage. Stokols argues that a wide range of environmental variables may influence health behavior and other health variables. Relevant geographical variables include climate, environmental pollution, and the restorative effect of natural environments. Architectural and technological variables include whether or not building designs are injury-resistant, water quality is good, and automobiles and roads are safe. Sociocultural influences include whether or not there is political stability, high-quality health media, health promotion legislation, and insurance incentives for healthful behaviors. Stokols (1992) challenges researchers to include measures of the physical and social environments in their studies and challenges practitioners to improve the way social and physical environments promote health.

Although the promise of ecological models for improving people's abilities to understand and improve health behavior is widely acknowledged, we note again that relatively little research attention has focused on environmental influences on health behavior. Stokols (1995) identifies this paradox in the context of environmental psychology and provides some possible explanations for the lack of growth in research on the interface between environment and behavior.

Models That Apply Ecological Concepts

Theoretical and conceptual advancement are critical steps in the development of new approaches to health promotion. However, it is necessary to make the difficult transition from theory to practice; to demonstrate how broad explanatory models help organize practitioners' understanding of specific problems and lead to effective innovations in health promotion practice. Two examples of models that apply ecological concepts to health promotion practice are reviewed here, though other writers have provided additional valuable perspectives (Baranowski, 1989; Ewart, 1990; Green and Kreuter, 1990; Karoly, 1985; Elder, Geller, Hovell, and Mayer, 1994; Winett, 1995).

McLeroy, Bibeau, Steckler, and Glanz (1988) propose an ecological model for health promotion that identifies the primary sources of influence on health behavior. The model is designed to guide researchers and practitioners to systematically assess and intervene on each source as appropriate. An underlying assumption is that a comprehensive approach is more effective than a one-level approach. The five levels of influence are *intrapersonal factors, interpersonal processes and primary groups, institutional factors, community factors,* and *public policy.* This model takes the general concept of levels of analysis, which is common to most ecological models, and identifies the levels most relevant for a range of health behaviors. The authors provide examples of the ways consideration of influences across the levels of analysis can be useful in explaining and changing health behavior.

A framework for integrating public health and psychology approaches for the purpose of creating more effective health promotion interventions was developed by Winett, King, and Altman (1989). Their framework incorporates the host-agent-environment model from public health, the ecological tradition from psychology, multilevel analysis from social ecology, and systematic planning from the PRECEDE model. A unique contribution of Winett, King, and Altman's book is that it provides detailed recommendations for comprehensive health promotion programs that address many key health behaviors of concern in industrialized societies. It presents a wealth of ideas about how to create environments that promote health and how to integrate ecological approaches with individual and small-group behavioral and educational interventions.

Principles of Ecological Approaches to Health Behavior Change

Based on our review of ecological concepts and models, we have developed a list of principles that we hope will be useful in guiding future research and practice in health promotion. Some of the principles are common features of ecological models, and other principles reflect our recommendations for strengthening the applicability of the models to the design of effective health promotion approaches.

1. *Multiple dimensions of influence on behaviors.* Ecological models specify that intrapersonal factors, social and cultural environments, and physical environments can influence health behaviors. The inclusion of all three categories, or dimensions, of influence sets ecological models apart from the theories in Parts Two and Three of this book that consider only intrapersonal and interpersonal variables.

2. *Interactions of influences across dimensions.* To be useful in designing studies and interventions, the model should not merely predict that the categories of determinants interact, the model should also state *how* they interact.

3. *Multiple levels of environmental influences.* Ecological models specify multiple levels of environmental factors that directly influence behavior. Intrapersonal theories describe numerous psychological, cognitive, and emotional influences, and these can be incorporated into ecological models. Levels of social and cultural influences—family, peers, organizations, communities, institutions, and public policies—have

been proposed. The unique contribution of ecological models is the identification of physical environment factors. Characteristics of the natural environment such as weather, climate, and geography may affect behavior. Various dimensions of constructed environments may also affect behavior. Examples of these environments are homes, architectural features, and local communities, and also information, entertainment, and technological environments.

4. *Environments directly influence behaviors.* Ecological models include the proposition that environmental factors directly influence behavior. This is a feature that distinguishes ecological models from intrapersonal theories, which sometimes hypothesize that selected environmental influences are mediated through psychological processes. An example of an ecological hypothesis is that factors in intrapersonal, social and cultural, and physical environments make unique contributions to the explanation of health behavior in addition to any health effects these environments may produce through interacting with one another.

5. *Behavior-specific ecological models.* Specific ecological models will be needed to guide research and intervention for each health behavior. Existing ecological models are general statements that multiple levels of environmental variables exert widespread influence on a variety of outcomes related to human health and welfare. The existing models argue that multiple levels of variables are believed to be important, describe some of the principles of environmental influence, and indicate the behaviors or outcomes likely to be influenced by environments. Authors of ecological models often suggest that research and intervention in various fields could be improved through application of an ecological model. However, the level of discourse in almost all writings on ecological approaches to health improvement is very general, reflecting an assumption that ecological principles apply in similar ways across behaviors.

Intrapersonal and interpersonal models of behavior are meant to generalize across behaviors, and many of these models can be readily adapted for a variety of behaviors. We do not believe that *general* ecological models will be similarly useful because environmental influences are much more behavior specific. Health behaviors are performed in many behavior settings, and each setting has numerous characteristics that may affect each behavior differently. Hypotheses about specific environmental influences are needed to guide research and intervention, but it is difficult to imagine specific environmental influences that will generalize across several behaviors. General statements that environments affect behavior do not tell researchers which behaviors are most likely to be influenced by changes in weather conditions, or crowded urban settings, or living in a wine-making or tobacco-growing region. Operationalizing the general principles of ecological models for specific behaviors is likely to be challenging, and model developers need to identify the environmental variables most relevant for each behavior so that researchers can be steered to study the most promising variables.

Applications of Ecological Models to Health Behavior

In this section, we present an overview of applying the principles of ecological models to studies of eating and physical activity in order to improve researchers and practitioners' ability to explain these behaviors and create more effective interventions. In some cases, we refer to studies that have already begun to explore the relation between environmental variables and behaviors. In other cases, we provide suggestions for improving research and practice by considering the influence of environmental variables.

Application to Eating Behavior

Unhealthful eating practices are linked to five of the top ten causes of death in industrialized nations: heart disease, some cancers, stroke, diabetes, and atherosclerosis (U.S. Department of Health and Human Services, 1988). Changes in dietary habits of individuals of all ages have been recommended as part of national efforts to promote better health, but recent data indicate that these dietary goals are not being met (U.S. Department of Health and Human Services, 1991; Commonwealth Department of Human Services and Health, 1994). For simplicity, we focus here on the target behavior of dietary fat consumption. We propose how application of ecological principles to the study of health-related eating behavior could lead to important improvements in public health. (An expanded discussion of an ecological approach to nutrition and a literature review was published recently by Glanz and others, 1995.)

Multiple Dimensions of Influence on Behaviors. Eating is a complex set of behaviors influenced by an array of factors. Each domain of influences is expected to make unique contributions to eating habits. It is not difficult to identify likely influences in each domain. Intrapersonal factors could include taste preferences, health beliefs, moods, and perceived ability to change. Eating habits of family, friends, and others in the social environment should have a major influence. At a higher level of social integration, culture is often expressed through food, and food and eating habits are used to communicate with the culture. For example, serving steak is a symbol of high status in many European American communities, but a high-status meal in an Indian culture may be defined by its elaborate preparation and use of expensive spices.

Despite the importance of intrapersonal and social and cultural factors, multiple aspects of the physical environment can also be influential. One simple way to think about environmental influences is that you cannot eat what you do not have. Everyone is familiar with the effects of droughts and floods on the food supply in some countries, but distribution systems that compensate for short-ages in particular areas are also important environmental influences on eating. Climate affects what is grown, so even with modern distribution, people in the tropics have better access to exotic fruits, and people near the sea find it easier to obtain seafood. Agricultural and economic policies also affect access to food: or-anges may be less expensive in Hawai'i than locally grown pineapples, most of which are shipped elsewhere to be sold. Cost of food is also an environmental fac-tor. A comprehensive ecological approach to changing diet might educate people about foods that are low in fat, show role models switching to and enjoying low-fat alternatives, and reduce environmental barriers by putting low-fat choices in nearby stores at attractive prices.

A paradoxical situation showing the complexity of changing eating behav-ior may arise if high-fat foods are targeted and *all* low-fat foods are then perceived as healthy, even those high in sugar and calories. When this happens, the em-phasis on eating low-fat foods may inadvertently contribute to excess body weight.

Interactions of Influences Across Dimensions. Although it should be obvious that educating people to change dietary habits that are not acceptable to their peer groups or to eat foods that they cannot afford is a questionable strategy, it is com-monly done in the health promotion field. We can illustrate this problem with a personal example. One of us (James Sallis) worked with others on a study designed to teach low-income Mexican American families to reduce their fat and sodium intake. Those engaged in this study attempted to teach these families to identify and select more healthful foods and helped them encourage and support other family members in doing so. A similar program was delivered to European Amer-ican families, who were more affluent. In general, the European American fami-lies, primarily the adults, changed their diets, and the Mexican Americans made few changes (Nader and others, 1989). There are several potential explanations for these differences, but one explanation shows how intrapersonal and environ-mental factors may interact. One study element was a survey of the availability of a long list of low-fat and low-sodium foods in areas where the study families lived. The survey showed that larger stores had many more healthful choices than smaller stores. However, in the low-income areas, there were no supermarkets. The small corner stores in the neighborhoods where the Mexican American fam-ilies lived simply did not have most of the items promoted in the intervention (Sal-lis and others, 1986). Families who wanted to eat healthful foods were more likely to be successful if those foods could be bought conveniently. The interactions among these different influences on dietary behavior are poorly understood.

Multiple Levels of Environmental Influence. Environmental determinants of eat-ing are not well researched (Glanz and others, 1995), but an ecological perspective suggests multiple levels of influence. Borrowing from the conceptualization of McLeroy, Bibeau, Steckler, and Glanz (1988), we propose some influences on eating at the institutional, community, and public policy levels. The institutional level is included here because food processing, distribution, purchasing, preparation, and consumption are often controlled by institutions. Because so much processed food is consumed in industrialized nations, the ingredients and preparation methods used by major food suppliers and restaurant chains are important factors in the diets of large populations. The respective promotion and advertising of low-fat and high-fat foods also needs to be considered. Even a casual viewer of television will notice that the foods advertised are likely to be high in fat. The effects of food company policies on dietary intake need to be studied by health behavior researchers. The preparation of school lunches affects millions of children and adults each day, so the effect on fat intake and health might be substantial if school lunches routinely met dietary guidelines (Farris, Nicklas, Webber, and Berenson, 1992).

Communities are affected by the interactions of organizations, institutions, and social networks (McLeroy, Bibeau, Steckler, and Glanz, 1988). An example of the complex interplay of factors that affects nutrition in communities can be found in the Torres Strait Islands, north of the Australian mainland. In past centuries, the islanders had to be self-sufficient, so they raised most of their own food. With development came new sources of food, so the islanders eventually became dependent on imported food and almost entirely stopped growing their own. Owing to the remoteness and the relatively small population of the islands, food shipments are infrequent, and three weeks is a typical transit time. These long delays affect the quality and price of some foods more than others. The most adversely affected foods are fresh fruits and vegetables. It was recently documented that not enough fresh fruits and vegetables reach the Torres Strait Islands to allow the residents to eat the recommended amounts (Lowson, Toolis, and Leonard, 1995). The community now suffers high rates of chronic diseases consistent with a diet high in fatty processed foods and deficient in fresh produce. This pattern can be seen in developing or recently developed countries in South America as well. Other communities are affected by the interplay of different environmental factors.

Governmental policies at the national, state, and local levels influence dietary behaviors. Prominent federal policies in the United States subsidize producers of many agricultural commodities. However, most of those policies are systematically more generous for unhealthful and high-fat products than for those considered more healthful (Milio, 1986), keeping prices of unhealthy foods artificially low. These policies also produce surplus amounts of fatty foods such as cheese and meat, and the surpluses are then given to schools and poor people. State and local policies that minimize funding for school lunches may pressure schools to rely on unhealthful donated commodities. Partly due to these policies, school lunches are higher in fat content than is recommended (Farris, Nicklas, Webber, and Berenson, 1992).

Environments Directly Influence Behaviors. Several intrapersonal models and Lewin's ecological psychology model (1936) posit that environments affect behavior indirectly, by way of psychological variables. We believe a model of indirect influence cannot explain most observations about eating behavior. For example, the perception of high prices for healthful food can be a barrier to purchasing them and is an example of an indirect environmental effect. However, the inability to purchase a specific healthful food because it is unavailable in the local community or because the price is truly too high for a poor person's budget is an example of a direct environmental effect.

Behavior-Specific Ecological Models. Research and practice will be served best by models that identify specific behavior settings and policies that influence the appropriate behavior. The climate and weather of a geographical area in which food is grown and a community lives are likely to affect consumption. The availability of refrigeration and storage facilities is also important. Food products availability is affected by the policies and practices of food-processing companies, schools, workplaces, restaurants, and advertising agencies. A different set of organizations and environments are relevant for other health behaviors. Governmental policies affect all behaviors, but relevant agencies differ according to the behavior. For eating behavior, policies of agriculture, environmental protection, finance, health, housing, and consumer protection should be considered. At the present time, each investigator studying environmental influences on eating must propose relevant variables because there is no existing definitive ecological model of eating behavior, no comprehensive conceptualization. Further, separate sets of variables may be needed when the concerns differ: for example, when food safety is a problem compared to when concern is about excessive intake of dietary fat.

Application to Physical Activity

Physical activity is now recognized as one of the most important health behaviors in industrialized nations because of its role in the etiology of major chronic diseases (Hahn, Teutsch, Rothenberg, and Marks, 1990). Substantial portions of the population report doing either no physical activity on a regular basis or insufficient activity to meet the guidelines adopted in many nations (Owen and Bauman, 1992; Stephens and Caspersen, 1994). Despite extensive study, the influences on physical activity are not well understood, and the interventions studied to date have not produced impressive or long-term increases in physical activity (Dishman and Sallis, 1994). Physical activity research and practice may benefit from the application of ecological models. An expanded discussion of an ecological approach to physical activity and a literature review were published recently by King and others (1995).

Multiple Dimensions of Influence on Behavior. Research on the correlates of physical activity has established that variables in all the domains (intrapersonal, social and cultural, and physical) are related to physical activity in adults (Dishman and Sallis, 1994) and youths (Sallis and others, 1992). Thus, the ecological model clearly applies to physical activity. Many psychological variables, such as intentions and self-efficacy, are consistent correlates, and specific social support behaviors appear to strongly influence physical activity. Physical environment characteristics have been least thoroughly studied, so it is a high priority to further explore the many possible environmental variables that could influence physical activity. Improving understanding of the effect of natural environmental factors such as weather and terrain on physical activity could aid in the design of interventions to help people overcome ones that are barriers. Constructed environments may have even more important effects. Very little is known about the effects of design of buildings, urban and suburban developments, and transportation systems on physical activity, but we believe the effects could be profound. Modern societies have invested heavily in infrastructures that allow very sedentary lifestyles. Consider how the infrastructures for automobile transportation, passive entertainment (television, movies, computer games), and labor-saving devices at home and work encourage sedentariness and discourage physical activity.

One of the benefits of taking an ecological perspective on physical activity interventions is that it may make expectations more realistic. Most of the physical activity interventions to date have used educational and cognitive-behavioral approaches to informing individuals about physical activity, but these programs do not produce long-term effects (Dishman and Sallis, 1994). An ecological explanation for the failure of the behavior to be sustained is that the environmental factors that led to the sedentary behavior in the first place are still in place. Educational programs do not provide new bicycle lanes, showers at work, homes within walking distance of workplaces, alternatives to sedentary entertainment, or incentives to be more physically active. Because the infrastructures for sedentary behavior are not changed, investigators should not expect physical activity promotion programs that emphasize changes in intrapersonal or even social variables to have long-term effects.

Interactions of Influences Across Dimensions. We illustrate the relevance of this ecological principle for physical activity with a commonly discussed problem. People who live in high-crime neighborhoods are often afraid for their safety if they walk or jog near their homes, and this is a legitimate concern. If these people are also poor, they may not have the money to join a private health club. The reduction in funding for public recreation centers in the United States leads to a situation in which a poor person does not have access to appropriate physical activity resources. For someone who does not intend to be active, lack of resources may be unimportant. However, if a poor person had strong intentions to be active, access to adequate resources might determine whether his or her attempt was successful. Thus, intention can interact with access to resources.

A similar example can be developed for children. In a study of physical activity promotion in fourth- and fifth-grade children, students set goals to be active outside of school each week. However, this intervention did not result in measurable increases in activity after school (Sallis and others, forthcoming). One of several explanations for the lack of effect may be that latchkey children are instructed to stay indoors at home every day after school until a parent returns. Because children are unable to be very active indoors, they are prevented from meeting their goals. Thus, social and environmental factors interact with individual goals and intentions.

Multiple Levels of Environmental Influences. McLeroy, Bibeau, Steckler, and Glanz's conceptualization (1988) of institutional, community, and public policy factors is applicable to physical activity. At the institutional level, schools influence physical activity through physical education, recess periods, and health education. Worksites have policies that can encourage or discourage physical activity. The health care and insurance industries are institutions that have potential for promoting physical activity.

In addition to the social influences within communities, community physical design may be important for physical activity. Suburbs are typically designed on the assumption that residents will have automobiles: shops and workplaces are not usually within convenient walking distance. Older inner-city neighborhoods are more self-contained, and many destinations can be reached on foot or by bicycle. Communities also vary in the availability of physical activity resources such as parks, recreation facilities, and walking or bicycling trails. It may be necessary to understand the safety, attractiveness, and convenience of these resources in designing any intervention.

There are probably a great many laws and policies that have indirect or unintended effects on physical activity. For example, policies that provide massive funding for roads and highways but little or nothing for walking and bicycle trails may unintentionally create barriers to physical activity. Budget cuts for parks and recreation departments may be rationalized as means to preserve money for health care for the poor, and cuts in school physical education may reflect a priority on preserving core academic programs without consideration of the effects on children's physical activity. Building codes that require stairwells to be bare and closed may compromise safety and convenience and discourage stair use. It is likely that many policies directed at education, transportation, urban and suburban design, building codes, and health care expenditures have effects on physical activity, and these effects need to be studied.

Environments Directly Influence Behaviors. At least one study showed the relevance of this principle for studying physical activity. In a large survey, *perceived* convenience of physical activity resources was not correlated with the probability of being an exerciser, leading to an interpretation that resources are unimportant. To extend previous findings, an inventory of facilities in the city was conducted, and the density of facilities around subjects' homes was calculated. Not only was the *objective* measure of convenience of facilities related to exercise status (after adjusting for demographic factors) but perceived and actual measures of the environment were generally unrelated to each other (Sallis and others, 1990). The latter study is interpreted as showing that the environment may have a direct effect on behavior that is not mediated by perceptions.

Behavior-Specific Ecological Models. An ecological model of physical activity will have to consider the effects of such settings as parks, health and fitness centers, neighborhoods, schools, workplaces, and shopping malls. Organizations and policies that affect transportation, health care, education, sporting goods availability, entertainment availability, urban design, and labor-saving devices need to be considered. The range of behavior settings and organizations with potential impact on physical activity suggests that a specific ecological model will be complex and that testing the model will be even more difficult than constructing it.

An Ecological Health Promotion Research Agenda

Ecological perspectives are now guiding health promotion policies and approaches internationally, but application has outpaced research. We are concerned that interest in ecological approaches will wane unless environmental interventions are informed by rigorous empirical research. In this section, we present some of the challenges of conducting ecological research and propose some research strategies and methods that we believe will be fruitful.

We contend that environmental variables have at least three functions that are important for health promotion researchers and practitioners. First, environmental variables are part of the complex web of causation that leads to healthful and unhealthful behaviors: most health behaviors will not be fully understood until environmental variables are considered. Second, environmental variables are likely to moderate the effects of health promotion programs; for example, programs that teach low-income mothers to prepare low-fat meals for their families will have limited success in environments in which the local food markets have few low-fat choices and the mothers do not have transportation to better-stocked markets. Third, environmental variables can be manipulated to achieve health promotion objectives.

There are unique challenges in studying environmental and social variables at higher levels of integration. We believe that these challenges discourage many researchers from pursuing investigations based on ecological models. Perhaps the most basic challenge is that many ecological variables are less subject to experimental control and manipulation than intrapersonal variables. On the one hand, it may take many years to change a health-related governmental policy, as it did to alter nutrition labeling in the United States. Obtaining more funds for bicycle trails, convincing food market managers to stock more low-fat items, and passing laws to ban cigarette vending machines may also be very difficult. On the other hand, workplace smoking bans have been introduced rapidly and have generated some compelling evidence of behavior-setting influences (Borland, Chapman, Owen, and Hill, 1990). Creativity, persistence, and teamwork will likely be required by health promotion professionals to achieve the types of environmental changes that warrant study. Changing environmental and policy variables often requires shifting the behavioral change target from the individual "consumer" to policy makers in corporations and governmental agencies. Many health promotion professionals have only limited experience in these areas, although antitobacco activists have broken a great deal of ground in recent years.

The very fact that environmental variables are ubiquitous and can have widespread effects on the population makes them difficult, if not impossible, to study. The measurement challenges are great, though some recent efforts have begun to move the field forward (Cheadle and others, 1992). When studying the effects of changes in behavior settings on health choices and actions, it is no longer possible to randomly assign *individuals* to experimental conditions. Larger units, or behavior settings, such as worksites, schools, and communities must be randomized. These studies are complex and expensive, and few of them will be conducted. Thus, the database on the effects of changing environmental variables grows slowly.

Despite the methodological and logistical challenges of ecological health behavior research, it is essential to expand the current database. The issues are somewhat different for various health behaviors, but we provide some general suggestions for conducting research on environmental influences.

1. Much more work is needed to conceptualize the relevant environmental and policy variables for each health behavior and develop objective measures of these variables. Research will not advance without progress in both conceptualization and measurement.

2. Descriptive research is needed to demonstrate that physical environment measures add variance to the explanation of behavior provided by intrapersonal and social and cultural domains. Thus, ecological research should include variables from all three domains.

3. Ecological models need to be tested with objective measures of environments. It cannot be assumed that measures of perceived environments alone accurately reflect actual environmental characteristics. Associations between perceived and objectively measured environmental variables should also be studied.

4. Multiple geographical and cultural settings may need to be studied to achieve sufficient variation in environmental and policy variables for investigators to study their associations with behavior. For some variables, it may be necessary and desirable to conduct studies in multiple countries. This strategy should apply to descriptive studies initially because intervention studies, if successful, will create variance in environmental characteristics.

5. Intervention research is needed to demonstrate that well-targeted environmental interventions are effective in changing behaviors. It is insufficient to document only changes in physical and social environments when the reason for promoting these changes was in fact to improve health behavior.

6. Intervention research is needed to demonstrate that well-targeted environmental interventions improve the effectiveness of programs targeting changes in intrapersonal or social variables. The implication of ecological models is that the most effective programs change relevant variables in all domains, including the physical environment.

7. As policies with the potential to influence health behavior are identified in the public and private sectors, the behavior of policy makers becomes a legitimate field of study. If the success of health promotion interventions depends on the actions of policy makers, then it is important to develop and evaluate programs to change policy makers' behavior. Although this shift of focus from consumers to policy makers may be uncomfortable for some health promotion professionals, this is a research topic with public health significance. Scientists and practitioners who are dedicated to improving public health cannot and should not overlook the potential impact of bringing their findings into the policy arena (Glanz, Rimer, and Lerman, 1996).

Conclusion

Theoretical work on ecological models has already had an impact on the practice of health promotion, and health promotion practice and policy are driving the development of innovative research. "Efforts to promote human well-being should be based on an understanding of the dynamic interplay among diverse environmental and personal factors, rather than on analyses that focus exclusively on environmental, biological, or behavioral factors" (Stokols, 1992). Too much of the energy and resources in health promotion research and practice remains narrowly focused on changing behavior through changes in intrapersonal factors such as knowledge, attitudes, and skills. Ecological models logically lead to health promotion approaches that supplement behavioral and educational programs with modifications in social climates, in policies, and in physical environments—modifications that encourage and support individuals to make healthy choices and take healthy actions in the conduct of their daily routines.

The database on environmental and policy influences on health behaviors will be incomplete in many key areas for years to come. This raises the important question whether health promotion practitioners should work harder to alter environmental variables and policies that ecological models suggest have influence on health behaviors or should wait for empirical documentation of the effects of a particular variable or policy before acting. Although we advocate empirically based health promotion practice, we think it would be shortsighted to discourage practitioners from trying to create environments that promote health just because data on the relationship between the environmental variable (or policy) and the behavior in question are limited. Ongoing dialogue between researchers and practitioners on these issues is crucial. Opportunities to evaluate innovations in practice deserve their collaborative attention.

Increasingly, health promotion practitioners and researchers are exhorted to focus on the settings in which people engage in health-related behavior. A better understanding of ecological models of health behavior and the explicit identification of the role of environmental variables in modifying health behaviors may lead to more effective approaches to health promotion.

References

Abrams, D. B., and others. "Social Learning Principles for Organizational Health Promotion: An Integrated Approach." In M. F. Cataldo and T. J. Coates, *Health and Industry: A Behavioral Medicine Perspective.* New York: Wiley, 1986.

Bandura, A. *Social Foundations of Thought and Action: A Social Cognitive Theory.* Englewood Cliffs, N.J.: Prentice Hall, 1986.

Baranowski, T. "Reciprocal Determinism at the Stages of Behavior Change: An Integration of Community, Personal, and Behavioral Perspectives." *International Quarterly of Community Health Education,* 1989, *10,* 297–327.

Barker, R. G. *Ecological Psychology.* Stanford, Calif.: Stanford University Press, 1968.

Borland, R., Chapman, S., Owen, N., and Hill, D. J. "Effects of Workplace Smoking Bans on Cigarette Consumption." *American Journal of Public Health,* 1990, *80,* 178–180.

Bronfenbrenner, U. *The Ecology of Human Development.* Cambridge, Mass.: Harvard University Press, 1979.

Cheadle, A., and others. "Environmental Indicators: A Tool for Evaluating Community-Based Health-Promotion Programs." *American Journal of Preventive Medicine,* 1992, *8*(6), 345–350.

Commonwealth Department of Human Services and Health. *Better Health Outcomes for Australians*. Canberra: Australian Government Publishing Service, 1994.

Dishman, R. K., and Sallis, J. F. "Determinants and Interventions for Physical Activity and Exercise." In C. Bouchard, R. J. Shephard, and T. Stephens (eds.), *Physical Activity, Fitness, and Health: International Proceedings and Consensus Statement*. Champaign, Ill.: Human Kinetics, 1994.

Elder, J. P., Geller, E. S., Hovell, M. F., and Mayer, J. A. *Motivating Health Behavior*. Albany, N.Y.: Delmar, 1994.

Ewart, C. K. "Social Action Theory for a Public Health Psychology." *American Psychologist*, 1990, *46*, 931–946.

Farris, R. P., Nicklas, T. A., Webber, L. S., and Berenson, G. S. "Nutrient Contribution of School Lunch Program: Implications for Healthy People 2000." *Journal of School Health*, 1992, *62*, 180–184.

Glanz, K., Rimer, B. K., and Lerman, C. "Ethical Issues in the Design and Conduct of Community-Based Intervention Studies." In S. Coughlin and T. Beauchamp (eds.), *Ethics in Epidemiology*. New York: Oxford University Press, 1996.

Glanz, K., and others. "Environmental and Policy Approaches to Cardiovascular Disease Prevention Through Nutrition: Opportunities for State and Local Action." *Health Education Quarterly*, 1995, *22*, 512–528.

Green, L. W., and Kreuter, M. W. *Health Promotion Planning: An Educational and Environmental Approach*. Mountain View, Calif.: Mayfield, 1990.

Hahn, R. A., Teutsch, S. M., Rothenberg, R. B., and Marks, J. S. "Excess Deaths from Nine Chronic Diseases in the United States, 1986." *Journal of the American Medical Association*, 1990, *264*, 2654–2659.

Karoly, P. "Ecobehavioral Assessment in Health Life-Styles: Concepts and Methods." In P. Karoly (ed.), *Measurement Strategies in Health Psychology*. New York: Wiley, 1985.

King, A. C., and others. "Environmental and Policy Approaches to Cardiovascular Disease Prevention Through Physical Activity: Issues and Opportunities." *Health Education Quarterly*, 1995, *22*, 499–511.

Lalonde, M. *A New Perspective on the Health of Canadians: A Working Document*. Toronto: Health and Welfare Canada, 1974.

Lewin, K. *Principles of Topological Psychology*. New York: McGraw-Hill, 1936.

Lowson, S., Toolis, R., and Leonard, D. "Store Food Studies in the Torres Strait." Paper presented at the annual meeting of the Public Health Association of Australia, Cairns, Queensland, Sept. 1995.

McLeroy, K. R., Bibeau, D., Steckler, A., and Glanz, K. "An Ecological Perspective on Health Promotion Programs." *Health Education Quarterly*, 1988, *15*, 351–377.

Milio, N. *Promoting Health Through Public Policy*. Ottawa: Canadian Public Health Association, 1986.

Moos, R. H. *The Human Context: Environmental Determinants of Behavior*. New York: Wiley-Interscience, 1976.

Moos, R. H. "Social-Ecological Perspectives on Health." In G. C. Stone, F. Cohen, and N. E. Adler (eds.), *Health Psychology: A Handbook*. San Francisco: Jossey-Bass, 1979.

Nader, P. R., and others. "A Family Approach to Cardiovascular Risk Reduction: Results from the San Diego Family Health Project." *Health Education Quarterly*, 1989, *16*, 229–244.

Ottawa Charter for Health Promotion. Ottawa: Canadian Public Health Association, 1986.

Owen, N., and Bauman, A. "The Descriptive Epidemiology of Physical Inactivity in Adult Australians." *International Journal of Epidemiology*, 1992, *21*, 305–310.

Sallis, J. F., and Hovell, M. F. "Determinants of Exercise Behavior." *Exercise and Sports Sciences Reviews*, 1990, *18*, 307–330.

Sallis, J. F., and others. "San Diego Surveyed for Heart-Healthy Foods and Exercise Facilities." *Public Health Reports*, 1986, *101*, 216–219.

Sallis, J. F., and others. "Distance Between Homes and Exercise Facilities Related to the Frequency of Exercise Among San Diego Residents." *Public Health Reports*, 1990, *105*, 179–185.

Sallis, J. F., and others. "Determinants of Physical Activity and Interventions In Youth." *Medicine and Science in Sports and Exercise*, 1992, *24*, S248–S257.

Sallis, J. F., and others. "Effects of a Two-Year Health-Related Physical Education Program on Physical Activity and Fitness in Elementary School Students: SPARK." *American Journal of Public Health*, forthcoming.

Skinner, B. F. *Science and Human Behavior.* New York: Macmillan, 1953.

Stephens, T., and Caspersen, C. "The Demography of Physical Activity." In C. Bouchard, R. J. Shephard, and T. Stephens (eds.), *Physical Activity, Fitness, and Health: International Proceedings and Consensus Statement.* Champaign, Ill: Human Kinetics, 1994.

Stokols, D. "Establishing and Maintaining Healthy Environments: Toward a Social Ecology of Health Promotion." *American Psychologist*, 1992, *47*(1), 6–22.

Stokols, D. "The Paradox of Environmental Psychology." *American Psychologist*, 1995, *50*, 821–837.

U.S. Department of Health and Human Services. *The Surgeon General's Report on Nutrition and Health.* DHHS publication no. PHS 91–50213. Washington, D.C.: U.S. Government Printing Office, 1988.

U.S. Department of Health and Human Services. *Healthy People 2000: National Health Promotion and Disease Prevention Objectives.* DHHS publication no. PHS 91–50213. Washington, D.C.: U.S. Government Printing Office, 1991.

Wicker, A. W. *An Introduction to Ecological Psychology.* Pacific Grove, Calif.: Brooks/Cole, 1979.

Winett, R. A. "A Framework for Health Promotion and Disease Prevention Programs." *American Psychologist*, 1995, *50*(5), 341–350.

Winett, R. A., King, A. C., and Altman, D. G. *Health Psychology and Public Health: An Integrative Approach.* New York: Pergamon, 1989.

CHAPTER TWENTY

SOCIOECONOMIC AND CULTURAL FACTORS IN THE DEVELOPMENT AND USE OF THEORY

Rena J. Pasick

"Barring occasional revolutions, science proceeds by replacing simpler truths with more complex ones," says Oechsli (1995). We see this borne out when we consider the effect that socioeconomic and cultural factors have, or ought to have, on theory and its applications.

The greatest burden of morbidity and mortality is disproportionately borne by people of color (Polednak, 1989) and by those in the lower socioeconomic strata of society (Aday, 1993; Susser, Watson, and Hopper, 1985; Kosa and Zola, 1975). Yet socioeconomic status and race and ethnicity often have been treated simplistically in the health literature, as context in health promotion and as variables to be controlled in epidemiology (Haan, Kaplan, and Syme, 1989; Marmot, Kogevinas, and Elston, 1987). As a result, many researchers and practitioners alike frequently express concern that the major health promotion theories are not derived from nor adequately tested among populations across socioeconomic classes and cultures.

This chapter illuminates steps we can take toward bridging this gap. Because race and class are important determinants of health, the underlying concepts and dimensions of these variables should become integral to theories of behavior and health promotion. Before this integration can be accomplished, several major challenges must first be understood and overcome. After a discussion of these challenges, highlights of past and current work illustrate both the challenges and some breakthroughs. Finally, this chapter makes recommendations that acknowledge the complex and multidimensional nature of socioeconomic and cultural factors, yet strive toward a manageable approach to understanding their influences on health and health behavior. Throughout, the implications for prioritizing, targeting, and tailoring health promotion interventions are emphasized.

Relevance of Socioeconomic Status and Culture for Theory

Theory is fundamental to health promotion as a means of understanding and predicting health behavior and informing interventions designed to promote and protect health. The extensive efforts to derive, test, and apply theory in health education and health promotion have been based on the tenet that there are commonalities across population groups in the factors that influence behavior and that there is consistency and predictability in the relationships among these factors. It is not that all concepts and patterns are considered the same for all people but that behavioral change propositions are considered applicable to population segments large enough to make the propositions very valuable in the pursuit of better health. Once such propositions are demonstrated under one set of circumstances, the questions then become: How generalizable are they to other conditions? And what, if any, are the most likely differences?

There are any number of circumstances under which theoretical relationships among factors affecting health behavior and health status might vary. But two that are particularly important are variations in socioeconomic conditions and in cultures. This is at least in part because, as a large body of evidence now shows, many health behaviors vary by socioeconomic status or by race and ethnicity (commonly used indicators of culture, as discussed later). For example, the now classic treatise on class and health known as the Black Report found that people's material conditions of life and their life positions in the social structure greatly affect their behavior, which in turn affects their health (Townsend and Davidson, 1988; Marmot, Kogevinas, and Elston, 1987). Similarly, culture has been described as "the milieu of attitudes and values [that] affects all choices" (Kreps and Kunimoto, 1994). The importance of socioeconomic status and culture is evident from the consistency with which each of these factors has been shown to predict behavior, morbidity, and mortality across a range of risk factors and health problems (Feinstein, 1993; U.S. Department of Health and Human Services, 1987).

Furthermore, the 1990 U.S. Census revealed a 30 percent increase from 1980 in the number of non-Anglos and persons of color (African Americans, Asians and Pacific Islanders, Hispanics, and others) who are residents of this country. The combined growth of these racial and ethnic groups is more than seven times the rate for non-Hispanic whites, leading to a new demographic reality for the twenty-first century, a country where whites will no longer form a majority of the population (Edmondson, 1991). Interwoven with this trend are sociocultural, economic, and political phenomena such as the growing number of children living in poverty (Children's Defense Fund, 1991; Aday, 1993), increasing homelessness, declining investments in education and social services (Skilnick, 1993), and the unprecedented disparity in income between rich and poor (Cutler and Katz, 1992). Thus, as people of color make up greater proportions of the population and as more people experience the deprivations associated with low income, we could expect that the health problems of these groups will at least persist and may be likely to increase. In fact, disparities in mortality between the poor and those with higher incomes increased dramatically over the past three decades (Pappas, Queen, Hadden, and Fisher, 1993). These are complex, multidimensional concerns. Development of theoretical models that can account for and address these issues must begin with recognition of the challenges that accompany this line of inquiry.

Key Concepts

This section defines some key terms and concepts and their relationship to measurement of outcomes.

Race, Ethnicity, and Culture

In the public health literature, the terms *race, ethnicity,* and *culture* are often used interchangeably. The implication appears to be that racial and ethnic categories define populations that are homogeneous in ways that are meaningful to health outcomes. However, a substantial body of scholarly work has demonstrated that race is a social construction with little direct biological significance and not a static genetically based characteristic (Kumanyika and Golden, 1991; Cooper and David, 1986; Williams, Lavizzo-Mourey, Warren, 1994; Betancourt and Lopez, 1993). In fact, there is more genetic variation *within* races than *between* them (Krieger and Bassett, 1986; Polednak, 1989). Furthermore, every major racial and ethnic group is composed of diverse subgroups whose experiences and values are substantially different. For the development and application of behavioral and health education theory, the concept of culture as distinct from race is more meaningful because it consists of a range of factors directly relevant to behavior. After all, behavior is the product of knowledge, attitudes, and beliefs arising in the context of life circumstances and experiences. When such beliefs or practices are learned, shared, and homogeneous within a group (not necessarily a racially defined group), they may be said to be cultural. While we cannot escape from the racial categories used in the presentation of important health data, our contributions to theory can be augmented by searching out the cultural similarities and differences within and across these groups. Toward this end, the following working operational definition of culture has been advanced. It is specific to the goals and methods of health promotion: culture is revealed through the unique shared values, beliefs, and practices that (1) are directly associated with a health-related behavior, (2) are indirectly associated with a behavior, or (3) influence acceptance and adoption of the health education message (Pasick, D'Onofrio, and Otero-Sabogal, forthcoming). For a review of other definitions of culture, see Orlandi, Weston, and Epstein, 1992.

An example of a cultural construct directly associated with a health behavior is the fatalistic outlook (*fatalismo*) reported among Latinos. It has been associated with denial of the potential for curing cancer and is a barrier to use of cancer screening tests (Perez-Stable and others, 1992). However, this fatalism is not unique to Latinos and has been observed among populations as diverse as Vietnamese immigrants and residents of Appalachia (Pasick and others, forthcoming; Garland, 1994). In an example of a cultural value indirectly associated with a behavior, Rimer and others (1991) have shown that physician reminders are important motivators for use of mammography. Thus, in cultures with a strong regard for physicians as authority figures, patients may be unlikely to request a mammogram if one has not been recommended by their doctor. Finally, culture can play a major role in the success or failure of an intervention by affecting the way people perceive and respond to a message or strategy. If a message appealing to each person's individuality is used in a highly collectivist culture (where it is the norm to give priority to the group and emphasize interdependence) (Triandis, 1994), the message will probably not be heard or attended to. Conversely, a health educator may influence someone in a culture that values family interdependence to accept cancer screening by presenting messages in terms of the importance of screening to a person's family.

Social Class and Socioeconomic Status

In general, *social class* is a theoretical concept "indicating the individual's location in the social stratification system and access to material resources, influence, and information" (Mechanic, 1989). *Socioeconomic status* (SES) is a constellation of variables used as indicators for social class. Typically, SES includes measures of income, education, and occupational status. The debatable aspects concern the extent to which these measures capture all the social, psychological, behavioral, political, material, and environmental factors suggested as links between social class and health. This is critical when the implication is that health-related behavior at the individual level is determined by a great number of interacting fac-tors at other levels (Sussman, 1992).

Some scholars have observed that many known risk factors often do not ex-plain very much of the observed health disparity between social classes (Krieger and others, 1993). Indeed, more and better research is needed to examine the role of behavior in the association between class and health and the socioeconomic determinants and consequences of health behaviors. Equally important is con-sideration of interventions that go beyond individual risk factors and deal with so-cioeconomic conditions that directly or indirectly influence health regardless of behavior. This might be achievable by defining target audiences based on so-cioeconomic and associated psychosocial characteristics, a definition that again raises the matter of the interaction between race and socioeconomic status.

Further, race and ethnicity can interact with SES but also have an indepen-dent influence on health. The extent of this relationship appears to depend on the psychosocial meaning that a particular racial or ethnic group has in society (Bunker, Gomby, and Kehrer, 1989). For example, it has long been observed that African American women are more likely than white women to be diagnosed at the later stages of breast cancer. A recent study found that history of mammog-raphy screening accounted for only 10 percent of this racial difference. After ac-counting for alternative explanations, the authors suggest that, because of race-linked differences in medical care and social factors, blacks may receive lower-quality screening services than do whites (Jones and others, 1995).

The available data suggest that the higher rates of disease among individuals in the lower socioeconomic strata are not simply a reflection of the higher per-centage of minority persons in those strata (Haan, Kaplan, and Syme, 1989). In fact, as several studies have noted, once income, education, and other socioeco-nomic variables are included in a model, race has little explanatory power for mor-tality (Logue and Jarjoura, 1990; Townsend, Davidson, and Whitehead, 1988). In other words, it may be SES that is most influential in accounting for disparities in disease rates.

This point is reinforced in a review of another enigmatic facet of the SES-health relationship, the graded association with health at all levels of socioeconomic status (Adler and others, 1994). This *gradient effect,* in which disparities in health be-haviors and outcomes are observed not only between rich and poor but between those better and worse off at every level of SES, most likely affords the best con-text for elucidating links between SES and health. Adler and colleagues (1994) pro-pose several analytical and conceptual steps toward this end, including examination of variables beyond the standard SES indicators, variables such as health behav-iors, psychological factors, and perceptions of social ordering. They further suggest that such analyses may point to higher-order variables such as the concept of control over existing life circumstances (Rodin, 1986). Further, they suggest that new conceptualizations and measures of control may be needed to capture this type of cross-domain influence. This recommendation illuminates still another paradox, the importance of measurement across diverse populations whose linguistic and cultural differences present challenges in every aspect of measurement.

Measurement

The development and testing of theory is highly dependent on the valid and reliable measurement of concepts. If a theory is to be tested across cultures and socioeconomic strata, the relevant variables must have comparable meaning across these groups, that is, they must have *cultural equivalence* (Berry, 1969). Also, the measurement tools must be culturally appropriate (Marín and Marín, 1991) and usable for multiple educational and literacy levels.

A concept that is likely to be culturally bound and subjective, such as sense of control, is difficult to measure across cultures. This dilemma is best approached by first establishing a body of knowledge on the cultural characteristics of target audiences. For example, to know if variables measuring a concept like perceived susceptibility (see Chapter Three) are comparable in different cultures and languages, extensive qualitative and quantitative testing is needed within each group. Next, cross-cultural testing can establish whether or not particular constructs have universal or culture-specific meaning (Triandis, 1994). If language differences exist, questions need to be translated so that comparable meaning is retained (Pasick and others, forthcoming). The research that is needed to ensure the quality and comparability of key theoretical variables is likely to be extensive and time consuming, much more so than the investigation generally planned for construct development with a single population.

Advances to Date

Much has already been learned in the course of research and practice that can inform the advancement of theory in the context of diversity. Noteworthy examples are highlighted here.

Audience Segmentation, Targeting, and Tailoring

The application of social marketing principles and methods to health promotion in general and to audience segmentation in particular (Kotler and Roberto, 1989) has contributed to a great diversification of research and a growing body of data on many different population subgroups. Integral to the social marketing concept is refinement of the terms *targeting* (the process of identifying a population subgroup by parameters relevant to program objectives) and *tailoring* (the adaptation of interventions that best fit the relevant needs and characteristics of a specified target population). For example, intra-ethnic segmentation reveals the heterogeneity within racial and ethnic classifications. In a study demonstrating the value of ethnic group disaggregation, Williams and Flora (1995) identified heterogeneous behaviors in mutually exclusive Hispanic subgroups that were meaningful both for health criteria (such as lipid levels and hypertension) and for intervention dimensions (such as income, education, communication channels, health practices, and diet and exercise self-efficacy). Williams and Flora's conclusion was that the subgroups are audience segments sufficiently different to warrant different messages in a communication campaign.

An important cultural variable on which to segment for intra-ethnic and cross-ethnic comparisons is *acculturation,* the cultural learning and behavioral adaptation that takes place among individuals exposed to a new culture (Padilla, 1980). Although this concept is complex to measure, particularly across cultures and languages, it has been repeatedly shown to modify significantly the effect of many health factors (Marín and Marín, 1991). An example appears in a later section.

Beyond Reaching the Hard to Reach

In health promotion and education from the mid-1960s through the mid-1980s, most research and programming were targeted to the predominantly white middle class. During that time, disparities in health practices and outcomes were widening, leading to the conclusion that populations of color and lower-class groups were "hard to reach" (Freimuth and Mettger, 1990). The tide appears to have turned dramatically on this point as there are now published reports of programs that bring AIDS education to prostitutes and injection drug users (Janz and others, 1996), strategies that increase breast and cervical cancer screening among inner-city black women (Lacey and others, 1993), programs that serve the homeless and drug addicted (Nyamathi, 1994), cancer control programs that are offered to American Indians (Michielutte, Sharp, Dignan, and Blinson, 1994), heart health education that is presented to Southeast Asians (Chen, 1989), communication strategies that are targeted to low-literacy adults (Plimpton and Root, 1994), and many more.

Increasing Acceptance of Qualitative Research

As already suggested, much that remains to be learned about the relationships between culture, socioeconomic status, and health eludes or pushes the bounds of standard methods of quantitative research. Even before the current widespread appreciation for social marketing principles and methods, professionals in health education and health promotion began to regard use of focus groups and other qualitative methods as valuable tools. Now, epidemiologists and health services researchers are recognizing the value of inductive reasoning, observation, unstructured interviews, and triangulation of qualitative and quantitative methods (see, for example, Pope and Mays, 1995).

The development of theory that explains behavior among persons of diverse SES and culture will likely have its origins in qualitative research. For example, Roe, Minkler, and Saunders (1995) studied the socioeconomic and cultural phenomenon of grandparent caregiving in the context of the crack cocaine epidemic. This is a unique population segment based not on race or any disease-specific risk factor but on a social condition with broad implications for health. Investigators used grounded theory (Strauss and Corbin, 1990), and sampling and concepts to be measured evolved as data were collected. While this was primarily a formative study, it used the data collection process to discover influential variables and to initiate family-, community-, and policy-level action. Ultimately, theories generated in this way will require cross-cultural testing using new or adapted methods of survey research.

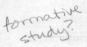

Examples from Current Research

Race- and ethnic-specific studies have been described as a second generation of health promotion research, the first being the body of work that did not differentiate racial and ethnic groups or was specifically confined to mainstream populations. The first generation of health promotion studies assumed similarities across groups, with not much focus on potentially important differences. The second generation has been immersed in the differences (Pasick, D'Onofrio, and Otero-Sabogal, forthcoming).

Research on single racial or ethnic groups should not be an end in itself but can serve as a tool that opens up new territory for exploration. For one thing, the diversity within a racial or ethnic population may perpetuate derivation of theory that is overly generic. Second, this approach diverts attention from some other cultural elements with relevance to behavior. Thus, second-generation research should be primarily preparation for a third generation that advances understanding of both behavioral influences and intervention elements that are universal and those that are culture-specific. More and better second-generation studies (those that study one ethnic group) should be designed and implemented with the specific intent to facilitate valid cross-ethnic comparisons.

Several studies at the Northern California Cancer Center suggest directions for third-generation inquiry. They address the problems of late-stage diagnosis of breast and cervical cancer, attributed to low use of screening among specific racial and ethnic and lower-SES groups. This research includes descriptive studies of the barriers and incentives to screening among Filipino women (McBride and Pasick, 1994–1997) and Chinese women (a Pathways project, Lee, 1992–1996). It also includes the Breast and Cervical Cancer Intervention Trial (BACCIS), a community-based randomized controlled intervention trial targeting multiple groups (Latina, African American, Chinese, and white) (Hiatt, 1991–1996), and intervention trials focusing on single racial and ethnic groups (Vietnamese and Latina) (Pathways projects, McPhee 1992–1996; Perez-Stable, 1992–1996). The following collection of experiences from these ongoing studies illustrates some of the key issues, advances, and problems described previously.

Application to Measurement

The identification and measurement of variables to inform and test theories across racial and ethnic groups was not a specific aim of the studies mentioned. However, those of us conducting the studies have attempted to integrate this question into the research for all of them. The BACCIS, Pathways, and Filipino studies used telephone or household surveys as the primary source of descriptive and evaluative data. In the development of each instrument, we faced a trade-off between adequately covering important elements of subjective culture and inclusion of variables to measure theoretic concepts. Funding and the constraints of survey research converged to limit our interview time to no more than forty minutes. Large sections of the instruments had to be devoted to key dependent and demographic variables, including measures of acculturation, screening practices, cancer history, access to medical care, source of care, and patient-provider communication. Thus, neither culture nor theory could be extensively explored. There was room only for a few variables from potentially relevant theories such the Health Belief Model and the Theory of Reasoned Action and for exploration of some PRECEDE model components.

Application to Audience Segmentation

Early in the BACCIS community intervention, we saw that there were no printed materials in Chinese on breast and cervical cancer screening. From our multi-ethnic, multilingual baseline survey ($n = 1,600$), we found the lowest levels of screening reported among monolingual Chinese women, regardless of age. For example, 51 percent of low acculturation level (indicated by non-English-speaking status)

Chinese women had never even heard of a mammogram. Sixty-eight percent had never had a mammogram, compared with 24 percent in the total BACCIS sample, and 30 percent in a national survey of whites, blacks, and Hispanics (Hiatt and Pasick, forthcoming).

We decided to focus specifically on the monolingual Chinese population. In this group ($n = 194$), factor analysis was used to identify factors that were key barriers to screening. These were (1) lack of access to medical care (due to inadequate insurance or lack of a regular source of care, for example); (2) low use of available providers (no routine doctor visits in the past year and no plans for a checkup among those with a regular source of care); and (3) lack of awareness of the value of screening (belief that a mammogram is not needed if nothing is wrong and if the doctor does not recommend it).

Further analysis of groups of respondents according to these factors revealed four clusters: (1) women with no access (the working poor: those who were employed but reported low income and no health insurance); (2) women with access but no use (slightly higher income: healthy women who have insurance but who do not feel the need for medical services); (3) women with access and use but low awareness (generally low-income elderly: women who were retired with insurance and who used medical care regularly); and (4) women with access, use, and awareness (relatively well off financially: those who were insured, and who had been screened). Clearly, the women in the first cluster were the neediest, and they became the targeted segment for a Chinese-language booklet. A translated version was developed for professional use, because Chinese women who speak only English represent a very different segment, one not addressed by this booklet.

Application to Intervention Design

In the design of community-based interventions informed by theory, we have had our most consistent success across cultures with combinations of elements from Social Cognitive Theory (see Chapter Eight), diffusion theory (see Chapter Thirteen), and The Transtheoretical Model of behavioral change (see Chapter Four). Although there have been cultural nuances in the applications, the general strategy of using role models from the community, trained for outreach and education, has been central to our interventions (Bird, Otero-Sabogal, Ha, and McPhee, forthcoming). We believe that an important next step will be grounded theory research (Strauss and Corbin, 1990) on the cultural dimensions of communication between lay health workers and their clients.

One of the primary tasks of the BACCIS lay health workers was to ascertain the adoption stage for mammography and Pap smear screening of women contacted in the course of outreach. The lay health workers then followed protocols for message tailoring and for reinforcement over time. Although collection of outcome data is currently under way, impact data for initial and follow-up adoption stages show significant improvements in stage of readiness over the course of the intervention for all racial and ethnic groups. Thus, elements of The Transtheoretical Model appear to have broad applicability both for informing the intervention and documenting its impact.

In addition to providing outreach to individuals, BACCIS worked with providers and other agencies to establish free screening resources in low-income communities. Still, organizational barriers persist in the form of long waits for appointments and the need for multiple visits to complete screening. Furthermore, only the lowest-income women are eligible for free services, and those whose residency status is undocumented face additional hurdles when tests require follow-up of an abnormality. These problems are likely to worsen as safety-net providers (county clinics and hospitals) fail in the competitive environment of managed care. So, although our research is producing interpersonal and organizational intervention strategies that appear effective across cultures, persistent sociostructural barriers continually require elucidation and multilevel intervention.

Conclusion and Recommendations

This section draws on the preceding discussion and applications to suggest ways that health promotion and health behavior practitioners and researchers can better incorporate cultural and socioeconomic diversity into their application of theories and conceptual frameworks.

Focus on Both Social Class and Culture

Professionals dedicated to improving health should strive to understand and address the social and political determinants of social class and their relationship to health. Even risk factor–specific strategies can be embedded in a broader context. In research and practice, social class should be considered an object of change rather than merely an independent variable. Both social class and culture are important factors in predicting behavior and defining meaningful audience segments, but social class warrants special attention as a determinant of behavior. When practitioners or researchers are trying to enhance the reach and appeal of interventions, culture is likely to be pivotal as well.

Synthesize and Build on What Is Known

The literature and experiences from the field could better inform theory if organized and presented with the aim of synthesizing and building on what is known. First, there exists a considerable body of knowledge about why diverse groups behave in certain ways, what strategies work, and under what conditions they work.

Practitioners who live and work among the target populations are the often untapped source of this information. Research should be encouraged that originates with inductive exploration of practitioners' experiences for the derivation of concepts and theories followed by empirical testing.

Second, far more detailed information is needed on the specifics of what works and what does not, as reports in the literature tend to focus more on outcomes than on how those outcomes were achieved. Published reports could be improved as a source of this detailed information. Two models are found in Shea, Basch, Wechsler, and Lantigua (1996) and Janz and others (1996). The former reports on a single study, detailing successful and unsuccessful program elements. The latter is a quantitative and qualitative review of thirty-seven AIDS prevention projects, describing the factors and mechanisms influencing the interventions. Of particular importance are the conclusions drawn about the effectiveness of specific program elements for different population segments.

Third, the current diffuse literature could be synthesized through a consensus-building process that informs a long-range research agenda. This synthesis might be initiated by convening a multidisciplinary, multi-ethnic team of experts from around the country to extensively review the health literature and the literature of other relevant social sciences such as cross-cultural psychology, education, and social welfare. Based on initial findings, a conference could foster dialogue on substantive and methodological topics, culminating in a state-of-the-science monograph. It will be important that such an endeavor truly delve into the empirical and conceptual literature, not merely amount to a discussion of the ideas held by experts and interested parties.

Test Existing Theory

Rather than attempting to fit the study of culture and social class into research with other primary aims, investigators need to conduct studies that specifically address comparative testing of theories across cultures, acculturation levels, and socioeconomic strata. This testing could be modeled on Mullen, Hersey, and Iverson's survey (1987) of a white, black, and Hispanic sample to compare the predictive power of the Health Belief Model, PRECEDE, and the Theory of Reasoned Action for four health behaviors. Their findings were comparisons of each theory's predictive power, relative parsimony, acceptability to respondents, and specificity for planning.

Expand the Field of Qualified Professionals

A long-standing lament throughout the health professions is the need for cultural diversity within their own ranks. This is true in practice but all the more so in the research that produces theory. Far more intensive efforts are needed to recruit graduate students and professionals from all backgrounds into the field of research on health and behavior. While individuals cannot presume to speak for entire cultural groups, there can be no substitute for the combination of innate knowledge of a culture and strong research skills.

References

Aday, L. A. *At Risk in America: The Health and Health Care Needs of Vulnerable Populations in the United States.* San Francisco: Jossey-Bass, 1993.

Adler, N. E., and others. "Socioeconomic Status and Health: The Challenge of the Gradient." *American Psychologist,* 1994, *49*(1), 15–24.

Berry, J. "On Cross-Cultural Comparability." *International Journal of Psychology,* 1969, *4,* 207–229.

Betancourt, H., and Lopez, S. R. "The Study of Culture, Ethnicity, and Race in American Psychology." *American Psychology,* 1993, *48,* 629–637.

Bird, J. A., Otero-Sabogal, R., Ha, N. T., and McPhee, S. J. "Lay Health Worker Interventions: The Vietnamese and Latina Pathways Programs." *Health Education Quarterly Supplement: Promoting Cancer Screening in Ethnically Diverse and Underserved Communities: The Pathways Project,* forthcoming.

Bunker, J. P., Gomby, D. S., and Kehrer, B. H. (eds.). *Pathways to Health: The Role of Social Factors.* Menlo Park, Calif.: Henry J. Kaiser Family Foundation, 1989.

Chen, M. S. "The Indigenous Model and Its Application to Heart Health for Southeast Asians." *Health Education,* 1989, *20,* 48–51.

Children's Defense Fund. *Child Poverty in America.* Washington, D.C.: Children's Defense Fund, 1991.

Cooper, R., and David, R. "The Biological Concept of Race and Its Application to Public Health and Epidemiology." *Journal of Health Politics, Policy and Law,* 1986, *11,* 97–116.

Cutler, D. M., and Katz, L. F. "Untouched by the Rising Tide: Why the 1980s Economic Expansion Left the Poor Behind." *Brookings Review,* 1992, *10,* 40–46.

Edmondson, B. *American Diversity.* American Demographics Desk Reference Series, no. 1. Ithaca, N.Y.: American Demographics, 1991.

Feinstein, J. S. "The Relationship Between Socioeconomic Status and Health: A Review of the Literature." *Milbank Memorial Fund Quarterly,* 1993, *71*(2), 279–322.

Freimuth, V. S., and Mettger, W. "Is There a Hard-to-Reach Audience?" *Public Health Reports,* 1990, *105,* 232–238.

Garland, B. "Appalachian Issues." Paper presented at the President's Cancer Panel Meeting on Cancer and the Cultures of America, San Francisco, Nov. 1994.

Haan, M. N., Kaplan, G. A., and Syme, S. L. *Socioeconomic Status and Health: Old Observations and New Thoughts.* In J. P. Bunker, D. S. Gomby, and B. H. Kehrer (eds.), *Pathways to Health: The Role of Social Factors.* Menlo Park, Calif.: Henry J. Kaiser Family Foundation, 1989.

Hiatt, R. A. "Breast and Cervical Cancer Intervention Study" (BACCIS). National Institutes of Health/National Cancer Institute Grant no. RO1-CA54605, 9/25/91–8/31/96.

Hiatt, R. A., and Pasick, R. J. "Unsolved Problems in Early Breast Cancer Detection: Focus on the Underserved." *Breast Cancer Research and Treatment,* forthcoming.

Janz, N. K., and others. "Evaluation of 37 AIDS Prevention Projects: Successful Approaches and Barriers to Program Effectiveness." *Health Education Quarterly,* 1996, *23*(1), 80–97.

Jones, B. A., and others. "Can Mammography Screening Explain the Race Difference in Stage at Diagnosis of Breast Cancer?" *Cancer,* 1995, *75,* 2103–2113.

Kosa, J., and Zola, I. K. (eds.). *Poverty and Health: A Sociological Analysis.* Cambridge, Mass.: Harvard University Press, 1975.

Kotler, P., and Roberto, E. L. *Social Marketing: Strategies for Changing Public Behavior.* New York: Free Press, 1989.

Kreps, G. L., and Kunimoto, E. N. *Effective Communication in Multi-Cultural Health Care Settings.* Thousand Oaks, Calif.: Sage, 1994.

Krieger, N., and Bassett, M. "The Health of Black Folk: Disease, Class and Ideology in Science." *Monthly Review,* 1986, *38,* 74–85.

Krieger, N., and others. "Racism, Sexism, and Social Class: Implications for Studies of Health, Disease, and Well-Being." *American Journal of Preventive Medicine,* 1993, *8,* 82S–122S.

Kumanyika, S. K., and Golden, P. M. "Cross-Sectional Differences in Health Status in U.S. Racial/Ethnic Minority Groups: Potential Influence of Temporal Changes, Disease, and Life-Style Transitions." *Ethnicity and Disease,* 1991, *1,* 50–59.

Lacey, L., and others. "Referral Adherence in an Inner City Breast and Cervical Cancer Screening Program." *Cancer,* 1993, *72,* 950–955.

Lee, M. "Pathways to Early Cancer Detection for Chinese Americans: A Developmental Study." (R. A. Hiatt, Project P.I.) National Institutes of Health/National Cancer Institute Grant no. PO1 CA55112, "Pathways to Cancer Screening for Five Ethnic Groups," 9/30/92–9/29/96.

Logue, E. E., and Jarjoura, D. "Modeling Heart Disease Mortality with Census Tract Rates and Social Class Mixtures." *Social Science and Medicine,* 1990, *31,* 545–550.

Marín, G., and Marín, B. V. *Research with Hispanic Populations.* Thousand Oaks, Calif.: Sage, 1991.

Marmot, M. G., Kogevinas, M., and Elston, M. S. "Social/Economic Status and Disease." *Annual Review of Public Health,* 1987, *8,* 111–135.

McBride, M. R., and Pasick, R. J. "Early Cancer Detection for Filipino American Women." U.S. Army, Department of Defense Grant no. DAMD17–94-J-4215, 10/1/94–9/30/97.

McPhee, S. "Pathways to Early Cancer Detection for Vietnamese." (R. A. Hiatt, Project P.I.) National Institutes of Health/National Cancer Institute Grant no. PO1 CA55112, "Pathways to Cancer Screening for Five Ethnic Groups," 9/30/92–9/29/96.

Mechanic, D. "Socioeconomic Status and Health: An Examination of Underlying Processes." In J. P. Bunker, D. S. Gomby, and B. H. Kehrer (eds.), *Pathways to Health: The Role of Social Factors.* Menlo Park, Calif.: Henry J. Kaiser Family Foundation, 1989.

Michielutte, R., Sharp, P. C., Dignan, M. B., and Blinson, K. "Cultural Issues in the Development of Cancer Control Programs for American Indian Populations." *Journal of Health Care for the Poor and Underserved,* 1994, *5,* 280–296.

Mullen, P. D., Hersey, J. C., and Iverson, D. C. "Health Behavior Models Compared." *Social Science and Medicine,* 1987, *24*(11), 973–981.

Nyamathi, A. M. "A Research Trajectory on Health Promotion Among Impoverished Women of Color." In *Wellness Lecture Series.* Vol. 2. Oakland: University of California/Health Net, 1994.

Oechsli, F. W. "Ethnicity, Socioeconomic Status, and the 50-Year U.S. Infant Mortality Record." Editorial. *American Journal of Public Health,* 1995, *85,* 905–906.

Orlandi, M. A., Weston, R., and Epstein, L. G. (eds.). *Cultural Competence for Evaluators.* DHHS publication no. 92–1884. Washington, D.C.: U.S. Department of Health and Human Services, 1992.

Padilla, A. M. (ed.) *Acculturation: Theory, Models and Some New Findings.* Boulder, Colo.: Westview, 1980.

Pappas, G., Queen, S., Hadden, W., and Fisher, G. "The Increasing Disparity in Mortality Between Socioeconomic Groups in the United States, 1960–1986." *New England Journal of Medicine,* 1993, *329,* 103–109.

Pasick, R. J., D'Onofrio, C. N., and Otero-Sabogal, R. "Similarities and Differences Across Cultures: Questions to Inform a Third Generation for Health Promotion Research." *Health Education Quarterly Supplement: Promoting Cancer Screening in Ethnically Diverse and Underserved Communities: The Pathways Project,* forthcoming.

Pasick, R. J., and others. "Problems and Progress in Development and Translation of Health Questions Across Race/Ethnic Groups: The Pathways Experience." *Health Education Quarterly Supplement: Promoting Cancer Screening in Ethnically Diverse and Underserved Communities: The Pathways Project,* forthcoming.

Perez-Stable, E. "Pathways to Early Cancer Detection for Hispanics." (R. A. Hiatt, Project P.I.) National Institutes of Health/National Cancer Institute Grant no. PO1 CA55112, "Pathways to Cancer Screening for Five Ethnic Groups," 9/30/92–9/29/96.

Perez-Stable, E., and others. "Misconceptions About Cancer Among Latinos and Anglos." *Journal of the American Medical Association,* 1992, *268,* 3219–3223.

Plimpton, S., and Root, J. "Materials and Strategies That Work in Low Literacy Health Communication." *Public Health Reports,* 1994, *109,* 86–92.

Polednak, A. P. *Racial and Ethnic Differences in Disease.* New York: Oxford University Press, 1989.

Pope, C., and Mays, N. "Reaching the Parts Other Methods Cannot Reach: An Introduction to Qualitative Methods in Health and Health Services Research." *British Medical Journal,* 1995, *311,* 42–45.

Rimer, B. K., and others. "Why Do Women Get Regular Mammograms?" *American Journal of Preventive Medicine,* 1991, *7*(2), 69–74.

Rodin, J. "Aging and Health: Effects of the Sense of Control." *Science,* 1986, *233,* 1271–1276.

Roe, K. M., Minkler, M., and Saunders, F. F. "Combining Research, Advocacy, and Education: The Methods of the Grandparent Caregiver Study." *Health Education Quarterly,* 1995, *22*(4), 458–475.

Sabogal, F., and others. "Printed Health Education Materials for Diverse Communities: Suggestions Learned from the Field." *Health Education Quarterly Supplement: Promoting Cancer Screening in Ethnically Diverse and Underserved Communities: The Pathways Project,* forthcoming.

Shea, S., Basch, C. E., Wechsler, H., and Lantigua, R. "The Washington Heights–Inwood Health Heart Program: A 6-Year Report from a Disadvantaged Urban Setting." *American Journal of Public Health,* 1996, *86,* 166–171.

Skilnick, A. "NMA Seeks Prescription to End Violence." *Journal of the American Medical Association,* 1993, *270,* 1283–1284.

Strauss, A. L., and Corbin, J. M. *Basics of Qualitative Research: Grounded Theory Procedures and Techniques.* Thousand Oaks, Calif.: Sage, 1990.

Susser, M. W., Watson, W., and Hopper, K. (eds.). *Sociology in Medicine.* (3rd ed.) New York: Oxford University Press, 1985.

Sussman, L. K. "Critical Assessment of Models." In D. M. Becker and others (eds.), *Health Behavior Research in Minority Populations.* NIH publication no. 92–2965. Bethesda, Md.: U.S. Department of Health and Human Services, 1992.

Townsend, P., and Davidson, N. (eds.). *Inequalities in Health: The Black Report.* Harmondsworth, England: Penguin Books, 1988.

Townsend, P., Davidson, N., and Whitehead, M. *Inequalities in Health.* Harmondsworth, England: Penguin Books, 1988.

Triandis, H. C. *Culture and Social Behavior.* New York: McGraw-Hill, 1994.

U.S. Department of Health and Human Services. *Report of the Secretary's Task Force on Black and Minority Health.* Washington, D.C.: U.S. Government Printing Office, 1987.

Williams, D. R., Lavizzo-Mourey, R., and Warren, R. C. "The Concept of Race and Health Status in America." *Public Health Reports,* 1994, *109*(1), 26–41.

Williams, J. E. "Using Social Marketing to Understand Racially, Ethnically, and Culturally Diverse Audiences for Public Health Interventions." In D. M. Becker and others (eds.), *Health Behavior Research in Minority Populations.* NIH publication no. 92–2965. Bethesda, Md.: U.S. Department of Health and Human Services, 1992.

Williams, J. E., and Flora, J. A. "Health Behavior Segmentation and Campaign Planning to Reduce Cardiovascular Disease Risk Among Hispanics." *Health Education Quarterly,* 1995, *22*, 36–48.

CHAPTER TWENTY-ONE

PERSPECTIVES ON USING THEORY

Karen Glanz

The chapters in Part Five describe models for using theories in combination, consider ecological models as an overarching perspective to guide health behavior and health promotion interventions, and examine how cultural and socioeconomic factors have been, and can be, integrated into theory development and application. Together, these chapters of *Health Behavior and Health Education* tackle the complexity of health behavior and health promotion at its multiple levels. A basic theme is that if intervention strategies are based on a carefully researched understanding of the determinants of behavior and environments, and if systematic approaches to tailoring, targeting, implementation, and evaluation are used, the chances are good that programs will be effective.

This chapter reviews highlights from each of the four chapters in this section, discusses emerging developments and challenges, and comments on the state of the art in the use of theory and on the role and influence of funding institutions on theory, research, and practice. The discussion aims to provoke thought and debate and to stimulate further reading rather than to provide definitive answers or prescriptions for the field.

PRECEDE-PROCEED Model for Health Promotion Planning

In Chapter Seventeen, Gielen and McDonald present an overview of PRECEDE-PROCEED, describe each of its phases, and apply the model in a case study of child injury prevention. They explicitly illustrate the ways that behavioral change theories can be applied and incorporated into a systematic planning process. They further note the challenges of using PRECEDE-PROCEED, which can be a demanding and laborious model for practitioners and community groups. When mastered, however, it can lead to the development of effective, appropriate health education programs. Computer technologies that employ expert systems have now been developed to assist with the data-gathering tasks of PRECEDE-PROCEED (Green, Gold, Tan, and Kreuter, 1994).

Although health behavior theories are critical tools, the health educator cannot substitute theory for planning or research. The role of theory is to help us interpret problem situations and plan feasible and promising interventions. It also assists us in program evaluation. Because it identifies the assumptions behind intervention strategies, theory helps us pinpoint intermediate steps that should be assessed in evaluation. These *mediating factors* clarify the reasons why programs achieve or fail to achieve our goals for success in changing behaviors or environments. The PRECEDE-PROCEED model has as its raison d'être the systematic application of theory and previous research to the assessment of local needs, priorities, circumstances, and resources (Green and others, 1994). Its owes its robustness in part to the fact that it is intuitively appealing and logical; in fact, though it has been widely used for more than fifteen years, similar models continue to be put forth today (Winett, 1995).

Theory is most likely to be informative during phase 4 of the planning process suggested by PRECEDE-PROCEED, the educational and organizational diagnosis. This phase examines factors that shape behavioral actions and environmental factors. Theories guide the examination of predisposing, enabling, and reinforcing factors. For example, the constructs of the Health Belief Model might help investigators understand why some women do not get mammograms (see Chapter Three). PRECEDE-PROCEED can also be used in conjunction with The Transtheoretical Model of Stages of Change to design stage-appropriate health education messages (Rimer, 1995; see Chapter Four). This type of analysis focuses on the specific leverage points that best influence desired behaviors. Levers are sought among such predisposing factors as motives, such reinforcing factors as rewards, and such enabling factors or barriers as health insurance or access to care. The concepts of priority, changeability, and community preferences should be considered along with analytical and empirical findings about health behavior determinants.

Social Marketing

Social marketing is a process to develop, implement, evaluate, and control behavioral change programs by creating and maintaining exchanges. It involves the adaptation of commercial marketing technologies to promote socially desirable goals.

As Lefebvre and Rochlin stress in Chapter Eighteen, social marketing takes a *consumer orientation:* success is most likely when health promoters accurately determine the perceptions, needs, and wants of target markets and satisfy them through the design, communication, pricing, and delivery of appropriate, competitive, and visible offerings. The process is consumer driven, not expert driven. It is consistent with principles of community organization, and its product development approach parallels the innovation development process of diffusion theory.

Like the PRECEDE-PROCEED model, social marketing provides a framework for identifying factors that drive and maintain behavior and that drive and maintain behavioral change. It also requires identification of potential intermediaries, channels of distribution and communication, and actual and potential competitors. Theories of health behavior can help guide the analytical process in social marketing and aid in the formulation of intervention strategies and materials. Due to the focus on understanding consumers (or target audiences) from the consumers' point of view, social marketing models are robust for use in diverse and unique populations, including disadvantaged groups and ethnic minorities (Lasater and others, 1992).

Social marketing techniques have been widely used to design complex and large-scale health promotion campaigns such as the Office of Cancer Communication's breast cancer education program. Individual-level models, network analyses, and communication theories all figure into the planning process. As Lefebvre and Rochlin point out, while there is a great deal of research *within* social marketing models, there is less research *on* the approach itself. Thus, it is not possible to say whether better programs are created with social marketing methods than with other planning processes, whether the process is efficient or unnecessarily demanding, and the like. Such evaluations should be included on health education's research agenda for the future.

Ecological Models

In Chapter Nineteen, Sallis and Owen discuss the aims and core concepts of ecological models for health promotion. As shown in Chapter One, the basic tenets of ecological perspectives—of multilevel determinants of behavior and environments and of transactions between individuals and their environments—are widely recognized as useful and appropriate orientations for contemporary health promotion. Sallis and Owen trace the historical development of ecological models and note, quite accurately, that applications of the models have outpaced research identifying either their demonstrable effects or the mechanisms by which their components parts operate. In 1992, Stokols recommended choosing among alternative strategies within a social ecological perspective for health promotion on the basis of their grounding in research, feasibility, likelihood of reaching a large segment of the target population, and consistency with community priorities and commitments. These recommendations resonate clearly with key elements of the program-planning processes advanced in the PRECEDE-PROCEED and social marketing models.

The contemporary focus on ecological models was highlighted by the recent publication of a special social ecology issue of the *American Journal of Health Promotion,* released after the completion of Chapter Nineteen. The tenor of some of the special issue articles echoes Sallis and Owen's sentiments that ecological strategies tend to be complex and cumbersome and that few, if any, rigorous program evaluations test the value of ecological approaches (Stokols, Allen, and Bellingham, 1996). In an adaptation for ecologically sustainable community planning and evaluation, Green and colleagues depict the compatibility of ecological approaches with the PRECEDE-PROCEED model (Green, Richards, and Potvin, 1996). An important and useful article in the collection contains Stokols's guidelines for translating social ecological theory into guidelines for community health promotion (Stokols, 1996). He identifies parallels between and distinctions among theoretical and research perspectives at the individual, community, environmental, and social ecological levels. He notes that combinations of active and passive interventions spanning individual, organizational, and community levels are most closely suggested by social ecology. Finally, he identifies procedural guidelines for applying various ecological principles, including examining links between multiple facets of well-being and environmental conditions; examining joint influences on behavioral responses to the environment; identifying points of poor person-environment fit and developing interventions to improve that fit; identifying leverage points for health promotion; and integrating biomedical, regulatory, behavioral, and environmental interventions. These guidelines, while fitting the ecological tradition most closely, overlap substantially with much of what has been suggested in other models and theories for health promotion. They also fit with the core principles explicated by Sallis and Owen.

The challenge to conduct better research on ecological interventions is a paradoxical one. Hypothetico-deductive scientific method may require a degree of simplification of ecosystems, making strategies seem artificially clear-cut when they are inherently complex (Green, Richards, and Potvin, 1996). A combination of the inductive and deductive methods, using both qualitative and quantitative approaches, is more likely to reveal the rich texture of ecological approaches while also allowing assessment of their impact on valued outcomes.

Cultural and Socioeconomic Factors

Pasick's chapter on socioeconomic and cultural factors in the development and use of theory provides the rationale for health behavior theory and health promotion that takes account of an increasingly diverse population. Pasick also defines key terms and addresses the challenges inherent in addressing diversity. The U.S. population is becoming increasingly diverse, minority group members are often economically disadvantaged, and disparities in health continue to be large and marked. Behavioral and health promotion researchers and practitioners are increasingly cognizant of these issues and beginning to address them with great vigor, but the state of the art provides few, if any, clear-cut answers to how best to proceed. The more we work with special populations, the more we discover how little we really know about them.

With respect to socioeconomic status (SES), a variety of mechanisms have been suggested for the graded association of SES with health at all levels: access to care, depression, psychological stress, effects of hierarchical positioning in society, and health behavior (Adler and others, 1994). Canadian researchers found that socioeconomic risk explained 87 percent to 92 percent of differences in health status and acute hospitalizations, suggesting interactions between intrapersonal factors and inequities in access to health care (Mustard and Frohlich, 1995). The multidimensionality of socioeconomic status, which includes the factors of income, education, and conditions of housing, and its multicollinearity with minority ethnic status suggest that many important variables are probably intertwined (Adler and others, 1994).

Many recently funded community intervention studies that are rooted in health behavior theories are ongoing in minority and disadvantaged populations (Glanz, forthcoming), but it will be several years until their results are available. Some existing evaluation data provide timely and practical lessons for health promotion: for example, that cultural sensitivity needs to be built into programs and not "tacked on" as an afterthought (Janz and others, 1996). Other studies underscore the disempowering effects of community violence in communities of color, and the need to consider these effects in new health promotion efforts (Sanders-Phillips, 1996). A review of interventions among Native Americans revealed the use of such appropriate strategies as involving tribal elders, storytelling, and participatory planning but indicated that barriers of distrust and lack of acceptance of outside interventionists persist (LeMaster and Connell, 1994).

Calls for more and better application of theory in programs and research are echoed in the literature with predictable regularity (Marín and others, 1995; Lasater and others, 1992). Still, some contemporary theories and models lend themselves well to diverse populations; for example, PRECEDE-PROCEED, The Transtheoretical Model, Social Cognitive Theory (Rimer and others, 1992), and social marketing (Lasater and others, 1992). Due to their disproportionate burden of disease, disability, and premature death, we will continue to see increased intervention research directed to minority and low-income communities, even though such research is made difficult by complex issues of equivalence of measurement, translation, and the like (Triandis,

1994). Community relations must also be considered. In order to produce high-quality, ethical health research in minority and disadvantaged communities, both researchers and funding institutions need to overcome objections that community partnerships introduce unacceptable biases and compromise methodological rigor (Glanz, Rimer, and Lerman, 1996).

Is Theory Being Used?

To what degree are professional health promotion and educational activities based on *theory*? Few empirical data on this question are available (Glanz and Oldenburg, 1996). In a review of theory use in the recent professional literature, the editors of this book found that slightly less than half of all articles relevant to health behavior and health promotion reported on explicit use of one or more theories (see Chapter Two). As to practitioners' use of theory, it has been suggested that many are most comfortable regarding "theory and practice as separate realms" (D'Onofrio, 1992). Practitioners may find the abstract thinking involved in applying theoretical constructs too demanding for their fast-paced work environments (Glanz and Oldenburg, 1996). Others may find that theory acts as a valuable reference point, maintaining their focus on key goals during turbulent times (Howze and Redman, 1992). Nevertheless, there is likely a small but significant proportion of health promotion professionals who consistently aim to use theory as a tool to untangle and simplify the complexities of human nature (Green and others, 1994).

Little research is available to confirm these observations, though one recent study provides partial support. A survey of 284 practitioners and researchers in nutrition education and consumer behavior showed that most respondents considered theoretically based concepts to be important but not readily accessible or routinely used. Researchers were more familiar with a range of theories than were practitioners, and the results indicated a perceived need for more active interchange between researchers and practitioners as well as literature to better guide translation of theories into practical methods (Glanz and Rudd, 1993). Increasingly, there are resources that make theory accessible to practitioners and introduce and reinforce it in clear, usable, problem-based formats. The chapters in Part Five of this book should be valuable to those who seek to use theory in their work.

Funding Sources, Health Promotion, and Applied Theory

Several chapters in this text have made reference to the role that funding plays in facilitating health promotion programs and research. Concerns have also been raised about the way in which funding circumscribes the type of health promotion strategies used and the specific health problem focus. Some have astutely suggested that categorical health funding (for example, for drug and alcohol abuse prevention, cancer control, diabetes, and so on) is antithetical to health promotion principles and strategies that encourage communities to define their own needs and problems. More foundations have departed from categorical funding in recent years, but most governmental and voluntary health organizations prefer to support work that is consistent with their missions. It remains for skillful practitioners and researchers to use funds wisely so that communities are served well and so that the cumulative body of knowledge in health behavior includes generalizable findings and lessons.

The availability, amount, and duration of funding profoundly affects applied behavioral research based on health behavior theories. As noted earlier, research involving minority and disadvantaged communities is not always well served by traditional investigator-driven scientific methods, though these are often most readily funded. Often, theoretically informed research answers tests a central hypothesis without adequately analyzing the extent to which the components of theory are supported by the data (Rimer and others, 1992). Funding institutions should support these analyses with supplemental grants for selected projects and by drawing together groups of investigators and projects whose work is amenable to secondary analysis, in order to answer important theoretical and practical questions that cut across individual projects.

Conclusion

After practitioners become familiar with some contemporary theories of health behavior, the challenge is to use them within a comprehensive planning process. Planning systems like social marketing and PRECEDE-PROCEED increase the odds of success by examining health and behavior at multiple levels. This ecological perspective emphasizes two main options: change people or change the environment. The most powerful approaches will use both of these options together. The activities most directly tied to changing *people* are derived from individual-level theories like the Health Belief Model, The Transtheoretical Model of Stages of Change, and the Transactional Model of Stress and Coping. In contrast, activities aimed at changing the *environment* draw on community-level theories. In between are Social Cognitive Theory, social support and social networks, and interpersonal communication models. Each of these focuses on reciprocal relations among persons or between individuals and their environments.

Theoretical frameworks are guides in the pursuit of successful efforts, maximizing program flexibility and helping investigators apply the abstract concepts of theory in ways that are most useful in diverse work settings and situations. A knowledge of theory and comprehensive planning systems offers a great deal. Other key elements of effective programs are a good program-to-audience match; accessible and practical information; active learning and involvement; and skill building, practice, and reinforcement. Theory helps investigators ask the right questions, and effective planning enables them to zero in on elements that relate to a specific problem. Effective use of theory for practice and research requires practice but can yield important dividends in efforts to enhance the health of individuals and populations.

References

Adler, N. E., and others. "Socioeconomic Status and Health: The Challenge of the Gradient." *American Psychologist,* 1994, *49*(1), 15–24.

D'Onofrio, C. N. "Theory and the Empowerment of Health Education Practitioners." *Health Education Quarterly,* 1992, *19*(3), 385–403.

Glanz, K. "Behavioral Research Contributions and Needs in Cancer Prevention and Control: Dietary Change." *Preventive Medicine,* forthcoming.

Glanz, K., and Oldenburg, B. "Relevance of Health Behavior Research to Health Promotion and Education." In D. S. Gochman (ed.), *Handbook of Health Behavior Research,* Vol. 4. New York: Plenum, 1996.

Glanz, K., Rimer, B. K., and Lerman, C. "Ethical Issues in the Design and Conduct of Community-Based Intervention Studies." In S. Coughlin and T. Beauchamp (eds.), *Ethics in Epidemiology.* New York: Oxford University Press, 1996.

Glanz, K., and Rudd, J. "Views of Theory, Research, and Practice: A Survey of Nutrition Education and Consumer Behavior Professionals." *Journal of Nutrition Education,* 1993, *25*(5), 269–273.

Green, L. W., Gold, R., Tan, J., and Kreuter, M. "The EMPOWER/Canadian Health Expert System." *Canadian Medical Informatics,* 1994, *1*(4), 20–23.

Green, L. W., Richards, L., and Potvin, L. "Ecological Foundations of Health Promotion." *American Journal of Health Promotion,* 1996, *10*(4), 270–281.

Green, L. W., and others. "Can We Build On, or Must We Replace, the Theories and Models in Health Education?" *Health Education Research,* 1994, *9*(3), 397–404.

Howze, E. H., and Redman, L. J. "The Uses of Theory in Health Advocacy: Policies and Programs." *Health Education Quarterly,* 1992, *19*(3; special issue: *Roles and Uses of Theory in Health Education Practice*), 369–383.

Janz, N. K., and others. "Evaluation of 37 AIDS Prevention Projects: Successful Approaches and Barriers to Program Effectiveness." *Health Education Quarterly,* 1996, *23*(1), 80–97.

Lasater, T., and others. "Task Group VI: Social Marketing Planning Model: An Approach to Programs and Research for Groups from Diverse Backgrounds." In D. M. Becker and others (eds.), *Health Behavior Research in Minority Populations: Access, Design, and Implementation.* NIH publication no. 92–2965. Bethesda, Md.: U.S. Department of Health and Human Services, 1992.

LeMaster, P., and Connell, C. "Health Education Interventions Among Native Americans: A Review and Analysis." *Health Education Quarterly,* 1994, *21*(4), 521–538.

Marín, G., and others. "A Research Agenda for Health Education Among Underserved Populations." *Health Education Quarterly,* 1995, *22*(3), 346–363.

Mustard, C., and Frohlich, N. "Socioeconomic Status and the Health of the Population." *Medical Care,* 1995, *33*(12), DS43–DS54.

Rimer, B. K. "Audiences and Messages for Breast and Cervical Cancer Screening." *Wellness Perspectives: Research, Theory and Practice,* 1995, *11*(2), 13–39.

Rimer, B. K., and others. "Task Group V: The Role of Theory in Health Behavior Research in Minority Populations." In D. M. Becker and others (eds.), *Health Behavior Research in Minority Populations: Access, Design, and Implementation.* NIH publication no. 92–2965. Bethesda, Md.: U.S. Department of Health and Human Services, 1992.

Sanders-Phillips, K. "The Ecology of Urban Violence: Its Relationships to Health Promotion Behaviors in Low-Income Black and Latino Communities." *American Journal of Health Promotion,* 1996, *10*(4), 308–317.

Stokols, D. "Establishing and Maintaining Healthy Environments: Toward a Social Ecology of Health Promotion." *American Psychologist,* 1992, *47*(1), 6–22.

Stokols, D. "Translating Social Ecological Theory into Guidelines for Community Health Promotion." *American Journal of Health Promotion,* 1996, *10*(4), 282–298.

Stokols, D., Allen, J., and Bellingham, R. "The Social Ecology of Health Promotion: Implications for Research and Practice." *American Journal of Health Promotion,* 1996, *10*(4), 247–251.

Triandis, H. C. *Culture and Social Behavior.* New York: McGraw-Hill, 1994.

Winett, R. A. "A Framework for Health Promotion and Disease Prevention Programs." *American Psychologist,* 1995, *50*(5), 341–350.

PART SIX

NEXT STEPS AND BEYOND

CHAPTER TWENTY-TWO

HEALTH BEHAVIOR
AND HEALTH EDUCATION

The Past, Present, and Future

David B. Abrams
Karen M. Emmons
Laura A. Linnan

If I have seen further . . . it is by standing on the shoulders of giants.
ISAAC NEWTON, LETTER TO ROBERT HOOKE, FEBRUARY 5, 1676

Just as Sir Isaac Newton's discoveries rested upon the work of his predecessors, the future of health promotion and education holds great promise as a result of the efforts of many—researchers and practitioners alike. This chapter addresses four primary objectives that remain to challenge researchers and practitioners. First, we explore the need for an overarching integrative framework. Second, we identify selected conceptual issues that cut across chapters. Our aim is to highlight constructs that have withstood the test of time and to demonstrate how cross-cutting comparisons can reveal differences, similarities, and new perspectives. An understanding of the different theoretical perspectives can identify boundary conditions and can lead to new insights as well as to the reevaluation of current wisdom.

Third, we identify practical realities that rise above theoretical concerns and pose barriers to the integration of theory into practice. It is our premise that failure

We thank Barbara Doll for doing outstanding work on the typing of this chapter. Preparation of this chapter is supported in part by National Cancer Institute Grants CA38309, CA27821, and PO1 CA50087 and by National Heart, Lung, and Blood Institute grant HL32318.

to acknowledge and contend with tensions between theory and practice slows the progress of improving the health of populations across the world, from developed to developing to impoverished nations. Fourth, we address our vision of the future for health behavior and health education. Exciting opportunities lie ahead for those involved in health behavior change. Interdisciplinary integration is central to advancing individual and population health behavior change research and practice. The lessons of the past and the current status of the field can guide us toward producing a new synthesis of concepts for the future. We will propose working toward a more unified and parsimonious approach to theory construction and toward a seamless melding of research with socially relevant real-world practice. The involvement of the target audience and practitioners in the process of theory construction moves all of us closer to the goal of participatory or action research. To move forward will also require our taking the high ground, rising above the insularity, rivalries, and self-protection within the current theoretical schools, disciplines, and practice constituencies. Our field needs less dogmatism and more openness to criticism, more testing of one theory against another, and a stronger commitment among constituencies to search for and find common ground in language, definition of constructs, measures, descriptions of samples, and intervention principles.

Integrative Conceptual Framework

This chapter as a whole is guided by an overarching conceptual framework that highlights the current need to focus on social imperatives (the socioeconomic, environmental, and individual factors that determine the scale and the pattern of disease), the need to take action, and the ways to best prioritize interventions and cost effectively allocate finite resources for the greatest long-term benefit to society.

Four major dimensions define the overarching contextual boundaries of health behavior change:

1. A continuum that ranges from individual to population *characteristics,* indicating vulnerability and motivational readiness to change, such as genetic susceptibility, knowledge, beliefs, resources and supports, and sociodemographics.
2. A continuum of *intervention characteristics,* indicating intensity and impact as determined by efficacy, reach (penetration), and cost. Impact is an example of a common metric of efficiency (as described later and in Table 22.1) that combines effectiveness and reach into a defined population (impact = efficacy × reach) per unit cost. Impact and cost effectiveness can be conceived as a function of

population characteristics and intervention types, modes, methods, and delivery channels.

3. A *temporal dimension,* reflecting the change process over time and in interaction with the first two dimensions. At the individual level, the temporal dimension is reflected in such predisposing factors as the intergenerational transmission of genetic vulnerability and the behavioral history of risk factors that interact with the environment and unfold over the lifespan from conception to death. At the population level, time is reflected in institutional norms, policies, and values in a specific society, that is, in a population's sociopolitical infrastructure. Predisposing factors at the population level include a nation's socioeconomic development status (with important differences between developed and developing nations of the world) and the historical and current values within defined populations such as states, communities, worksites, and school systems.

4. A continuum from wellness to illness, along which the population is proportionally distributed as determined by interactions among the other three dimensions.

This four-dimensional conceptualization of the key dimensions needed to describe a health behavior change process also provides direction and focus; it serves as a contextual compass and a road map for action. As an overarching framework, it places each element of a specific health education approach, theory, or measure in a contextual perspective. It can be envisioned as a pyramid within whose area one can locate the position of a specific type of intervention or conceptual model; target a particular individual or population within a relevant developmental time frame and within the history of predisposing individual, group, community, or national developmental factors; and produce a particular pattern and type of variation along the continuum of health status from illness to wellness (see Figure 22.1).

Contextual Boundaries in Health Education

Health education and health behavior have evolved over the years as an interdisciplinary field, dedicated to understanding and changing the tripartite "bio-psycho-social" factors that determine health and illness (Weiss, 1987). Different segments of populations can be targeted for change by the various intervention delivery strategies of the biopsychosocial model: (1) the biomedical disciplines (for example, the basic biological sciences such as genetics, molecular biology, neuroscience, and the medical model); (2) the individual cognitive and behavioral disciplines (for example, behavioral medicine, clinical nutrition, and the psychosocial

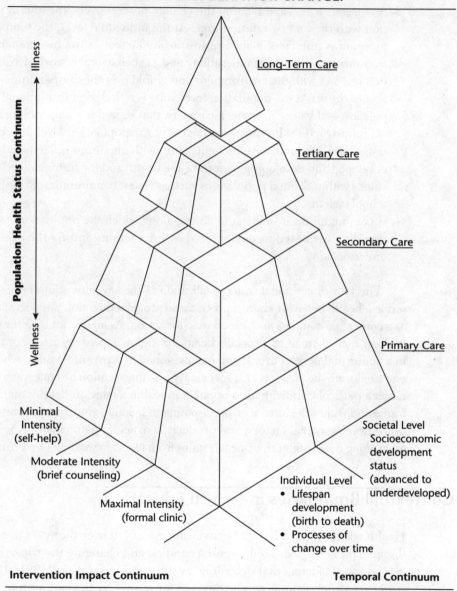

**FIGURE 22.1. FOUR-DIMENSIONAL FRAMEWORK
FOR HEALTH BEHAVIOR CHANGE.**

models of individual change); and (3) the disciplines that study groups or populations, reflecting the sociocultural, normative, economic, epidemiological, and political arenas (for example, mass communications, community organization models of change, and health policy and other public health models). The common metric of impact (efficacy × reach) and of cost per unit of impact (for example, cost of obtaining a 5 percent cessation rate among 30 percent of all the smokers in a worksite over one year) can be mapped onto the domain of a continuum of care from primary prevention through secondary and tertiary care to rehabilitation and long-term care (see Figure 22.2). As interventions vary from least effective and least intensive to most effective and most intensive, their reach ranges from larger to smaller proportions of a population, and the cost per unit of change in intervention impact will generally range from low to high cost.

The inside area of the triangle in Figure 22.2 represents any type of a defined population (for example, a worksite, a school, a community, or a nation). The distribution of health and disease among the individuals and groups within this defined population is proportional to the horizontal bands in the triangle. For an economically advanced (Western industrialized) population, the majority of the population is made up of younger and healthier members, represented in the largest band, at the base of the triangle. The middle band of the triangle represents the increasingly high-risk proportions of the population, such as the genetically susceptible and the older, higher risk, and lower socioeconomic status members. At the apex of the triangle is the much smaller proportion of those already acutely, chronically, or terminally ill. The largest health care needs, costs, and demands for intensive specialty services are made by this small minority. This is the domain of traditional medicine as it focuses on the treatment of illness.

The biopsychosocial model depicted in Figure 22.2 illustrates with greater specificity the relationship among interventions and population characteristics shown in the overarching pyramid structure of Figure 22.1. Within the biopsychosocial model, researchers and practitioners need to better integrate biomedical, cognitive-behavioral, and public health theories in order to optimize the design, delivery, and prioritization of interventions across the continuum of health care from primary, secondary, and tertiary care to rehabilitation and long-term care. For example, linkages are needed across similar levels as they are addressed by such different disciplines as public health education, public policy, community medicine, and occupational health and safety at the societal primary prevention level and family practice, pediatrics, and primary care medicine at the individual primary prevention level. Then, linkages are also needed between different levels: for example, between the two primary prevention levels and such more traditional medical care levels as specialty, hospital, and emergency treatment for

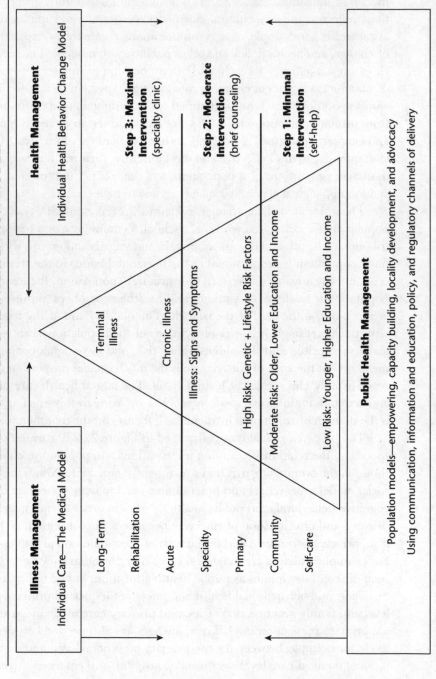

FIGURE 22.2. A STEPPED-CARE INTERVENTION MODEL.

Illness Management

Individual Care—The Medical Model

Long-Term

Rehabilitation

Acute

Specialty

Primary

Community

Self-care

Terminal Illness

Chronic Illness

Illness: Signs and Symptoms

High Risk: Genetic + Lifestyle Risk Factors

Moderate Risk: Older, Lower Education and Income

Low Risk: Younger, Higher Education and Income

Health Management

Individual Health Behavior Change Model

Step 3: Maximal Intervention (specialty clinic)

Step 2: Moderate Intervention (brief counseling)

Step 1: Minimal Intervention (self-help)

Public Health Management

Population models—empowering, capacity building, locality development, and advocacy

Using communication, information and education, policy, and regulatory channels of delivery those members of society who require acute care and between rehabilitative medicine and long-term care and those areas of the health care system such as home care and hospice care that deal with the management of terminal illness. Rose (1992) states, "The primary determinants of disease are mainly economic and social, and therefore its remedies must also be economic and social. Medicine and politics cannot and should not be kept apart." To medicine and politics, we would add behavior, since over 50 percent of chronic disease is potentially preventable, as it is attributable to such lifestyle factors as smoking, poor diet, lack of physical activity, and failure to obtain regular screening tests (McGinnis and Lee, 1995).

The major intervention domains (primary, secondary, and tertiary) to improve the health status of populations should be more strongly linked together, but finite costs and limited resources make rational allocation difficult to accomplish in practice. Linkages of services can be accomplished using three broad levels, or steps, in a *stepped-care* approach that allocates interventions across populations according to their cost and impact, that is, their value to society in the long run. Relatively low-cost public health interventions (for example, mass media and self-help materials) can be widely disseminated to populations (step 1: minimal intensity). Such programs generally have very low efficacy, but they do have broad reach. Programs with somewhat greater levels of intervention intensity constitute step 2 (moderate intensity). These programs focus on reaching individuals or groups rather than whole populations, and they do so through specific delivery channels. However, they can still reach relatively large numbers of persons. Some of the attractive specific channels are community organizations, schools, worksites, and primary care physicians' offices. Over 70 percent of Americans visit a physician at least once a year. Thus, step 2 interventions are more effective, intensive, specialized, and tailored to individual (or channel-specific) needs—*and* more costly than step 1 interventions. For example, a step 2 intervention through the primary care channel might consist of brief physician advice, nicotine replacement therapy, and follow-ups by a nurse-educator to assist a currently healthy forty-five-year-old smoker to quit smoking during a routine office visit for bronchitis. Because step 2 interventions are brief, they remain a good value in terms of impact and cost. They can still reach relatively large proportions of the population with moderate efficacy, so they may be considered the single most important set of interventions within the continuum of care.

Step 3 interventions are clearly more specialized, expensive, and targeted toward high-risk individuals who are hard to treat, already have signs or symptoms of chronic disease, or are in tertiary care: rehabilitation and long-term care. Step 3 interventions target individuals at highest risk and with the most serious psychological, biological, and environmental complications. It would be difficult or impossible for these individuals to improve their lifestyles with only step 1 or step 2 levels of care. Individuals who need step 3 care generally have multiple risk factors, may have comorbidity in the form of psychiatric disorders (for example, the alcoholic who is sedentary, has a poor diet, smokes heavily and has a family history of major depressive disorder) and may experience other severe environmental barriers to changing behaviors and accessing preventive care (poverty, lack of transport, or lack of health insurance or child care). Step 3 care is very specialized and expensive and has an extremely limited reach. Compared to steps 1 and 2, step 3 has the greatest efficacy but only modest *impact* because of its narrow reach and high cost. Table 22.1 uses the stepped-care classification of interventions and the concept of reach to directly compare impact and efficiency and hence cost effectiveness (see also Glanz and Seewald-Klein, 1986). This three-step approach to improving the health status of a population guides the integration and optimization of health education resources across the continuum of care for the greatest societal benefit.

With the dawning of the twenty-first century there is a crucial need for better allocation of finite resources and for better continuity in health care delivery strategies to improve the health of the population. The bottom-line criterion for selection of an optimal intervention strategy is its benefit to society at large, measured in terms of intensity, reach, efficacy, and the like. This criterion is best communicated by a standard metric—a measure of societal "value" such as impact (Abrams and others, forthcoming), cost effectiveness (Warner and Luce, 1982) or quality-adjusted life-years saved (Zeckhauser and Shepard, 1976).

TABLE 22.1. THE EFFICACY, REACH, AND IMPACT OF STEPPED STRATEGIES.

Intervention Intensity	Efficacy (E) (percent)	Reach (R) (percent)	Impact (R × E)
Step 1: minimal (self-help)	5	80	4.0
Step 2: moderate (brief counseling)	15	70	10.5
Step 3: maximal (specialty clinic)	40	10	4.0

This table illustrates the use of impact as a common metric to compare the efficiency of individual-clinical and population–public health strategies. Impact is defined on a 100-point scale (in arbitrary units) and reflects a combination of efficacy and reach (impact = efficacy x reach); where efficacy is the percentage of a population that meets an outcome criterion (for example, stops smoking) and reach is the percentage of penetration into the population (for example, 10 percent of all eligible smokers were aware of the intervention and had access to it).

The Importance of Good Theory in Health Education and the Issue of Proliferation

Perhaps the most important guideline for good theory is the law of parsimony, which states that a theory must be reduced to its simplest and fewest essential principles. Evaluation of new theories (or of proposed extensions to existing ones) should determine (1) whether the new definitions of terms, models, or constructs do or do not overlap with existing ones; and (2) whether the new model has any incremental value for the field. The recommended solution to the discovery of overlap or redundancy in a theory is surgery—the application of Occam's razor—to reduce the theory to its essential, simplest, necessary, and sufficient (parsimonious) elements.

Descriptive classifications, or taxonomies, based on observation of differences among known groups (for example, sociodemographics or stages of change) can be useful. Taxonomies can also be based on empirical distinctions, as in the case, for example, of using a cluster analysis of a population to reveal important subgroups that may benefit from different intervention approaches (that is, the matching of individuals or subgroups to treatments). Moreover, developing a descriptive classification system does not necessarily create a new theory or model. It often takes decades before the elements in a new model can be prospectively tested.

Weinstein (1993) cautions against the proliferation of theories. Expanding the scope of a coherent, integrative theory is distinctly different from creating minor variations on an existing theory or putting together conglomerates from different theories. There is little to be gained from a proliferation of redundant theories. Part of the problem with proliferation is that the field of health education does not have a common core of widely agreed upon universal principles or truths about human behavior.

Weinstein (1993) also observed that few reviews offer detailed comparisons between models. He pointed out what to look for when seeking the differences between models, such as the differences in the rules used to combine independent variables when predicting behavioral outcomes, the differences in the principle mediating and moderating the variables involved, whether the rules are additive or multiplicative, and whether appropriate weightings of variables are applied. This detailed level of scrutiny can lead us to a better understanding of the strengths and weaknesses of existing theories. A similar comparison of models was completed recently for applications to mammography (Curry and Emmons, 1994); others would be useful as well. Cummings, Becker, and Maile (1980) recommended an empirical approach to comparing theories of health behavior. They suggest that the actual number of truly distinct concepts needed to explain health-related actions is considerably smaller than the large number of variables typically employed in research studies. They presented fourteen models to a panel of expert judges, asking them to create a parsimonious taxonomy of the common factors affecting health behavior. From the ninety-nine variables included in the selected models, *only six variable* categories were extracted.

Common Roots and Cross-Cutting Themes among Individual, Group, and Community Theories

Many theories derive from common psychological, sociological, and biological principles. The goal of this section is to highlight selected key theoretical constructs that have made important contributions to the field and have withstood empirical scrutiny. Some of these constructs may be candidates for an inventory of rules or core principles that guide health behavior change processes. Selected examples of interventions are provided here that integrate or cut across theories and across the sections in this book.

The chapters by Strecher and Rosenstock (Chapter Three) and Baranowski, Perry, and Parcel (Chapter Eight) espouse the historical importance of the sciences of psychology and sociology in health education and remind us of our roots in the first half of this century in Lewin's field theory, along with Thorndike's, Watson's, Pavlov's, and Skinner's cognitive, stimulus-response, classical, and operant learning theories, respectively. The models derived from these theories incorporate several universal principles that cut across our latest theories and have stood the test of time.

Individual theories, such as Skinner's theory of operant conditioning (1953), contain several valuable cross-cutting principles: one is that positive reinforcers shape new behavior and are preferable to punishments that simply suppress behavior (for example, a zero-tolerance drug policy may simply suppress behavior while a more open harm-reduction philosophy could reinforce (behaviorally shape) individuals for any small positive steps toward reducing risky behavior) (Marlatt and Tappert, 1993). Another Skinnerian principle is that an immediate certain reward is more powerful than a delayed or uncertain reward. Proximity of cues and consequences is also important—proximity can be temporal, physical, social, environmental, biobehavioral, or cognitive or emotional (Miller, Shoda, and Hurley, 1996). A smaller immediate reward is usually more powerful than a larger delayed reward. Immediate, personal, tailored, biological, cognitive, emotional, and behavioral constructs can be used as powerful motivators of change or as cues to action (Green and Kreuter, 1991). Using biomarker feedback for smokers (which tells them such things as their pulmonary function and carbon monoxide levels) or recently discovered markers of genetic susceptibility for breast cancer such as BRCA1 and BRCA2 (Lerman and others, 1996) allows personalized tailored feedback to an individual about personal vulnerability using his or her own biological data.

Building on the foundation laid by Skinner and the learning theorists, Bandura (1986) and others developed Social Learning Theory in the early 1960s. They incorporated the cognitive and interpersonal processes into behavioral change mechanisms. One of Bandura's earliest contributions was to recognize the importance of learning very complex behaviors by observing the behavior of others (role models). Simply watching a violent role model increased violent behavior (punching an inflated doll) among children. This powerful principle of human behavior has not been lost on the tobacco advertising industry—Joe Camel is more popular among preteen children than Mickey Mouse. One cross-cutting social-learning construct concerns the importance of outcome expectations (Bandura, 1986), which reflect a person's beliefs about the likelihood of a specific negative health outcome. These beliefs have most often been labeled *perceived vulnerability* or *perceived susceptibility.* This construct can be found in the Health Belief Model, The Transtheoretical Model, the Theory of Reasoned Action, and the Theory of Planned Behavior.

The large amount of research conducted on self-efficacy highlights the robustness of the self-efficacy construct. Self-efficacy is an individual's level of confidence that he or she has the skills and persistence to accomplish a desired goal. Beliefs about personal efficacy (Bandura, 1986) and the newer concept of a *collective* or group sense of self-efficacy (Abrams and others, 1986) now occupy a pivotal role in several theories. Self-efficacy may be labeled differently by some theorists, for example, it is referred to as "the temptations" scale in The Transtheoretical Model of smoking behavior (Velicer, DiClemente, Rossi, and Prochaska, 1990). Self-efficacy expectations predict future behavior across a wide variety of lifestyle risk factors (Clark and others, 1991). Self-efficacy also explains persistence in the light of setbacks on the path to change (Bandura, 1986). Intervention programs are now routinely designed to enhance self-efficacy for change.

Another cross-cutting social-learning construct relates to the process of self-regulation or self-control (Bandura, 1986). Self-regulation involves imagining future outcomes, setting small achievable (proximal) goals, acquiring knowledge and coping skills, building self-efficacy and then self-observing one's progress, correcting errors, and providing self-directed reinforcement for progress made toward goal attainment. Individual goal setting, making plans to change a behavior, or intention, is also a central part of the Theory of Reasoned Action and the Theory of Planned Behavior (Chapter Five). The self-regulatory process probably underlies the movement through the stages of change (concept of motivation) that are part of The Transtheoretical Model (Chapter Four). Intentions and goal-setting constructs can also bridge individual, group, organizational, and population change levels, as illustrated by the reciprocal interaction between self and environment that is also part of the self-regulation process (Leventhal, Zimmerman, and Gutmann, 1984) and appears in early models of organizational and community change (Abrams and others, 1986).

Many of the theories used in health education (for example, the Health Belief Model and The Transtheoretical Model) focus on the individual. Reciprocal determinism (Bandura, 1986) holds that change and learning is a function of a three-way (and bidirectional) interaction among a person's cognitive self-regulatory mechanisms, his or her behavior, and the social and physical environment. Reciprocal determinism can be considered the guiding principle behind the current trend toward simultaneously intervening on multiple levels of behavioral influence (see Chapter Nineteen, on ecological models). Examples include interventions at the patient, provider, and health care system levels and community programs that target for change both individuals and their proximal (for example, family) and distal (for example, worksite) social and physical environments (Abrams and others, 1986, 1991, 1994). Reciprocal determinism also draws attention to the temporal and dynamic process of change across multiple levels of social influence over time. Groups of individuals change over time, moving from lower to higher motivation, and a critical mass develops. The process of change through a social network, in turn, contributes to the rate of diffusion (the S-curve) at the population level (Rogers, 1983; see Chapter Thirteen).

The chapters in this book on group and organizational theory research and practice (Chapters Eight to Sixteen) incorporate reciprocal determinism. Examples include (1) models for optimizing school and worksite health promotion programs (Flay, Phil, Petraitis, and Hu, 1995); (2) strategies for reducing community cardiovascular disease risk factors; and (3) calls for better integration of interventions that target multiple risk factors within and across individuals over time, factors such as alcohol, tobacco, diet, and sedentary lifestyle and also mental health factors such as depression (Abrams, Marlatt, and Sobell, 1995; Emmons and others, 1994). Oldenburg, Owen, Parle, and Gomel (1995) used a composite score of multiple risk factors to conduct a cost-effectiveness evaluation of a worksite cardiovascular risk reduction intervention.

This selective review of underlying concepts that cut across disciplines is not exhaustive. Space constraints preclude coverage of all the concepts worthy of consideration. Moreover, as we shall see in the next section, the translation of theory and its best principles into practice, and even the use of multiple theoretical perspectives and cross-cutting concepts, appears to have resulted in only modest improvements in the overall impact and cost effectiveness of most intervention trials to date, especially those dissemination studies targeted to communities (Fisher, 1995; see Chapter One).

Practical Realities in the Integration of Theory into Practice

Practical realities face both researchers and practitioners in their quest to improve the impact of interventions. Although health educators are admonished to employ theoretical approaches in their program development and evaluation (D'Onofrio, 1992), the barriers to doing so are infrequently addressed. Failure to acknowledge conflicts or tensions between theory and practice will result in missed opportunities and will slow the field's progress. Tensions are ever present in any field and are a healthy sign of dissatisfaction with the status quo. As writers in this field, we recognize that our depiction of such tensions as extremes oversimplifies complex issues. Nonetheless, it may be helpful to showcase the extremes because some tensions may be obvious but others are more subtle. A specific context or situation may mask tension or pull investigators' attention in a particular direction so that other options are overlooked, resulting in less than optimal allocation of finite public health resources. For example, an investigator planning an antiviolence strategy, out of political urgency to "do something now," might choose to spend the entire allocated budget on a short-lived, but very visible, mass media campaign, when an alternative might have been to focus on the root causes of violence and to employ grassroots community coalition building, using a locality development model. In the long run, the locality development perspective may be more participatory, cost effective, and enduring, embedded in the cultural values of community members and owned by them rather than imposed on them (see Chapter Twelve).

Value of Theory for Practice

Health educators are told that theory will strengthen practice, but strategies for operationalizing theory for application are seldom emphasized (D'Onofrio, 1992). Theory can be overwhelming at times, resulting in myths and false assumptions that undermine the value of theory in practice. Some myths about theory include the belief that the body of theory in health education is unique, that theory is immutable truth and should perfectly explain problems in the field, and that theory provides foolproof recipes for practice (D'Onofrio, 1992). Some practitioners also assume that theory is not current and has little relevance for contemporary social problems. Challenging these myths is important. The interactions between practitioners and researchers play a key role in the development of better theories, as theoretical postulates are challenged, tested, and modified by both real-world experience and empirical research.

Examples of Combining Theory-Driven Interventions

Interventions derived from a single intervention model or from within only one level of social structure (individual, group, or organizational) have inherent limitations in overall efficacy (see Lichtenstein and Glasgow, 1992; Shiffman, 1993). Program strategies that combine levels have also had mixed results; examples are the Working Well worksite trial, based on The Transtheoretical Model and organizational models (Sorensen and others, forthcoming); the community smoking cessation trial (Community Intervention Trial for Smoking Cessation Research Group, 1995a, 1995b); and community heart disease prevention trials (for example, Carleton and others, 1995; Farquhar and others, 1990; Mittlemark, Hunt, Health, and Schmid, 1993; see Chapter One). A number of reasons for the limited effects of worksite and community-based trials have been proposed (Susser, 1995; Fisher, 1995). They include (1) an insufficient allocation of time (for either intervention or evaluation) to permit sufficient diffusion of the intervention into the worksite or community and (2) the challenge of targeting a defined population that usually comprises a majority of individuals low in motivation (Abrams and Biener, 1992). Thus, the larger proportion of individuals, those who are low in motivation, do not change, resulting in aggregate change of small magnitude. There are also problems of limited power to test small effect sizes over and above secular trends and the associated limitations of research design, such as when using cross-sectional surveys of a small number of communities or worksites as the unit of randomization and of analysis. There are problems with the sensitivity and specificity of self-report measures and with competing priorities for people's time and for their attention to other pressing organizational or community issues. Current theories are not powerful enough to capitalize on potentially synergistic interactions, even when combined into intuitively appealing blueprints for action. In summary, researchers in these trials expected too much from theory and from practice, given the designs, time frames, and measures that were feasible.

We all need to return to our roots in the basic science of behavior change, and focus research questions on the gaps in our knowledge about mechanisms that enhance change and dissemination. If we are to achieve larger population impacts, we need refined models for proactive intervention, clearly specified mediators, and examination of process-to-outcome relationships that hint at promising synergistic interactions. This kind of translational research will help us bridge the gap between individual and clinical models of health education and population (public health) models. For example, more emphasis can be placed on new technologics such as interactive multimedia expert systems and the information superhighway (Strecher and others, 1994) and on health services delivery and usage research. Researchers rarely measure their programs and process mechanisms adequately and then link processes and levels of change to outcomes in repeated measures longitudinal cohort studies.

Strategies for screening individuals at high risk (such as younger women with a family history of breast cancer or older black males who are at high risk for prostate cancer) must also attend to powerful sociocultural and normative contextual factors as well as to the ways such factors interact with cognitive coping styles, risk perception, and decision making under conditions of uncertainty (Lerman and others, 1995; Miller, Shoda, and Hurley, 1996; see Chapters Six and Twenty). Promising cognitive models are being developed to illustrate how specific *schemata,* or cognitive styles (for example, the style of blunters, who minimize their fears of getting cancer), interact with counseling and educational messages.

Temporal Dimension

Change can be sudden or gradual and incremental at any level of a living system, from the micro (for example, cellular, molecular, individual) to the molar (for example, community or society). Three temporal factors that are key to theory and practice are (1) choosing an appropriate unit of time to measure change, (2) considering time as a key dependent variable, and (3) being aware of the importance of timing in planning for change. The unit of time can range from nanoseconds to decades depending on the research question. The time it takes to move from low motivation to taking action can be viewed as a dependent measure.

An awareness of temporal factors alerts us to the importance of natural cycles, trends, and developmental phases and should help us determine the most appropriate intervention plan. At the individual level, chronological age (for example a child's age compared to an adult's age) greatly influences the range of measures considered normal and the types of lifestyle intervention that could be beneficial. At a more molar level, consideration of time alerts health educators to the different priorities that can be set in, for example, an advanced industrialized nation as compared to an impoverished Third World country with little formal governmental infrastructure and few financial resources (see Figure 22.1). Consideration of the temporal dimension forces a stronger focus on global and local social imperatives and on the urgency with which underserved individuals and developing nations should be approached, lest tens of thousands die prematurely of preventable causes.

Time can be used as a dependent variable (for example, in survival analysis) or to evaluate when change might be expected. Choosing realistic outcome measures requires knowledge of how long it will take for processes of change to unfold among individuals, proximal (small) groups, and larger groups (communities). To use tobacco as an example, determining a smoker's degree of nicotine dependence is a task that focuses on a temporal dimension of hours to days. This focus on short-term withdrawal severity measures an individual smoker's level of dependence and helps a health educator determine if nicotine replacement therapy is needed. To investigate psychosocial (cognitive-behavioral) predictors of smoking relapse requires a longer time frame, three to six months. Policy change and population prevalence reduction in smoking may take decades. For most people who develop lung cancer from smoking, the disease develops between ten and thirty years after smoking begins. The pyramid in Figure 22.1 can remind scientists and practitioners about the importance of considering the dimension of time and the developmental cycles of individuals and populations.

Individual Versus Population-Based Approaches

A sense of clarity about the issues central to the debate over whether we should be taking an individual high-risk approach or a more population-based approach can be found in Rose's seminal book (1992). Rose points out both the advantages and disadvantages of each approach as it relates to prevention strategies. High-risk intervention strategies, where individuals considered most at risk for deleterious health outcomes are targeted, serve best as interim actions that protect susceptible individuals, given that the underlying causes remain unknown or uncontrollable. Rose argues, however, that our priority needs to be on the discovery and control of the ultimate causes of disease, rooted in economics and sociopolitical structures, an argument that strongly emphasizes the population-based approach.

While the authors of this chapter are in general agreement with Rose, it may be necessary to examine his perspective in the light of how long it takes to achieve change in a population and in light of recent advances in biotechnology. If a solely population-based approach is taken, then considerable illness and suffering will be experienced by individuals at high risk. One possible solution is to bridge the gap between the extremes of an individual and high-risk approach and a population and public health approach. A bridging strategy could take the form of the approach that combines stepped care with treatment matching. A stepped-care model includes a range of interventions that start with public health and self-change strategies with broad reach and relatively low cost. As the degree of risk or of ill health increases, interventions of moderate or high intensity are provided and are matched to the smaller numbers of individuals who need them (Figure 22.2). This strategy provides for rational allocation of intervention resources and helps resolve the tension between the individual/clinical medicine constituencies and the public health and policy proponents in the field of health education.

Many would argue that policy, legislation, and political issues are the most important factors in advancing an agenda of social change. Our position is that policy change is an important component of a broader intervention approach designed to produce interactions between individual, group, and population strategies over time. Indeed, policy change does not usually occur out of the blue but either is triggered by an obvious public health danger (for example, exposure to carcinogens, radioactivity, or drinking water polluted by parasites or chemicals) or grows out of a grassroots movement (for example, advocacy for more research funds for AIDS or for breast cancer). Examples of policy interventions that can play a key role in behavioral change are increased tobacco taxes to reduce youth experimentation (Warner, 1987) and the earmarked tobacco taxes that have dramatically accelerated reductions in smoking prevalence in California (Pierce and others, 1994). Research on secondhand smoke exposure (Emmons and others, 1992, 1994) has accelerated the federal Environmental Protection Agency's regulations. Smoking is now banned on airline flights and in many buildings and worksites. Research on illegal purchase of cigarettes by minors is an outstanding example of how beneficial it can be to integrate policy and behavioral change, research, and practice within a community around an issue with a clear social imperative (Altman, Foster, Rasenick-Douss, and Tye, 1989).

Basic Science, Clinical, and Public Health Research Priorities

There will likely always be a tension between basic science research and clinical and public health applications. The need for closer collaboration between theory and practice parallels the need for better integration and collaboration among basic, clinical, and population scientists. When this happens, exciting advances can be made by interdisciplinary teams (for example, teams including specialists in molecular epidemiology, behavioral genetics, psychoneuroimmunology, behavioral medicine, health psychology, medical economics, clinical epidemiology, medical sociology, and medical anthropology). The discovery of genetic mutations that are the basis for screening high-risk women for hereditary breast cancer predisposition illustrates the necessity and the potential value of collaboration between molecular biology and the clinical, behavioral, and public health sciences (Lerman and others, 1995).

Practitioner Versus Researcher

Practitioners working in the community know which problems need to be addressed. They are part of the community. They are the doers. Researchers are questioners, often not part of the community that they approach, using agency-directed funds or personal creativity to specify the goals of the program before any collaborative relationship or contact is made with the community. Researchers need results to get additional funding so that they can continue to do research. Tensions often build between researcher and practitioner and between researcher and community (Altman, 1995). Although practitioners, too, are often interested in the theoretical constructs being tested, they live in the immediate world where problems need expedited solutions. By the time a theoretically based research proposal is planned, written, reviewed, funded, and ready for implementation, the target community may feel it was abandoned in its hour of need or may now have a host of new or competing priorities.

Researchers are encouraged to use the community-building strategies outlined by Minkler and Wallerstein (Chapter Twelve), with an up-front goal of "sustainability" as described by Altman (1995). Although it may not eliminate tensions, involvement of practitioners and consumers at the earliest stage of research is essential. Such participatory or action research has great ecological validity and practical relevance. It is also likely to ensure that there is a plan for maintaining successful components of intervention efforts, institutionalizing them into the fabric of the social system. If trusting, respectful, and effective long-term relationships are fostered between communities and researchers, the benefits may accrue over time to all parties. Such collaborative alliances can result in advancing the field. The result can be a partnership that fully embraces the social context and social imperatives of the population that the investigator seeks to serve, and makes theory and research valuable tools for attaining societal goals.

Process Versus Outcome

In the first edition of this book, Rosenstock (1990) commented on the importance of both process and outcome evaluations in health education research, saying: "while one should properly decry the paucity of well-controlled evaluations of health promotion activities, it is equally problematic to evaluate a program before its time. The ultimate goal of all health programs is to maintain or improve health status, but not all health programs can be properly evaluated against that criterion at any given point in time." We need to think more about what questions to ask and how to answer them. When results are modest, as, for example, they were in the large community trial COMMIT (Community Intervention Trial for Smoking Cessation Research Group [1995a, 1995b], it is critical to have an understanding of what really happened, to whom, and why. For example: Why did women, minorities, or less-educated members of society not participate? What types of intervention activities attracted which subgroups of the target population? What types of intervention components actually worked and attracted the most interest? What cognitive styles within individuals resulted in distortions in their risk perception (optimistic-pessimistic bias) and then interacted with a mass media campaign to help explain some unexpected result? What components of the interventions were most cost effective? Without appropriate process-to-outcome evaluations, we cannot effectively and completely explain our results or advance our knowledge of theory and mechanisms. This, in turn, makes research less relevant to the practitioner.

Qualitative research methodologies have gained new, and well-deserved, respect. Technological advances have moved qualitative research methodologies along at a rapid pace (Weitzman and Miles, 1995). As we focus more attention on low-literacy populations and audiences who may have language or cultural barriers to participating in an intervention, qualitative research techniques may be of particular help when used alone or in combination with other, more quantitative methodologies (see Chapter Twenty).

Insularity Versus Interdisciplinary Collaboration

Health educators represent multiple academic and practice perspectives. True *interdisciplinary* collaboration occurs when scientists and practitioners seek to produce a new synthesis that accounts for more predictive power or more variance or that has greater generalizability than was possible to produce from within the constituent disciplines or the theories themselves. Often, interdisciplinary collaboration is confused with *multidisciplinary* collaboration or theoretical eclecticism, where the perspectives of several disciplines may be used piecemeal or added onto a single discipline. However, a true interdisciplinary model, in contrast, involves a new synthesis of ideas, advancing the field and passing such tests of good theory as the law of parsimony and the criterion of potential falsification by empirical testing.

An example of an interdisciplinary collaboration resulting in a new synthesis is the work of Flay, Phil, Petraitis, and Hu (1995). These authors provide empirical evidence for a multilevel, multivariate structural model to explain adoption of risky behavior among adolescents. The model includes (1) the broad sociocultural milieu that surrounds the behavior (distal sociocultural influences); (2) the more immediate (proximal) situational context in which the behavior occurs; (3) the characteristics and predispositions of the individual performing the behavior (personality and genetic vulnerability); (4) the behavior itself and closely related behaviors (for example, drinking, cigarette smoking, and risky sex); and (5) the interactions among all of the previous items, embracing the notion of reciprocal determinism. Change is also seen as a process unfolding over time and hence needing a cohort sampling frame with multiple repeated measures over time. The Flay, Phil, Petraitis, and Hu model also uses the latest statistical innovations such as multipanel structural equation modeling over three time points in a longitudinal cohort analysis.

Future Directions in Health Promotion and Education

As we move into the next decade, many exciting and challenging opportunities lie ahead for researchers and practitioners in health promotion and education. As indicated throughout this chapter, theories usually address either individual-level, group- and organization-level, or community-level factors. Planning models, such as ecological models or the PRECEDE-PROCEED model, offer an opportunity to incorporate different theoretical levels (Green and Kreuter, 1991; see Chapter Seventeen). Although such planning models are frequently used in program planning and practice, they are less frequently used in research efforts to measure key mediators and processes. Wider use of such overarching theoretical approaches that address multiple levels of influence can make a significant contribution toward advancing the field.

Another important area for further study is the routine use of empowerment concepts (Zimmerman, 1996) for program design and evaluation. For program planners, practitioners, and researchers, conducting participatory or action research can be challenging. For example, researchers often approach communities with a particular preconceived agenda such as heart disease or cancer prevention. The predetermined agenda can limit the success of the partnership, especially if it does not reflect the community's own priorities. One possibility is for health education practitioners and researchers to form coalitions through which to approach community groups and conduct broad community assessments. When they do so, the effort and expense involved in developing community collaborations can be minimized while the likelihood that the community's priorities can be identified and addressed is increased. Again, the idea of participatory research is paramount.

Dissemination of health information and delivery of interventions involves channels, modes, methods, and organizations whose relationships to a particular community or target group may vary. Physician-delivered health behavior interventions are common. However, the uninsured and underserved have limited or no access to primary care. Thus, those who need prevention the most cannot benefit from this important delivery channel. Further, as technological innovations (such as interactive multimedia) continue to be developed, it is important to assess their appropriateness for diverse populations. An investigator should consider, for example, whether such technology-based interventions as computer expert systems and telephone counseling (Orleans, 1993; Strecher and others, 1994) meet the needs of culturally diverse populations. Further, in disenfranchised populations, such as the urban poor, interventions that lack human contact may be less desirable than efforts that include building trust through respectful and consistent regular human interactions.

Mass media and related technologies are playing an increasingly important role in the development and delivery of health messages. Finnegan and Viswanath (Chapter Fifteen) describe communication theories of special relevance to public health and health behavior change and highlight research findings concerning media message production and media effects and consequences. Today, more than ever, target audiences have the opportunity to be active participants in the exchange of information. For example, radio call-in shows and network or cable television talk shows are proliferating. The Internet has opened an entirely new channel for health message exchange that gives individuals instantaneous medical facts, distance learning opportunities, and support groups for almost any physical or mental health problem. Future health education efforts will need to keep pace with technological advances while maintaining the quality and integrity of the messages themselves.

An underresearched area that deserves attention is the study of multiple risk factors. Trends to improve this situation can be seen, for example, in recent worksite health promotion programs that attempt to integrate occupational risk, safety, health promotion, mental health, and employee assistance programs (Sorensen and others, 1995). The same trend is emerging in addiction programs, which are adding the treatment of tobacco dependence to the treatment of alcohol and substance abuse (Abrams, Marlatt, and Sobell, 1995). Emmons and others (1994) point out a need to develop models to address multiple risk factors within the same individual over time. Most health behavior theories do not adequately address multiple risk factors and the behavioral clustering of lifestyle risk factors, psychiatric co-morbidity, and physical illness within individuals. Therefore, empirical investigation of how to extend behavioral theories to address change in multiple risk factors could be very fruitful. For example, the idea of risk perception may be relevant. Given multiple health behaviors, we are beginning to learn how some disease risks carry an optimistic bias (heart disease) and others seem to carry a pessimistic bias (cancer) when compared to an individual's actual risk status.

Will we rise to accept the challenges of working toward a better synthesis of knowledge, toward a more unified and parsimonious strategy of theory building, with a common language, a shared operational definition of concepts, intervention strategies, and measures of outcome? There is a continuing need for the bridging of theory, research, and practice if we are to address social imperatives. To move forward requires that we take the high ground, rising above insularity, rivalries, and protectionist motives within theoretical schools, working across disciplines and with practice constituencies. The field of health promotion and education may advance more rapidly if there is a stronger ethic among all constituencies to search for and find common ground and build a new interdisciplinary set of universal operating concepts for health behavior change. One double-edged sword in this struggle to improve is competition—stimulating scientists to new heights on the one hand and impeding progress through jealously guarded secrets on the other hand. A balance between cooperation and competition is needed. Striking such a balance requires a willingness to openly criticize theories and models that compete with each other, subjecting them all to replication or falsification. Researchers also need to be more open to incorporating social values into their research agendas from the earliest stages of idea development, values such as full partnership with practitioners and target populations and dedication to carefully choosing priorities that support research that is cost effective and valuable to the community being served.

It is of central importance that theory, research, and practice bridge gaps between (1) the micro level, (2) the clinical treatment level, and (3) the macro level of the systems that constitute a society, and that they attend more strongly to the temporal dimension, matching the characteristics of the target population, the intervention, and the measures to appropriate time frames. Specific challenges include overcoming our use of different languages and jargon rather than a universal taxonomy of common constructs and avoiding a focus on relatively narrow univariate models. Other concerns are our lack of standards for measurement of final outcomes, our field's tendency to focus on dramatic short-term impacts to meet political agendas, the dominant research practice of regarding the randomized controlled clinical trial as the sole gold standard for rigorous research, the lack of due consideration for the appropriate longitudinal cohort and temporal dimensions needed to measure population change, and the tendency to view mechanisms as the proverbial black box whose inner workings are shielded from us. All these limitations can lead us to unrealistic expectations about what theory can do for practice, about how much benefit our practice can produce, and about how fast that benefit can be realized.

Future progress will result from a thorough appreciation of the past and of the contributions of the present era, especially when we stand back and examine their strengths and limitations. Occasional bursts of innovation will move our field significantly ahead. But moving knowledge and practice forward is both an awesome and a humbling experience. We look back and see our naïveté, our inability to move beyond common wisdom known for centuries. Yet we should be encouraged by knowledge acquired since the turn of this century and be hopeful for the future. Health promotion and education are moving forward, striving to create a better world, through individual and collective insights, research, and action. We are indeed making progress even though there have been no dramatic or revolutionary breakthroughs in health behavior and health education since the first edition of this book in 1990. Yet the authors of this book have seen a little further, by standing upon the shoulders of giants.

Their ideas raise more questions than we have answers. How can we develop more effective theories and interventions with greater benefits for society? What is truly new and important? What should be discarded as erroneous or misleading? How can we balance individual with collective interests, local with national concerns, and national with global world needs? What evidence is there that we are really able to change individual behavior or communities through planned programs and beyond the secular trends? Some of these questions may never be answered fully. Such is the nature of the scientific process as it unfolds over time.

Theory, research, and practice are reciprocally interrelated. Many disciplines contribute to health promotion and education and health behavior. The skilled academic and the skilled practitioner are at their best when empirical research confirms the value of a theory-driven intervention in actual real-world practice. Empowered individuals, groups, and societies can and should become active and equal partners in setting our agendas, in developing theory, and in designing blueprints for intervention and for dissemination. Health promotion and education practitioners can and should confidently question theory in the light of practice and actively join in the development of better theories to address the most pressing social issues in both the developed and the developing nations of the world.

References

Abrams, D. B., and Biener, L. "Motivational Characteristics of Smokers at the Worksite: A Public Health Challenge." *International Journal of Preventive Medicine*, 1992, *21*, 679–687.

Abrams, D. B., Marlatt, G. A., and Sobell, M. G. "Overview of Section II: Treatment, Early Intervention, and Policy." In J. Fertig and R. Allen (eds.), *Alcohol and Tobacco: From Basic Science to Policy*. NIAAA Research Monograph, no. 19. Washington, D.C.: National Institute of Alcoholism and Alcohol Abuse, 1995.

Abrams, D. B., and others. "Social Learning Principles for Organizational Health Promotion: An Integrated Approach." In M. F. Cataldo and T. J. Coates, *Health and Industry: A Behavioral Medicine Perspective*. New York: Wiley, 1986.

Abrams, D. B., and others. "Tobacco Dependence: An Integration of Individual and Public Health Perspectives." In P. E. Nathan, J. Langenbacher, B. S. McGrady, and W. Frankenstein (eds.), *Annual Review of Addictions Research and Treatment*. New York: Pergamon, 1991.

Abrams, D. B., and others. "Smoking Cessation at the Workplace: Conceptual and Practical Issues." In R. Richmond (ed.), *Interventions for Smokers: An International Perspective*. Baltimore, Md.: Williams & Wilkins, 1994.

Abrams, D. B., and others. "Integrating Individual and Public Health Perspectives for Treatment of Tobacco Dependence Under Managed Care: A Combined Stepped Care and Matching Model." *Annals of Behavioral Medicine*, forthcoming.

Altman, D. G. "Sustaining Interventions in Community Systems: On the Relationship Between Researchers and Communities." *Health Psychology*, 1995, *14*(6), 526–536.

Altman, D. G., Foster, V., Rasenick-Douss, L., and Tye, J. B. "Reducing the Illegal Sale of Cigarettes to Minors." *Journal of the American Medical Association,* 1989, *261,* 80–83.

Bandura, A. *Social Foundations of Thought and Action: A Social Cognitive Theory.* Englewood Cliffs, N.J.: Prentice Hall, 1986.

Carleton, R. A., and others. "The Pawtucket Heart Health Program: Community Changes in Cardiovascular Risk Factors and Projected Disease Risk." *American Journal of Public Health,* 1995, *85*(6), 777–785.

Clark, M. M., and others. "Self-Efficacy in Weight Management." *Journal of Consulting and Clinical Psychology,* 1991, *59,* 739–744.

Community Intervention Trial for Smoking Cessation Research Group. "Community Intervention Trial for Smoking Cessation (COMMIT): I. Cohort Results from a Four-Year Community Intervention." *American Journal of Public Health,* 1995a, *85,* 183–192.

Community Intervention Trial for Smoking Cessation Research Group. "Community Intervention Trial for Smoking Cessation (COMMIT): II. Changes in Adult Cigarette Smoking Prevalence." *American Journal of Public Health,* 1995b, *85,* 193–200.

Cummings, K. M., Becker, M. H., and Maile, M. C. "Bringing the Models Together: An Empirical Approach to Combining Variables Used to Explain Health Actions." *Journal of Behavioral Medicine,* 1980, *3*(2), 123–145.

Curry, S. J., and Emmons, K. M. "Theoretical Models for Predicting and Improving Compliance with Breast Cancer Screening." *Annals of Behavioral Medicine,* 1994, *16*(4), 302–316.

D'Onofrio, C. N. "Theory and the Empowerment of Health Education Practitioners." *Health Education Quarterly,* 1992, *19*(3), 385–403.

Emmons, K. M., and others. "Exposure to Environmental Tobacco Smoke in Naturalistic Settings." *American Journal of Public Health,* 1992, *82,* 24–28.

Emmons, K. M., and others. "Mechanisms in Multiple Risk Factor Interventions: Smoking, Physical Activity, and Dietary Fat Intake Among Manufacturing Workers." *Preventive Medicine,* 1994, *23,* 481–489.

Farquhar, J. W., and others. "Effects of Community-Wide Education on Cardiovascular Disease Risk Factors: The Stanford Five-City Project." *Journal of the American Medical Association,* 1990, *264,* 359–365.

Fisher, E. B., Jr. "The Results of the COMMIT Trial." (Editorial.) *American Journal of Public Health,* 1995, *85,* 159–160.

Flay, B. R., Phil, D., Petraitis, J., and Hu, F. B. "The Theory of Triadic Influence: Preliminary Evidence Related to Alcohol and Tobacco Use." In J. Fertig and R. Allen (eds.), *Alcohol and Tobacco: From Basic Science to Policy.* NIAAA Research Monograph, no. 19. Washington, D.C.: National Institute of Alcoholism and Alcohol Abuse, 1995.

Glanz, K., and Seewald-Klein, T. "Nutrition at the Worksite: An Overview." *Journal of Nutrition Education,* 1986, *18*(1, supp.), S1–S12.

Green, L. W., and Kreuter, M. W. *Health Promotion Planning: An Educational and Environmental Approach.* (2nd ed.) Mountain View, Calif.: Mayfield, 1991.

Lerman, C., and others. "Effects of Individualized Breast Cancer Risk Counseling: A Randomized Trial." *Journal of the National Cancer Institute,* 1995, *87,* 286–292.

Lerman, C., and others. "A Randomized Trial of Breast Cancer Risk Counseling: Interacting Effects of Counseling, Education Level and Coping Style." *Health Psychology,* 1996, *15,* 75–83.

Leventhal, H., Zimmerman, R., and Gutmann, M. "Compliance: A Self-Regulation Perspective." In D. Gentry (ed.), *Handbook of Behavioral Medicine.* New York: Guilford Press, 1984.

Lichtenstein, E., and Glasgow, R. E. "Smoking Cessation: What Have We Learned over the Past Decade?" *Journal of Consulting and Clinical Psychology*, 1992, *60*, 518–527.

Marlatt, G. A., and Tappert, S. F. "Harm Reduction: Reducing the Risks of Addictive Behaviors." In J. S. Baer, G. A. Marlatt, and R. J. McMahan (eds.), *Addictive Behaviors Across the Life Span*. Thousand Oaks, Calif.: Sage, 1993.

McGinnis, J. M., and Lee, P. R. "Healthy People 2000 at Mid Decade." *Journal of the American Medical Association*, 1995, *273*, 1123–1129.

Miller, S. M., Shoda, Y., and Hurley, K. "Applying Cognitive-Social Theory to Health-Protective Behavior: Breast Self-Examination in Cancer Screening." *Psychological Bulletin*, 1996, *119*(1), 70–94.

Mittlemark, M. B., Hunt, M. R., Health, G. W., and Schmid, T. L. "Realistic Outcomes: Lessons from Community-Based Research and Demonstration Programs for the Prevention of Cardiovascular Disease." *Journal of Public Health Policy*, 1993, *4*, 437–462.

Oldenburg, B., Owen, N. G., Parle, M., and Gomel, M. "An Economic Evaluation of Four Worksite-Based Cardiovascular Risk Factor Interventions." *Health Education Quarterly*, 1995, *22*(1), 9–19.

Orleans, C. T. "Treating Nicotine Dependence in Medical Settings: A Stepped-Care Model." In C. T. Orleans and J. Slade (eds.), *Nicotine Addiction: Principles and Management*. New York: Oxford University Press, 1993.

Pierce, J. P., and others. *Tobacco Use in California. An Evaluation of the Tobacco Control Program, 1989–1993*. La Jolla: University of California, San Diego, 1994.

Rogers, E. M. *Diffusion of Innovations*. (3rd ed.) New York: Free Press, 1983.

Rose, G. *The Strategy of Preventive Medicine*. New York: Oxford University Press, 1992.

Rosenstock, I. M. "The Past, Present, and Future of Health Education." In K. Glanz, F. M. Lewis, and B. K. Rimer (eds.), *Health Behavior and Health Education: Theory, Research, and Practice*. San Francisco: Jossey-Bass, 1990.

Shiffman, S. "Smoking Cessation Treatment: Any Progress?" *Journal of Consulting and Clinical Psychology*, 1993, *61*, 718–722.

Skinner, B. F. *Science and Human Behavior*. New York: Free Press, 1953.

Sorensen, G., and others. "A Model for Worksite Cancer Prevention: Integration of Health Protection and Health Promotion in the Wellworks Project." *American Journal of Health Promotion*, 1995, *10*(1), 55–62.

Sorensen, G., and others. "Working Well: Results from a Worksite-Based Cancer Prevention Trial." *American Journal of Public Health*, forthcoming.

Strecher, V. J., and others. "The Effects of Computer-Tailored Smoking Cessation Messages in Family Practice Settings." *Journal of Family Practice*, 1994, *39*(3), 262–270.

Susser, M. "The Tribulations of Trials—Intervention in Communities." (Editorial.) *American Journal of Public Health*, 1995, *85*, 156–158.

U.S. Public Health Service. Office of the Surgeon General. *Reducing the Health Consequences of Smoking: 25 Years of Progress. A Report of the Surgeon General*. DHHS publication no. 89–8411. Washington, D.C.: U.S. Department of Health and Human Services, Public Health Service, Centers for Disease Control, Office of Smoking and Health, 1989.

Velicer, W. F., DiClemente, C. C., Rossi, J. S., and Prochaska, J. O. "Relapse Situations and Self-Efficacy: An Integrative Model." *Addictive Behaviors*, 1990, *15*, 271–283.

Warner, K. E. "Selling Health Promotion to Corporate America: Uses and Abuses of the Economic Argument." *Health Education Quarterly*, 1987, *14*, 39–55.

Warner, K. E., and Luce, B. R. *Cost-Benefit and Cost Effectiveness Analysis in Health Care: Principles, Practice, and Potential.* Ann Arbor, Mich.: Health Administration Press, 1982.

Weinstein, N. D. "Testing Four Competing Theories of Health-Protective Behavior." *Health Psychology,* 1993, *12*(4), 324–333.

Weiss, S. M. "Health Psychology and Other Health Professions." In G. C. Stone and others (eds.), *Health Psychology: A Discipline and a Profession.* Chicago: University of Chicago Press, 1987.

Weitzman, E. A., and Miles, M. B. *A Software Source Book: Computer Programs for Qualitative Data Analysis.* Thousand Oaks, Calif.: Sage, 1995.

Zeckhauser, R. J., and Shepard, D. S. "Where Now for Saving Lives?" *Law and Contemporary Problems,* 1976, *40*(4), 5–45.

Zimmerman, M. A. "Empowerment Theory: Psychological, Organizational, and Community Levels of Analysis." In J. Rappaport and E. Seidman (eds.), *Handbook of Community Psychology.* New York: Plenum, 1996.

NAME INDEX

A

Abelson, R. P., 86, 110
Abrams, D. B., 143, 146, 155, 156, 159, 175, 409, 422, 453, 460, 463, 464, 466, 473, 475
Adams, J., 290, 311
Aday, L. A., 425, 427, 437
Adhikari, G., 247, 268
Adler, N. E., 6, 12, 15, 429, 437, 445, 448
Affleck, G., 119, 132
Ajzen, I., 23, 33, 38, 40, 86, 87n, 88, 90–91, 93, 94, 96, 110, 111, 140, 142, 146, 147, 276, 281, 284, 374, 381
Alagna, S. W., 183, 186, 204
Alinsky, S. D., 243, 245, 246, 249, 259, 265
Allard, R., 52, 53, 54, 57
Allen, J., 444, 449
Alter, C., 295, 296, 297, 298, 306–307, 309
Altman, D. G., 408, 411, 424, 469, 470, 475–476
Amezcua, C., 228, 234
Anderman, C., 95, 112
Andersen, B. L., 129, 132
Anderson, C., 272, 284
Anderson, D. M., 73, 81
Andreasen, A. R., 384, 385, 401
Antoni, M. H., 130, 132

Antonovsky, A., 115, 116, 123, 132
Antonucci, T. C., 185, 187, 190, 201, 202
Arean, P., 258, 265
Argyris, C., 290, 293, 309
Aristotle, 19
Armsden, G., 12, 15
Armstrong, K., 78, 83
Arnold, R., 255, 265
Ash, A., 210, 225
Aspinwall, L. G., 52, 53, 54, 57, 121, 132, 181, 204
Avery, B., 244, 265

B

Babbie, E., 22, 24, 25, 33
Bachman, J. G., 300, 310
Backer, T., 350, 355
Baker, S. A., 85, 111
Baker, S. P., 372, 381
Balch, G. I., 391, 392, 402
Balshem, A., 125, 135
Bandura, A., 23, 33, 43, 46, 47, 51, 57, 65, 81, 93, 110, 119, 132, 153, 155–156, 158, 159, 160–161, 162, 163, 164, 165, 172, 175, 181, 201, 276, 281, 284, 319, 335, 336, 350, 354, 366, 382, 407–408, 409, 422, 463, 464, 476
Baranowski, T., 149, 153, 155, 156, 159, 169, 174, 175, 177, 178, 227, 410, 422, 462

Barker, C., 329, 336
Barker, R. G., 404, 407, 422
Barndt, D., 252, 265
Barnes, J. A., 182, 201
Baron, R. M., 123, 132
Barton, S., 26, 33
Basch, C. E., 271, 272, 282, 283, 284, 436, 439
Basen-Engquist, K., 52, 54, 57
Baskerville, J. C., 51, 58
Bass, J. L., 372, 283
Bassett, M., 427, 438
Bauman, A., 416, 423
Bearman, N., 307, 309
Becker, M. H., 23, 27, 33, 35, 38, 40, 41, 42, 44, 47, 48, 49, 50, 52, 53, 57, 58, 119, 137, 140, 141, 146, 147, 172, 178, 214, 225, 228, 235, 368, 382, 461–462, 476
Beecher, H. K., 211, 225
Beigel, A., 6, 17
Bell, C., 255, 266
Belle, D., 231, 234
Bellingham, R., 444, 449
Bellis, J. M., 78, 82
Ben-Sira, Z., 215, 224
Beniger, J. R., 318, 336
Benoliel, J., 85, 111
Bensley, L. S., 232, 234
Benson, H., 127, 132
Berelson, B., 324, 337, 339
Berenson, G. S., 415, 423

479

SUBJECT INDEX